Anti-Semitism and Psychiatry

H. Steven Moffic • John R. Peteet
Ahmed Hankir • Mary V. Seeman
Editors

Anti-Semitism and Psychiatry

Recognition, Prevention, and Interventions

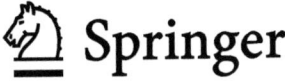 Springer

Editors
H. Steven Moffic, MD
Private Practice and Retired Tenured
Professor of Psychiatry
Medical College of Wisconsin
Milwaukee, WI
USA

Ahmed Hankir, MD
South London and Maudsley
NHS Foundation Trust
London
UK

John R. Peteet, MD
Department of Psychiatry
Brigham and Women's Hospital
Boston, MA
USA

Mary V. Seeman, OC, MDCM
Department of Psychiatry
University of Toronto
Toronto, ON
Canada

ISBN 978-3-030-37744-1   ISBN 978-3-030-37745-8   (eBook)
https://doi.org/10.1007/978-3-030-37745-8

This Springer imprint is published by the registered company Springer Nature Switzerland AG
The registered company address is: Gewerbestrasse 11, 6330 Cham, Switzerland

Editors' Introduction

Chutzpah!

Though chutzpah is not at all an everyday word used in scholarly psychiatry, it may be the best one word introduction to this edited volume. Indeed, producing this edited volume could be called an act of chutzpah.

Chutzpah originally was a Hebrew word that was adapted into Yiddish, Yiddish being the common language of Jews in Eastern Europe before the Holocaust of World War II. From Yiddish, it was adopted into English and everyday usage, especially in America, in recent times. It has been variously defined, as in Merriam-Webster, as "audacity, nerve, and supreme self-confidence." It even has an interesting pronunciation, with a hard "ch" that seems to reflect the hardness of its meaning, as heard in https://www.youtube.com/watch?v=Ot-81hJHIDY. Given its extreme implications, having chutzpah can turn out to be fantastic or destructive but generally not in between and/or blah.

Alan Dershowitz, the controversial and well-known twentieth-century American lawyer, wrote a best-selling book titled *Chutzpah* about 30 years ago. He tried to make the case that it's possible for a Jew to be 100% loyal to one's country as well as to Israel. In retrospect, this perspective may have been ahead of its time in regard to the current increase in anti-Semitism, its connection to anti-Zionism – or hostility toward Israel – and the lack of agreement on how to address this development. In line with his argument, Dershowitz recommended that Jews should stop trying to maintain a low profile in America.

This first attempt in decades to address the psychiatric aspects of anti-Semitism is upping the ante and profile. Is that chutzpah? Is it also chutzpah to go against one view of psychiatry – the view that psychiatry should just mind its own traditional business of direct patient care and stay away from social problems? Perhaps, but it is definitely chutzpah to think that our book might be able to help to significantly reduce anti-Semitism, given that it is the longest-running prejudice in history.

Since history also tells us that religions are often at conflict or war, it could also be an act of chutzpah to have a multi-faith team of editors for this volume, as well as a multicultural group of chapter writers. We have a male and female Jewish psychiatrist, a Christian psychiatrist, and a Muslim psychiatrist as editors. We also have a diverse representation of chapter writers, most of whom live currently in the United States but also in Canada, France, India, Israel, and the United Kingdom.

Moreover, their familial, emotional, and historical ties, always important for psychological insights, include such far-flung countries as Argentina, Egypt, Germany, Ireland, Lebanon, Libya, Poland, Romania, and Russia. One of the striking examples is a non-Jewish psychiatrist, with an expertise in community resilience, who had a family member who was an American prisoner of war (POW) in Nazi Germany. There were many such unanticipated connections of would-be authors to anti-Semitism, indicating how widespread its relevance may be, not only for Jews but also for many others.

This heterogeneous approach may be politically correct or incorrect, but we are confident that it is psychologically correct. We hope that this ethnic and religious diversity and interaction may serve as an exemplar on how we can effectively challenge societal problems such as anti-Semitism. Indeed, we are confident because we had a similar multi-faith collaboration of editors and writers for a prior Springer volume on Islamophobia and psychiatry, a book that has already received substantial positive feedback and review.

This new volume can be thought of as a sequel of sorts. It came to fruition when the same editorial representative from Springer who had acquired the *Islamophobia and Psychiatry* volume noticed the worrisome related rise of anti-Semitism in New York City and suggested we cover this risk to the mental health of Jewish people and to the anti-Semites themselves and prevent the inevitable spread of hatred to other cultural groups. One difference between the terminologies of these two groups is that "anti" tends to mean hate or against, as in this case, the long-term ebb and flow toward Jews. Phobia, instead, implies unrealistic fear, as (for the most part) in the more recent case of Muslims. The wisdom of this request seemed confirmed when at the May 2019 Annual Meeting of the American Psychiatric Association in San Francisco, a colleague came to the crowded Springer booth highlighting new books, saw the book on Islamophobia and psychiatry, and asked the person manning the stall if a textbook on anti-Semitism and psychiatry existed? The answer was, of course, that it is on its way! It will be the first book of its kind in a generation, a generation which wrongly assumed that anti-Semitism had virtually disappeared.

We cover various anti-Semitic topics and tropes and have grouped them into sections covering general interest, psychiatric implications, specific clinical challenges, and social psychiatric implications. There are several chapters of personal reflections of anti-Semitism in the lives of various psychiatrists, which turn out to engage with emerging research on the potential power and ability of such personal narratives to change attitudes. Many chapters discuss issues that one would expect to find in such a book, but some are on rarely addressed topics that also need our attention, including:

- The biological determinants of bigotry
- Updated clinical considerations concerning transference and countertransference
- A visual portrayal of anti-Semitism
- A reconsideration of Jung's anti-Semitism

- Two chapters with a modern psychoanalytic perspective, one from France and one from the United States
- Testimonies from people connected to the Pittsburgh synagogue shooting, derived from interviews by a native Pittsburgh psychiatrist
- Anti-Semitism in the Deep South considered by a psychiatrist who has worked there
- Original research on anti-Semitism in Argentina from 1976 to 1983 and its repercussions for Jewish children
- Anti-Semitic cults
- The influence of the Holocaust on the development of psychiatry in the United States
- The role of Jewish institutions in combatting anti-Semitism
- The unique role of film in combatting anti-Semitism
- Is anti-Semitism essential to Jewish identity?
- And perhaps the ultimate chutzpah, "Can anti-Semitism be cured?"

This is what psychiatrists and other mental healthcare professionals uniquely can – and should – do. When a psychological problem is not being solved, look for unexpected places where crucial information may be hidden, whether in one's mind or society.

Unfortunately, and unpredictably, there is no doubt or question that anti-Semitism, both covert and overt, is once again rearing its hateful face in the United States and many other countries around the world. Is it chutzpah to suggest that the missing perspective that could lead to its elimination, or at least more permanent reduction, is psychiatry?

Psychiatrist Rollo May in his 1975 book, *The Courage to Create*, wrote: "If you do not express daring ideas, …you will have failed to try to make a difference." This book is a work of chutzpah, in other words, of courage and audacity, and we trust that it will make a difference.

Milwaukee, WI, USA	H. Steven Moffic, MD
Boston, MA, USA	John R. Peteet, MD
London, UK	Ahmed Hankir, MD
Toronto, ON, Canada	Mary V. Seeman, MD

Contents

Contributors

Neil Krishan Aggarwal, MD Columbia University Medical Center, New York, NY, USA

New York State Psychiatric Institute, New York, NY, USA

Mary C. Boys, MA, Ed.D Union Theological Seminary in the City of New York, New York, NY, USA

Jon Caven-Atack Independent Scholar, Nottingham, UK

James L. Fleming, MD Psychiatric Medical Care, Kansas City, MO, USA

Jacob L. Freedman, MD Tufts University School of Medicine, Boston, MA, USA

Stanley J. J. Freeman, MSc, MD, FRCP(C) Professor Emeritus, Department of Psychiatry, University of Toronto, Toronto, ON, Canada

Sigalit Gal, PhD Faculty of Arts, Social Sciences, McGill University, Montreal, Canada

Rama Rao Goginene, MD Department of Psychiatry, Cooper University Hospital and Health System, Camden, NJ, USA

Ahmed Hankir, MD South London and Maudsley NHS Foundation Trust, London, UK

Madeline W. Harford, MD Private Practice, Dallas, TX, USA

University of Texas Southwestern Medical School, Dallas, TX, USA

Steven Hassan, MEd, LMHC, NCC The Program in Psychiatry and the Law. Massachusetts Mental Health Center, a teaching hospital of Harvard Medical School, Boston, MA, USA

Elizabeth C. Henderson, MD Henderson Clinic & Consulting, Hickory, MS, USA

Elana Kahn, MA Jewish Community Relations Council, Milwaukee Jewish Federation, Milwaukee, WI, USA

Andrew (Nachum) Klafter, MD Cincinnati Psychoanalytic Institute and University of Cincinnati Residency Training Program, Cincinnati, OH, USA

Saul Levine, MD University of California at San Diego (UCSD), Del Mar, CA, USA

Kate Miriam Loewenthal, PhD Department of Psychology, Royal Holloway, University of London, Egham, UK

Aryeh Maidenbaum, PhD New York Center for Jungian Studies, New York, NY, USA

Barry Marcus, MSW Bainbridge Island, WA, USA

Andrew J. McLean, MD, MPH Department of Psychiatry and Behavioral Science, University of North Dakota School of Medicine and Health Sciences, Fargo, ND, USA

H. Steven Moffic, MD Private Community Psychiatrist, Milwaukee, WI, USA

Rabbi Evan Moffic, MAHL Makom Solel Lakeside Congregation, Highland Park, IL, USA

Sharon Packer, MD Mount Sinai Beth Israel, New York City, NY, USA

John R. Peteet, MD Department of Psychiatry, Brigham and Women's Hospital, Boston, MA, USA

Jessica M. Rabbany, MD Sackler School of Medicine – NY State/American Program, New York, NY, USA

Omar Reda, MD Providence Health & Services, Portland, OR, USA

Mary V. Seeman, OC, MDCM Department of Psychiatry, University of Toronto, Toronto, ON, Canada

Shridhar Sharma, MD Department of Psychiatry, National Academy of Medical Services & Sciences Institute of Human Behavior and Allied Sciences, Delhi, India

Jean-Claude Stoloff, MD Société Psychanalytique de Recherche et de Formation (SPRF France), International Psychoanalytical Association (IPA), Paris, France

John S. Tamerin, MD Weill Cornell School of Medicine, New York, NY, USA

Suzanne Vogel-Scibilia, MD, DFAPA Chatham University, Pittsburgh, PA, USA

Part I

General Issues

A Short History of the Jewish People and Anti-Semitism

1

Rabbi Evan Moffic

Why does the world seem to hate the Jews? What accounts for the long history of anti-Semitism? Why does this hatred persist? How has it changed? This chapter addresses these historical questions. It does so by looking at various eras and the kinds of charges leveled at the Jewish people. These charges bristle with theological, psychological, and sociological justifications. They all, however, center on the Jews and Judaism. First, some definitions.

Who Are the Jews? Where Do They Live?

Jews are an ethnic-religious group, currently numbering about 14 million people. About 45 percent of the population lives in America. Another 45 percent live in Israel, and the remaining 10 percent are scattered throughout Canada, Europe, Australia, New Zealand, Mexico, and parts of Africa and Central and South America. They constitute about 0.02 percent of the world population.

Although the history of the Jewish people is long and complicated, there are some key events that stand out [1]. The origins of the Jewish people—who were initially known as Israelites—lies in what is now the state of Israel. While the exact origin date is unknown, the first literature reflects the period of about 2000 B.C.E. After about 2000 years of living primarily in the land of Israel, Jews were displaced by larger powers and began the diaspora, the dispersion of Jews around the world. The diaspora grew after the destruction of the Jerusalem Temple by the Romans in 70 C.E. and the subsequent expulsion of Jews from Jerusalem. In the late nineteenth century, a movement known as Zionism arose in Europe as a response to growing anti-Semitism, which is defined as hostility toward Jews and Judaism. The Zionist movement promoted a Jewish return to the land of Israel and

R. E. Moffic (✉)
Makom Solel Lakeside Congregation, Highland Park, IL, USA
e-mail: emoffic@gmail.com

© Springer Nature Switzerland AG 2020
H. S. Moffic et al. (eds.), *Anti-Semitism and Psychiatry*,
https://doi.org/10.1007/978-3-030-37745-8_1

the establishment of a modern nation-state there. The movement grew substantially in the early twentieth century, and the modern state of Israel came into being in 1948 after the horrific murder of six million Jews by the Nazis during the Second World War. This event is commonly known as the Holocaust and sometimes as the Shoah. After the Holocaust and the establishment of the state of Israel, many Jews believed anti-Semitism would decline. While it did decline through the 1990s, anti-Semitism has grown again in the post-2000 world. After first reviewing the history of anti-Semitism, we will review this recent resurgence.

What, Exactly, Is Anti-Semitism?

Anti-Semitism, as we noted, can be characterized as hostility toward Jews and Judaism. It is evident in behavior, words, political policies, economic transactions, and religious practice. Anti-Semitism can arise even in regions where Jews are absent, as was the case in Japan during the 1820s and 1830s, when the Japanese expressed hostile views of Jews even though they had never met one. In addition, certain beliefs, statements, and actions can be unintentionally anti-Semitic. For example, someone can say "the Jews killed Jesus," thinking they are saying something factual with no intended hostility. But as we will see, this belief has had destructive and deadly consequences.

It should also be noted that the term "anti-Semitism" is not technically the right term for referring to persecution of Jews because Jews are not the only Semitic people. Others throughout the Middle East are technically Semites. But we will use the phrase anti-Semitism throughout the book because it has come to be widely understood as referring to hostility toward Jews.

While a clear prejudice, anti-Semitism is not synonymous with bigotry or racism. Judaism is not a race because a person can convert into Judaism, but it is, in part, an ethnicity because Jews consider a person to be automatically Jewish if their mother is Jewish. Thus, anti-Semitism is not simply a traditional form of racism or religious bigotry. It is both and more.

Ancient Origins

Anti-Semitism does not seem to be present in the Hebrew Bible (also known as the Torah or Old Testament). The tension and wars between Israelites and other nations, such as the Egyptians, described in the Bible reflect normal political rivalries and conflict. Jews were not different from other nations of the time. Rather, anti-Semitism begins after the Jewish people start to live as a minority among other nations.

The person often considered the first anti-Semite was a third-century (B.C.E.) Egyptian named Manetho. Manetho wrote a history of Egypt under the rule of the Pharaohs. Even today his work is a valuable guide to ancient Egypt. But what makes Manetho the first prominent anti-Semite is that he offers a very different version of the Exodus story than we find in the Bible. His version establishes Jews as a deceitful people dedicated to undermining society wherever they live.

According to Manetho, Jews are a combination of two peoples—shepherds who invaded Egypt and lepers who were driven out of Egypt by the Pharaoh. The shepherds invaded Egypt from the North (which would be modern-day Israel) sometime during the seventeenth century B.C.E. They succeeded in conquering Egypt and ruling them with oppressive laws until they were driven out after about 100 years later.

Then, after native Egyptians retook control, a terrible plague infected the land. The Pharaoh received a dream in which he was told to isolate the sick lepers and imprison them in the city where the shepherds once lived. In that city, however, the lepers came under the influence of a renegade Egyptian priest who proclaimed a belief in one God and rejected the traditional Egyptian gods. This priest went to Jerusalem where he made an alliance with the shepherds who had fled there. Together these two groups united and conquered Egypt.

According to Manetho, they made the lives of the Egyptians miserable, setting fires to their cities and destroying their sacrifices. They forced the Egyptian priests and prophets to sacrifice animals sacred to them and stripped leaders of their titles and honor. Eventually, however, the Egyptians revolted and drove out the shepherd/lepers. These shepherd/lepers were the Jews, the people of Israel, because that is the land to which where they fled after both expulsions from Egypt.

Manetho's account proved influential and enduring. It established the Jews as impure and impious. They were lepers who destroyed all of Egypt's gods. They are were seen as brutal and tyrannical, as evidenced in the way they subjugated native Egyptians. They were a mortal threat to all other peoples. Writing in 2014, Professor David Nirenberg concluded that Manetho's views "proved so useful that they continue to provide cornerstones for ideologies up to the present day" [2]. Manetho's accounts and influence make him the first prominent anti-Semite.

Why did Manetho's writing emerge when it did? What was it about in the third century B.C.E. that provided a fertile context for anti-Semitism? Two critical explanations stand out. They remain charges leveled at Jews today. The first is assimilation. By the third century B.C.E., Jews were adopting much of Hellenistic culture. They lived in cities, spoke Greek, traded, and took on Greek names. The extent to which they assimilated Greek culture can be seen in the first major translation of the Hebrew Bible into another language. In the third century B.C.E., the Bible was translated into Greek—today, we refer to that translation as the Septuagint. Manetho's rewriting of the Exodus story may have been sparked by this translation because the biblical Exodus was now accessible to the Greek-speaking public. But the creation of the Septuagint is also important for understanding assimilation because it suggests that some Jews could not read the Bible in Hebrew. They could only read it in Greek. But Jews did not assimilate fully. They maintained a belief in one God and continued to eat certain foods and pray in particular temples.

In other words, Jews were both part of and apart from the wider culture. That created tension because it suggested to other groups who had adopted Hellenism more fully that the Jews thought of themselves as somehow unique and superior.

The notion of cultural pluralism we have today did not exist in the third century. The pressure to conform to the culture of the ruling power was immense. When Jews resisted it, they became targets.

Christian Anti-Semitism

The second major fuel of anti-Semitism came with the rise of Christianity. The relationship between Jews and early Christians is a complicated one, primarily because the early followers of Jesus saw themselves as Jews. It is when Christianity became a separate religion—sometime around 100 C.E.—that a new kind of anti-Semitism developed. It rested on the idea that Jews are responsible for the death of Jesus. This accusation became known as "deicide," the charge of having killed (−cide, as in homicide) God (deus). The most cited text held up in support of this is Matthew 27:24–25, "When Pilate saw that he was getting nowhere, but that instead an uproar was starting, he took water and washed his hands in front of the crowd. 'I am innocent of this man's blood,' he said. 'It is your responsibility!' All the people answered, 'His blood is on us and on our children!'"

The last sentence in particular stands out. "All the people" refers to a group of Jews witnessing Jesus' execution. They seem to accept responsibility and suggest that responsibility extends to their children as well. In other words, one can read this verse as the text by which Jews become responsible for killing Jesus, even though it was, of course, Romans who killed Jesus, and because Matthew says that Jesus' blood is on the Jews then present "and our children," the guilt for Jesus' death—his blood—is on the Jews of the first century and their descendants for all time.

Not all Christians throughout history have interpreted this verse this way. Some theologians say the speakers symbolize all of sinful humanity. But many early Church fathers and later theologians like Augustine and Martin Luther did see this verse as an indictment of the Jews: Jews caused the death of God. Indeed, numerous other biblical verses suggest Jewish responsibility for Jesus' death. Matthew, however, is the one most cited and significant because the text directly assigns blame to future generations of Jews as well. The deicide charge is accompanied by two other influential theological claims.

Supersessionism

The second claim is known as "supersessionism" or "replacement theology." Supersessionism is the idea that the Church and Christians have "superseded" and replaced Jews and Judaism as God's covenantal partner. In this view, God has removed His favor from the followers of the laws of the Torah and bestowed his favor instead upon followers of Jesus.

The superseded old covenant rested on Abraham's circumcision and the giving of the Law at Mount Sinai. It has been replaced by the new covenant, marked by belief in the death and resurrection of Jesus. The new Israel—those who believe

Jesus is Christ—has replaced the old Israel as God's chosen people. The new covenant is also superior to the old because it is open to all, not only those who practice Judaism, and it is marked by the spirit (faith) and not the flesh (ethnicity).

The Book of Hebrews articulates this view most clearly, "In speaking of a new covenant, he (God) makes the first one obsolete. And what is becoming obsolete and growing old is ready to vanish away" (Hebrews 8:13). Many scholars suggest the destruction of the Jerusalem Temple by the Romans in 70 C.E. lent credibility to the supersessionist thesis because it illustrated that God's favor and protection had left the Jewish temple and the Jewish people.

Historical Suffering

A third, related, charge Christians have often made against Jews is that they suffer and warrant punishment because of their rejection of Jesus. The Jews refused to accept the new covenant. They persecuted one of their own, who delivered God's message first to them. Therefore, their suffering—first signaled by the destruction of the Temple—is God's ongoing punishment and evidence for the truth of Christianity.

The most articulate and influential proponent of this view is Augustine of Hippo, also known as St. Augustine. His theology deeply shaped the Western church for centuries—it is to Augustine, for example, that the church owes the doctrine of heritable original sin.

Augustine's thinking about Jews was also deeply influential. He emphasized Jewish responsibility for the death of Jesus. He argued that Pilate wanted to save Jesus but he gave in at the insistence of the Jews, who truly believed Jesus had blasphemed God by claiming he was the son of God. The Jews did not understand who Jesus was, and feeling threatened by his growing power, they had him murdered.

Augustine then tried to explain why God did not destroy the Jews altogether in punishment for their act of deicide. He concluded that the survival of the Jews is part of God's ongoing plan to teach the truth of Christianity. They show Christianity's ancient roots. Their suffering and scattering around the world demonstrate the consequences of blindness to God's truth. They suffer because they refuse to accept Jesus. Their crime of deicide, Augustine says, justifies their murder, but God's mercy prevails, and their existence forever reminds Christians of the consequences of disobedience.

The Crusades

Beliefs about supersessionism and deicide were just that—beliefs. But Christian history has also been riddled with actual violence done by Christians to Jews (often, though not always, in the name of deicide charges). This section is a difficult one because we will review several of the most persistent Christian expressions of anti-Semitism with an eye toward understanding how thoroughly the fabric of Christianity has been permeated with violent fantasies about Jews and how often those fantasies have enabled actual violence.

Prior to the Holocaust in the twentieth century, the most horrific period of Jewish persecution was the Crusades. In 1096 Pope Urban II issued a call for Christians to reclaim the Holy Land from the Muslims, who had conquered it in 1071. Between 20,000 and 30,000 Christians responded to the Pope's call and set off from Western Europe on horseback and in groups. On the way they marched through dozens of Jewish towns.

While Pope Urban II targeted Muslims, the crusaders committed themselves to destroying infidels more generally. They were fighting a war for Christ, and anyone deemed against Christ was the enemy. As historian Leon Poliakov noted, the crusaders "were God's avengers, appointed to punish all infidels, whoever they might be… What could be more natural than to take revenge along the way upon the various infidels living in Christian territories?" [3]. Jews were the first and most frequently encountered infidels crusaders saw along the way. Thus, between 1096 and 1099, tens of thousands of Jews in the Rhineland were murdered. Scholars do not know the complete number, but entire Jewish sections of towns were destroyed.

The attacks on Jews were often not directly made by the crusaders. Crusaders' calls for Christian victory ignited passions in hundreds of local villages. Dozens of accounts exist of ordinary villagers entering and attacking synagogues and surrounding streets inhabited by Jews. Sometimes local bishops would try to stop the mobs from attacking the Jewish quarter. But they were usually unable to do so. Indeed, the murder of Jews became a self-perpetuating loop, suggesting to Christians that God's patience with these infidels had run out, thus feeding yet more violence.

In addition to the number of Jews killed, an important consequence of the Crusades was the blurring of the line between mob action and official Church-sanctioned policies. This blurring of the lines reached its apex during the Inquisition, during which the church targeted Jews and those Christians who had converted from Judaism and still maintained Jewish practices. They were often imprisoned and executed.

While prominent bishops and even Popes condemned the murder of Jews, virtually none of the murderers were punished after the events happened, and many bishops simply looked on as their Jewish communities were destroyed. This fuzzy line between authority and mass hysteria appears and reappears in the violent history of anti-Semitism: legal authorities were complicit in the pogroms (murderous attacks of Jews) in Russia and the Ukraine in the late nineteenth century and even in the 1913 lynching of Leo Frank in Atlanta. Leo Frank was a Jew from New York who had married into an Atlanta Jewish family who owned a pencil factory. He managed the factory, and a young woman was murdered there. Authorities accused Frank, even though the evidence was minimal and pointed to the factory's custodian. While Frank was awaiting trial, he was broken out of prison and murdered. His body was hung on an oak tree where it remained for several days. Accounts of the Leo Frank murder point out that among those who organized the jail break and hanging were prominent citizens.

Jews and the Devil

This violence did not occur in a vacuum. It embedded itself within Christian practices. Indeed, inseparable from many acts of violence was a long history of Christians speaking about or visually depicting Jews as a violent "other." For example, in the Middle Ages, meditating upon the Crucifixion was important to many Christians' piety. And in the prayerful meditations Christians used as a devotional aid and in the theatrical renditions of the Passion Play, many gathered to watch. Jews were depicted in horrible terms—as enacting unspeakable violence upon Jesus as he walked to his death and as relishing the violence.

Christian preaching and art also portrayed Jews in league with the devil. John 8:44, for example, reads, "You [the Jews] belong to your father, the devil, and you want to carry out your father's desires. He was a murderer from the beginning, not holding to the truth, for there is no truth in him. When he lies, he speaks his native language, for he is a liar and the father of lies."

This equation of the Jews with the devil solves an important theological question: who was wicked enough to murder God? Only the devil. Therefore, Jews are the devil incarnate. This view helps explain other aspects of Christian anti-Semitism that we do not have the space to further explore, including the views of Martin Luther and the blood libel—where Jews are accused of using Christian blood to make Passover matza.

Jews and Money

One of the charges leveled against Jews in the Middle Ages—that of greed and devilish powers with money—persists into today. Up until the nineteenth century, many European countries forbid Jews to own land. They could not join professional guilds either. They could, however, lend money because the Catholic Church forbid Christians from doing so. Thus, a tiny but influential group of Jews became bankers. While moneylending helped save lives and support the Jewish community, it came with a dark side. When economies experienced downturns, Jews were often blamed.

The economic charges combined with religious prejudice to stir violent hatred and anger toward Jews during times of crisis. When the Black Plague spread throughout Europe in the fourteenth century, for example, Jews were blamed for the deaths in their communities, and they were targeted by mobs, who stole from them, sometimes forced them to be baptized, and sometimes murdered them. It seemed like it was the money that led to killing the Jews, for if they had been poor and if the feudal lords had not been in debt to them, it would seem that they would not have been burnt.

Middlemen Minority

Another psychological dimension behind economic anti-Semitism comes from Jews frequently occupying the role of what Professor Thomas Sowell calls "middlemen minority" [4]. The middlemen minorities fuel the relationship between the producers and the consumers. They are the retailers selling goods produced somewhere else to local consumers. They are the bankers lending money to both producers and consumers, thereby facilitating economic exchange between the two groups.

Middlemen minorities do not only serve this intermediary economic role. They also serve as an intermediary between different social groups and frequently between different socioeconomic classes within a country. In Catholic Poland, for example, Jews were the intermediaries between the small group of wealthy landowners and the large group of peasants who paid taxes to these landowners.

This economic role had some advantages. It allowed Jews (and other minorities like the Lebanese in Africa or the Chinese in Indonesia) to maintain their identities. Being different from the larger culture—being a minority— made the middlemen more effective in their role because the different classes or groups were able to relate more effectively through a third party.

Serving as an intermediary, however, also presents acute dangers. First, when prices are high or an economy is in decline, the middlemen are often blamed. They are simply closer and more visible to the people who are suffering. Secondly, because the middlemen minority are, by definition, a minority, they are more susceptible to anger from the masses. They provide a unifying target.

A third and more subtle danger lurks in the perception that middlemen are earning a profit without producing anything of concrete value. That perception can quickly translate into violence. Sowell points out [4] that those who earned their livings without visible toil, with clean hands, and by simply selling things that others had produced at higher prices than the producers had charged became easy targets of resentments, especially when they enjoyed a higher standard of living than those who worked in factories or on farms. Actually, those nearby on the socioeconomic scale are often more hotly resented than richer people. In other words, resentment did not come because Jews were richer than the larger population. It came because of the role they played and their proximity to the consumer.

Modern Anti-Semitism

In 1789, as the effects of the French Revolution and American Revolution began to manifest themselves, many Jews felt a sense of hope. Perhaps the walls built by ancient prejudices would fall as reason and enlightenment emphasized our common humanity. While some Jews did integrate into modern life, anti-Semitism took on new forms. It mutated rather than dissolved.

At first, as the nineteenth century began, life improved. Jews left the ghettos and settled in better neighborhoods with stable jobs. They entered universities previously closed to them. They became citizens of the states where they had once been barely tolerated aliens. The era promised intellectual and political freedom. The French Revolution proclaimed equality, brotherhood, and liberty, and enlightened thinkers like Voltaire critiqued the religious prejudices that had been part of European life for centuries.

And for many Jews, this promise was realized. My great-grandparents would not have been able to leave Poland and Austria had not thinkers like John Locke and Thomas Jefferson articulated the ideas that led to the American Constitution. The intellectual and political movements for reason and freedom—known respectively as the Enlightenment and the Emancipation—changed Europe and the religious groups residing there.

But for Jews, there was also an underbelly. Freedom in theory did not mean equality in practice. Deep-seated hatreds did not disappear with a new form of government. And as more Jews interacted with Christians, more justifications for anti-Semitism arose. In the nineteenth century, the Christian threads that had held anti-Semitism together for so many centuries remained, but they were stitched into new forms of political and social scapegoating and sequined with faux science. This scapegoating gave energy to the most destructive expressions of anti-Semitism in history: the Holocaust.

The concept of Judaism as a race became more salient as racial and ethnic identity became the foundations for the emerging nation-state in the eighteenth and nineteenth centuries. If Jews were a race, then they could never be truly German, French, or British. This meant Jews who assimilated into modern society—even those who converted to Christianity—could still be hated because they were inherently Jewish by blood, with all the attendant prejudices that Christians across Europe had imbued for centuries. And that is what happened as nationalism spread across Europe and a new anti-Semitism emerged.

The nineteenth century also saw the rise of an anti-Semitism grounded in the eugenics movement. Eugenics, popular in the United States in the early 1900s, sought to be the "science" of ethnicity. In the wake of Charles Darwin's work on evolution and survival of the fittest, it gained much attention and support in the nineteenth and early twentieth centuries. It looked for a scientific basis for physical and mental traits associated with a group. Scientists tried to connect body types and intelligence levels with various ethnicities. At various times they differentiated supposed racial types such as white European, American Indian, Black Africans, Asians, and a catch-all miscellaneous group called "monstrous." They assigned various traits to these groups like laziness, miserliness, or craftiness.

Jews were one of the most frequent targets of examination. A representative document from 1938 called "The Racial Biology of the Jews" claimed to analyze the finger prints, blood types, and susceptibility to various diseases among Jews. To this purported analysis was added the claim that Jews have "hooked noses, fleshy lips, ruddy light yellow, dull-colored skin, and kinky hair. They have a slinking gait and a 'racial scent'." This seemed to be anti-Semitism disguised as science.

The term "anti-Semitism" itself emerged out of the pseudoscience of eugenics. A writer named Wilhelm Marr coined it [5]. He argued that Jewish Semites lacked within themselves the Christian-German spirit. It was simply not within their make-up, no matter how long they had lived in Germany. The Jewish spirit of intellectualism and greed was in conflict with the German folk spirit, and the Jews were winning because political emancipation had brought them into wider society. The Jews, he argued, were beginning to control German finance and industry, and if the German folk did not fight back, they would die as a people. Marr also formed the "League of Anti-Semites." It was committed exclusively to fighting the Jewish threat to German society and expelling Jews from the country.

It might seem surprising that the terms anti-Semite and anti-Semitism did not arise until the late nineteenth century. As we have noted earlier, hatred of Jews is one of the world's oldest and most persistent prejudices. But the word anti-Semitism marks a significant change because it marries religious and racial prejudice. It targets Jews not on the basis of what they believe but on who they are. Jews are not just different. They are inherently inferior.

What made this new type of anti-Semitism even more dangerous was that a "scientific" theory of anti-Semitism allowed for a "scientific" solution to it. Science is the language of cause and effect, of problem and solution. For Wilhelm Marr, the Jews were a problem that could only be solved by total assimilation or expulsion from Germany. They were immutably different from other Germans. Hitler and the Nazis took up this perspective. As we will see, they brought a technological and scientific precision to their solution to the "Jewish problem."

Indeed, the intertwining, in the eighteenth, nineteenth, and twentieth centuries, of philosophy, science, and hatred of the Jews makes clear that education and reason are not the solution to prejudice. The Enlightenment ushered in a philosophical anti-Semitism alongside racial and religious anti-Semitisms. Its adherents envisioned a world free of prejudice while remaining blind to one they maintained. They believed the mind could solve all the prejudices lodged within our psyche. Instead, the technologies they helped create gave new powers to the ancient hatred they helped sustain. Some of the most horrific views about the Jew came from the most intelligent people. Indeed, the scientific theories of the Enlightenment gave anti-Semites a new language and justification: Jews are subhuman. Their superstitious faith, so the argument went, impedes the development of humanity, which is the goal of the modern world. Moreover, they are clannish. They are a cancer on society. The only way to defeat the cancer and save the patient is to eliminate the cancer. Thus, Hitler's Final Solution—the murder of all the Jews of the world—seemed like a logical next step in the evolution of enlightened anti-Semitism.

Hitler's Science

Scholars debate whether the Holocaust was an expression of religious anti-Semitism. Were the Nazis acting out the ultimate expression of the anti-Jewish hatred that had been taught in churches for centuries? Or was the Holocaust an expression of the modern racial, pseudoscientific anti-Semitism? While both played a role, the second explanation is more persuasive. The Nazis were predominantly secular. Yes, many Nazi leaders came from Christian backgrounds, as did most Germans. And yes, some churches and pastors supported the Nazis. But the Nazis revered the state and the Führer above all. Pseudoscientific racial theories were part of their party platform. The death camps were organized through rational bureaucratic procedures. They employed scientific processes and perspectives. Doctors, for example, used torture in conducting tests on blindness and in determining differences between identical twins. They documented every finding as a scientist would. Some of their papers are still consulted today. The Holocaust was not a chaotic expression of pent-up religious hatred. It was organized, bureaucratic, and systematic genocide. Jews were not human beings created in the image of God. They were leeches on society who could be drained for all they were worth and then eliminated. Care was taken to be as cost-efficient as possible in doing so. Even the gold fillings from murdered Jews' teeth were extracted before their bodies were cremated. Such genocide was possible only because the Nazis and their allies saw Jews as less than human. And that conception was only possible because of the history of anti-Semitism, which shrank Jews to a physically inferior, slavish people.

Another reason the Holocaust is more of a secular than a theologic expression of anti-Semitism is captured by Yale historian Timothy Snyder [6]. According to Snyder, Hitler saw the natural order as one of survival of the fittest. Species and ethnicities compete with one another. The strongest survive. Equality, mercy, and kindness are not part of this order. Rather, conflict is the norm. Jews, however, introduced a different kind of order. Genesis 1:26 says every human being is created in the image of God. Thus, Jews brought a notion of human dignity and equality into creation. Snyder argues that with these concepts, Jews introduced a level of abstraction to human existence. Life was not simply about fighting for your tribe's survival. It was about living according to transcendent values. For Hitler, that was unnatural. That went against the dictates of nature.

In other words, basic empathy and respect for others is unnatural. Treating others as we ourselves would want to be treated has no place in the real world. "Doing unto others"—when the "other" is a Jew or alien—allows unfit, weak species and peoples to stay alive and thereby challenges the natural dominance of the strongest. By articulating the idea that everyone equally bears God's image, Jews brought disorder and alarming instability into society.

Hitler's anti-Semitism differs significantly from the traditional Christian anti-Semitism. Augustine and Martin Luther believed Jews committed the sin of murdering Jesus and thereby lost God's favor. Hitler believed Jews introduced human dignity into the world and thereby upset natural hierarchies. To simplify it further, we could say Christians hated Jews because Jews took God (in the form of Jesus) from the world. Hitler hated Jews because they brought God (in the form of the claim that all people are created in God's image) into the world. As such, Jews are a permanent stain on the world that must be eviscerated. This view justified the Holocaust.

Today

The Holocaust ended 75 years ago. Most of its survivors have passed away. The Jewish population also recently achieved a milestone in reaching again its pre-Holocaust level. Yet, while anti-Semitism declined markedly in the immediate decades following the Second World War, it has grown recently. So-called hate crimes against Jews seem to have tripled. In October 2018, a man walked into a Pittsburgh synagogue on a Sabbath morning and murdered eight Jews at prayer. Exactly 6 months later, a man walked into a San Diego synagogue and murdered a 60-year-old woman and shot the rabbi through the hand. These are only the most visible of a series of incidents of the last year. While I have written an entire book on this resurgence [7], as have others [8, 9], here I will simply summarize its three primary manifestations from my perspective.

Type 1: Right-Wing

The first type of modern anti-Semite sees Jews as sinister, dangerous, power-hungry globalists. The gunmen in Pittsburgh and in San Diego typified this view.

Jews, they say, manipulate the media, Hollywood, Wall Street, and even the White House. They do so to enrich themselves. They are constantly scheming to steal and hurt others.

Anti-Semites with these views present the most immediate violent danger. Their ideology promotes violence. It predominates in white supremacist circles and the alt-right.

The anti-Semitism demands vigilance. While it has existed for a long time, it diminished during the economic prosperity of the 1990s, but it has crept up again in the wake of the Great Recession and rise of right-wing populism.

Type 2: From the Middle East

The second type of anti-Semitism comes from extremist expressions of Islam. Its adherents see Israel as a Western colonial power occupying Arab land. The historical irony behind this form of anti-Semitism is that until the twentieth century, Islamic countries were generally much more welcoming to Jews than Christian countries. Today, however, mainstream newspapers in many Arab countries feature anti-Semitic myths developed in Christian Europe. This anti-Semitism wants Israel erased from the map.

Type 3: From the Left

The third type of anti-Semitism comes from the extreme political Left.

Recent examples abound. At the University of California at Berkeley, students recently echoed an increasingly popular claim that the Israeli army trains American police departments on how to better kill African-Americans. In May of 2018, the *New York Times* printed a cartoon with the Israeli Prime Minister on the face of a dog that could easily have appeared in a Nazi newspaper.

While the first type of anti-Semitism presents the most immediate danger and potential for violence, this left-wing anti-Semitism worries me the most because it supports a narrative that turns Israel and the Jewish community into moral villains. It pits Jews and Judaism against justice and peace. This tendency continues to intensify on college campuses and some political circles.

Times of crisis and social anxiety usually coincide with a rise in anti-Semitism. We saw this in the 1930s. We saw it again in the mid-1960s. We are seeing it again today. A society that can't come together soon begins to fall apart.

Conclusions

The longevity of anti-Semitism suggests its origins may lie in something essential to human nature. In the last century, the fields of psychiatry and psychology emerged, potentially to add new insights into anti-Semitism and how to reduce it. The remaining chapters in this edited volume convey the most cutting-edge psychological ideas on anti-Semitism.

References

1. Moffic E. What every Christian needs to know about Judaism. Nashville: Abingdon Press; 2020. (in press).
2. Nirenberg D. Anti-Judaism: the western tradition. New York: W.W. Norton; 2013. p. 14.
3. Poliakov L. The history of Anti-Semitism: from the Time of Christ to the Court Jews. New York: University of Pennsylvania Press; 2003. p. 41 and 56.
4. Sowell T. Black rednecks and white liberals. New York: Encounter Books; 2005. p. 70.
5. Zimmerman M. Wilhelm Marr: the patriarch of Anti-Semitism. New York: Oxford University Press; 1986.
6. Snyder T. Black earth: the holocaust as history and warning. New York: Tim Duggan Books; 2016.
7. Moffic E. First the Jews: combating the World's longest-running hate campaign. New York: Abingdon Press; 2019.
8. Lipstadt D. Antisemitism: here and now. New York: Schocken; 2019.
9. Weiss B. How to fight Anti-Semitism. New York: Crown; 2019.

Prejudice: Intra- and Interpersonal Aspects

2

Andrew J. McLean

Introduction

Prejudice is often considered an individual issue, while racism or other "isms" pertain to groups, however large. Intrapersonal aspects refer to the self, one's internal dialogue. Interpersonal aspects involve interactions with others—whether one to one, in-group, or out-group.

Historically, particular theories pertaining to prejudice have waxed and waned in popularity and have become interwoven (individual, social, biological, evolution) in a fashion not unlike other theories in psychology/psychiatry.

From an evolutionary standpoint, it is theorized that humans learned to categorize as an efficient cognitive tool—to simplify the processing of information/situations quickly. In Gordon Allport's seminal work, "The Nature of Prejudice" [1], he defined prejudice as "an antipathy based upon a faulty and inflexible generalization," while noting that "The human mind must think with the aid of categories." As Augustinos and Every [2] observed, categorization, while useful, is a distortion of the truth, as people are seen as prototypical group members and not viewed as individuals. Generalizations occur, then stereotypes, as part of this categorization. Stereotypes can be both malleable and fixed [3]. Despite our denial that we are unbiased, suppositions can become automatic and outside of our conscious awareness. We then can easily move to pre-judging (prejudice) and then to discrimination and from there to "isms," specific negative categorizations. As such, our human cognitive construct is paved with ever-increasing opportunities to see people not as real individuals but as members of assumed groups.

Duckitt [4] reviewed the varying psychodynamic processes and theories implicated in racism and prejudice, including displacement of hostility, projection,

A. J. McLean (✉)
Department of Psychiatry and Behavioral Science, University of North Dakota School of Medicine and Health Sciences, Fargo, ND, USA
e-mail: andrew.mclean@und.edu

© Springer Nature Switzerland AG 2020
H. S. Moffic et al. (eds.), *Anti-Semitism and Psychiatry*,
https://doi.org/10.1007/978-3-030-37745-8_2

frustration, and scapegoating. And within that work, while there is no "prejudiced personality" that explains all, there is a framework for understanding the formation of prejudice, whereby individual prejudicial processes become fostered through social and group dynamics.

Jews over millennia have been treated in different ways by different cultures and governments. Throughout history, it is rare to find evidence of local Jews being treated as equals with all the rights of citizenry and little discrimination. Often they have been tolerated, at times allowed partial rights. If Jewish people were seen through the lens of culture or religion rather than race, there was less animosity. The more progressive societies were those which dealt with the Jewish population from a perspective of culture. There have been times defined as "philo-Semitism," in which cultures have overtly supported Judaism. The Golden Age of Jewish culture in Spain, where religion, economy, and culture were supported, occurred during the Middle Ages. For centuries, Poland had welcomed persecuted Jews, and in the sixteenth century, Holland became the first European country to provide "civil emancipation" for Jews. The articulation of support by respected thinkers such as John Locke [5] was influential in enhancing Jewish rights.

On the continuum of stereotype/prejudice/anti-Semitism, there is also another factor of overtness, or degree of prejudice. The psychiatrist Chester Pierce [6] coined the term "microaggression." Sue and colleagues [7] elaborated on this term, defining microaggressions as "brief, everyday exchanges that send denigrating messages to certain individuals because of their group membership." Types of microaggressions include microinsults, microinvalidations, and microassaults, with the perpetrator often unconscious of the former two. Commonly seen in Christian majority countries is one category of religious aggression described by Nadal et al., the "Assumption of One's Own Religious Identity as the Norm" [8]. For example, this might manifest during December as microinvalidations of Jewish people when, although there is to be "separation of church and state" (the word "church" itself is a microinvalidation), references to Christmas seem ubiquitous in government buildings and throughout the public square.

More overtly, when aspects of "race" arise, soon the categorization of "pure" and "impure" follows. This has certainly been the case with anti-Semitism as well as other types of hate. At such times, hate becomes a faith—and religions often require devils. Faith is a conviction without requirement of reason or evidence. History has shown us that in times of social and economic unrest, aspects of prejudice increase. When prejudice moves beyond private beliefs to action with the virulence noted above, hate crimes occur.

Perry's definition of a hate crime entails the following: "It involves acts of violence and intimidation, usually directed toward already stigmatized and marginalized groups. As such, it is a mechanism of power, intended to reaffirm the precarious hierarchies that characterize a given social order. It attempts to recreate simultaneously the (real or imagined) hegemony of the perpetrator's group and the 'appropriate' subordinate identity of the victim's group" [9].

It is difficult to write a chapter on prejudice, in a book about anti-Semitism (especially from a psychological standpoint), and not reference Adolf Hitler, particularly as there are available treatises on the analysis of his personality. Hitler stated, "We must distrust the intelligence and the conscience and must place our faith in our instincts." "If a people is to become free it needs pride and will-power, defiance, hate, hate and once again hate" [10]. Waite [11] felt Hitler's own likely Jewish heritage (grandfather) was part of his projected guilt and subsequent move toward removing this "blemish" from history as well as his own psyche. For the Jewish population, this resulted in pogroms (organized massacres) and the Holocaust. In nation upon nation, this type of hate has resulted in genocide, where both ethnocentrism and xenophobia have been driving factors.

It is a timeless question as to whether we all have the capacity to subscribe to such hate. Carl Jung in "On the Psychology of the Unconscious" [12] wrote, "It is a frightening thought that man also has a shadow side to him, consisting not just of little weaknesses and foibles, but of a positively demonic dynamism. The individual seldom knows anything of this; to him, as an individual, it is incredible that he should ever in any circumstances go beyond himself. But let these harmless creatures form a mass, and there emerges a raging monster." [Jung himself dealt with controversy as to whether he was an anti-Semite and a Nazi sympathizer. In her biography of Jung, Deirdre Bair [13] notes that while there were missteps in the early days of power of Nazi Germany, Jung was sympathetic to the Jewish cause. He was involved in two plots to remove Hitler having become a secret agent for the OSS (predecessor to the CIA).]

Lewis in "Semites and Anti-Semites" [14] describes three types of hostility associated with prejudice: in the first, hostility is essentially against policy or government—political. The second, "conventional" or "normal" prejudice, is the type that one inherently finds between competing tribal groups. The third type of hostility goes beyond simple prejudice. This enmity is seen in anti-Semitism. There is often a dehumanizing approach and, at its worst, in both individual and broad (genocidal) interactions, a need for annihilation. For entities hostile to Jews, perceived risk of existential loss has been manifested by many iterations over the centuries. Under the guise of loss of racial purity, fear of cultural depletion, fear of eternal loss, fear of subversion, and fear of being overpowered, groups have directed their fear toward Jews in anti-Semitic hatred and attack.

The impact of hate crimes can be felt both individually and group-wide. This indeed can be an efficient way to spread fear, an effect which Weinstein coined in terrorem [15], whereby an entire group can be intimidated by victimizing one or more of its group members. This appears to be the current approach by many hate groups or individuals purporting to represent them. While the Anti-Defamation League (ADL) [16] reported decreases in anti-Semitic rhetoric and behavior over the past few decades, there has been an up-tick in the past few years. This is occurring not only in the USA but also globally. Anti-immigrant (essentially anti-Brown/Black), Islamophobic, and anti-Semitic events have become more pronounced.

Plous reviewed various theories of prejudice, [17] including "the authoritarian personality," a work by Theodor Adorno, who had escaped Nazi Germany. While similar to Duckitt's review of the "prejudiced personality" from the 1950s, negating an overt personality type, Plous's determination was that there are three individual traits that correlate with prejudice: "right-wing authoritarianism," social hierarchical views (social dominance orientation), and rigid categorical thinking.

Intrapersonal Aspects

Though there are no defined "prejudiced personalities," certain intrapersonal aspects are cited among the variables in play which align with both individual and group prejudice.

Psychological Theories

Within the psychological literature, particularly in the area of psychodynamics, theories have emerged relating to how individuals "protect" themselves against thoughts, feelings, and behaviors which might be unpleasant. These are considered to be unconscious, natural mechanisms ranging from primitive to mature. Examples of common primitive defense mechanisms particularly related to the topic at hand are denial (self-explanatory) and projection. Projection plays a role in many aspects of prejudice.

In his treatise on Hitler, written during the height of World War II, Langer wrote, "Hitler's outstanding defense mechanism is one commonly called PROJECTION. It is a technique by which the ego of an individual defends itself against unpleasant impulses, tendencies or characteristics by denying their existence in himself while he attributes them to others." Hitler's drive for world dominance was juxtaposed with the propaganda that it was Jews who plotted universal ascendancy through control of the global finance system.

More developmentally mature though not necessarily more copacetic defense mechanisms include rationalization and intellectualization. Rationalization allows for one's actions to be cognitively acceptable. Such justifications are often tied to faith or religion. Consistent with Plous's content, a meta-analysis by McCleary et al. [18] found that religious fundamentalism correlates with certain psychological variables, including prejudice. Intellectualization removes one's emotion from the task. Intellectualization is somewhat related to objectification: seeing others as objects. One lacks empathy for another, and thus one's ego is defended. (If I relate to your feelings, I risk harm to myself.)

Research has shown that those with high self-esteem display more in-group bias than those with lower self-esteem. And, individuals who have a decrease in self-esteem are more likely to exhibit prejudicial attitudes and behavior. One classic experiment by Fein and Spencer [19] reflected specific prejudice toward Jews vs. another select population when criticism or reduction in self-esteem of subjects occurred.

There have been eras in which frustration, even humiliation of previous "in-groups," resulted in displacement of hostility onto certain out-group populations. Sartre articulated this in "Anti-Semite and Jew" [20] when he stated, "If the Jew didn't exist, the anti-Semite would create him."

Dissociation has, in psychodynamic terms, been described as a disconnection from the world, often seen in the aftermath of trauma. More recently it has been used to describe disengagement or lack of empathy as a protective mechanism. A somewhat related mechanism is compartmentalization, the ability to maintain separate sets of values without yielding to or being aware of internal conflict. Specific to prejudice, Devine's dissociation model [21] purports stereotypes to be cognitive structures learned early in life (and frequently automatically activated), whereas overt racial attitudes (prejudice) are learned later. However, other researches have found racial prejudice in children as young as 2 ½ years of age [22].

Cognitive Dissonance

As we review psychological determinants of prejudice, we note not only psychodynamic defenses in which we "protect" our egos but also cognitive aspects by which we attend to, perceive, and think about ourselves and others. "Cognitive dissonance" is the internal disquiet that occurs when retaining psychologically incompatible thoughts or beliefs. The natural tendency is to avoid this from occurring or to reduce the discomfort.

One way of dealing with cognitive dissonance is to use defense mechanisms discussed above such as denial (including denial by fantasy), intellectualization, and rationalization. Hitler stated that conscience was a "Jewish invention," and "… only when the time comes when the race is no longer overshadowed by the consciousness of its own guilt then will it find internal peace." He rationalized away morality as a tool of the enemy, giving permission to himself and others to "distrust the intelligence and the conscience."

Emerging from object relations theory is the concept of "splitting," an ego defense mechanism which relates to cognitive dissonance as well as projection. While racial prejudice was not initially considered within its formulation, "splitting" is often described in popular nomenclature as "Black-and-White" thinking. "All or nothing." We cannot tolerate our own, often unconscious internal conflict, and thus we project our intolerable traits onto others. As one cannot tolerate "gray," one might see another (individual or group) in an undervalued fashion and others as overvalued. For the devalued out-group or individual, we hear terms such as dirty, filthy, or impure. Cognitive dissonance—we cannot mix.

Object relations theory proposes that a "good enough environment" allows infants and children to learn to transform "part objects" from their environment (including people) into whole objects, thus being able to tolerate ambiguity. The individual moves beyond "splitting" good and bad, to endure the ambivalent feelings regarding another and to eventually develop the necessary human trait of empathy. Empathy is the capacity to understand another's experience (thoughts/feelings/attitude) from their perspective. Humanity is a sufficient requirement for sympathizing; for empathizing, it is a necessary one. Empathy allows us to see "the other" in humane ways.

A healthy concept of "the other" is seeing others as separate from me/us, yet much more similar than different. And, their differences are of value. They are seen as individuals, persons, linked to me/us in numerous ways. Their value does not diminish mine—it is not "zero sum."

An unhealthy concept of "the other" is that not only are they separate but they also are of less value and are to be belittled and feared. They are "objects," to be avoided or overcome (or in the extreme, exterminated). We could never consider "the other" as potentially "us." Always "them."

Humanity, or Lack Thereof

Why is it that certain populations are targeted, not simply to be controlled, but destroyed? Aldous Huxley, the English writer and philosopher, wrote of the propaganda tool of dehumanization: its use is "to persuade one set of people that another set of people are not really human and that it is therefore legitimate to rob, swindle, bully and even murder them" [23].

In "Less than Human—Why We Demean, Enslave and Exterminate Others" [24], Smith describes the dehumanizing of others as a way of allowing such atrocities to occur.

Groups targeted for annihilation are seen as subhuman, un-human. During times of genocide, in Armenia, Rwanda, Germany, Russia, Cambodia, and many other places, victims would be labeled as "parasitic, blood-sucking, vermin." Along the evolutionary chain, we have microbes, parasites, and leeches (takers, removing not illness and toxins but essence and life—draining the purity). Untamed and primitive: dogs, monkeys, and subhuman "beasts in human form" (the latter is a quote from Himmler's *The Subhuman Magazine*—a publication literally for the German public during WWII). "Mongrel races" is a common phrase used by White Nationalist groups.

It is important to not assume that holding racist beliefs equates to lack of intellect. Some of the most intelligent people in the world have held prejudicial and racist views, while using their own reality to justify actions. Leading up to WWII, many US leaders supported the writings of Madison Grant (who wrote Hitler's favorite book, *The Passing of the Great Race*). As noted by the Southern Poverty Law Center, William Shockley, the 1956 Nobel Laureate in Physics, once stated the following to support his views on White Supremacy [25]: "Prejudice that is not supported by strong facts is both illogical and not in accordance with truth. The general principle that truth is a good thing applies here. Some things that are called prejudice, which are based on sound statistics, really shouldn't be called prejudice. ... It might be easier to think in terms of breeds of dogs...".

Stories, Myths, and Conspiracy Theories

Theologian Karen Armstrong has described myth as "the history of the human psyche." Myths are vitally important to people. They allow us to make meaning of our circumstances and to deal with our fears, including existential ones. In the preface to *The Case for God* [26], she writes, "When Freud and Jung began to chart their scientific search for the soul, they instinctively turned to these ancient myths. A myth was never intended as an accurate account of a historical event; it was *something that had in some sense happened once but that also happens all the time.*" She delineates between logos (reason) and mythos (myth) and emphasizes mankind's need for both. Unfortunately, misapplications of these different truths occur and are often utilized to further prejudice.

The term "Semite" comes from Shem, Noah's eldest son, whose descendant was Abraham, the Patriarch of Arabs and Hebrews and, according to Matthew, the progenitor of the lineage of Joseph and Jesus. Somehow, "Semite" has come to commonly refer only to those of Jewish lineage and not other descendants of Abraham. And, there have been many legends relating to the other sons of Noah—Ham and Japheth. The popular mythology of Aryan origins via alleged Japhethic lineage has played a role in Western racial ideology [27]. Ironically, those who claim Jewish deicide dismiss the Roman (Japhethic) aspect of the story.

A mechanism by which truth and reason are held at bay is through logical fallacy—circular reasoning. A fascinating version of this, seen often in the support of prejudice as well as confirmation bias, is the conspiracy theory. One might see an individual's tendency toward this in the same vein as Klein's object relations paranoid-schizoid position.

Conspiracy theories have attributed at times bizarre and outlandish behaviors toward a hated individual or out-group. This has been seen multiple times over centuries in attribution to Jewish people, often with the focus on "blood libel," the fallacy of Jews using Christian children's blood in ritual. Another claim is the "hidden world": Jews with special powers. Jews = evil; evil = Jews. Jews controlling the film industry, the financial markets, etc. An example of perpetuated anti-Semitic propaganda pertaining to Jewish global domination plans is the publication *Protocols of the Elders of Zion.*

There have been hate crimes including murders at synagogues. One of the alleged perpetrators in a 2019 US (Pittsburgh) slaying posted a conspiracy theory promulgated among hate groups that "there is an attempt to replace white Americans with immigrants" and that this is a Jewish-led effort [28]. Included was also the age-old "blood libel" commentary. Conspiracy theories defy counterbalancing, as those who attempt to do so are automatically suspect.

Jost et al. have noted in their system-justification theory [29] that conspiracy theories reflect many psychological needs including the desire for certainty, security, and positive image of self/group. Some research [30] indicates that exposure to conspiracy theories actually reduces people's sense of autonomy and control. Einstein and Glick have shown that experiments of exposure to conspiracy theories decrease trust in government and scientists [31].

As Lewendowsky et al. note [32], reliance on misinformation differs from ignorance. False beliefs are held with conviction. They note four features people tend to use to evaluate the true value of information: (1) Is it compatible with what I believe? (2) Is the story coherent (organized, compelling, "a good story")? (3) Is the source credible? (4) Do others believe it? In terms of battling misinformation, these same researchers note that only three factors have been identified that can increase the effectiveness of retractions: (a) warnings at the time of the initial exposure to misinformation, (b) repetition of the retraction, and (c) corrections that tell an alternative story that fills the coherence gap otherwise left by the retraction.

Berger notes [33] that emotional arousal increases the passing on of information. When there are plausible yet conflicting facts or answers to the mental model of a story or event, the gap in the theory (now less complete) leads to discomfort (i.e., cognitive dissonance). Thus people continue to choose the incorrect model rather than the now incomplete model.

Interpersonal

Social Theories

Janis [34] described a phenomenon of peer pressure termed "groupthink." The group discards or discourages dissent to reach consensus, despite faulty decisions that at times can reflect dehumanization. A known tendency of "groupthink" is polarization: movement of opinions gravitating to extremes.

How do in-groups maintain a healthy "pro-us" position without becoming "anti-them?" Social identity theory (SIT) elaborates on the psychological importance of differentiation between groups. However, such delineation should not threaten the identity of the other. Positive differentiation of the intergroup might be very "other-oriented." However, as Ellemers and Haslam report [35], these dimensions often develop into aspects of privilege, superiority, and dominance. When the in-group believes in absolutism and there is no tolerance, it is a recipe for violence.

Jones and colleagues [36] elaborate on the way that power differentials between in-groups/out-groups pave a road from prejudice to racism, with subsequent racist social practices. Social dominance theory purports that the dominant group position is an objective one and that laws and resources are based on the correctness of this power differential [37]. Those in the majority do not understand their privileged position, as they have not experienced what it is to be in the non-dominant group [38]. Consequently, social policies continue to be weighted toward the privileged. And, being blinded to the reality of inequity provides no incentive to change; in fact, it at times provides incentive not to change.

The world is filled with individuals who believe that everyone "gets what they deserve," particularly when there is a negative attribution to those in "out-groups." Examples of this "causal attribution" include social caste systems, the plight of the poor, trauma, etc. Whether unconsciously or intentionally, the outcome is the same. As Niebuhr wrote, "…it has always been the habit of the privileged groups to deny the oppressed classes every opportunity for the cultivation of innate capacities and then to accuse them of lacking what they have been denied the right to acquire" [39].

As we discuss defense mechanisms relating to anti-Semitism, we are primarily (though not exclusively) focusing on the beliefs, emotions, and behaviors of non-Jewish people. Many non-Jewish people, however, are not aware of the variety of groups and ideologies within Judaism, that there are multiple cultures within the religion, and that there is in-group/out-group discrimination within Judaism.

Researches by Goldstone [40] and others have inferred that in-group differences tend to be down-played, while differences from other groups are over-emphasized. Plous reflects that we tend to assume that those within their respective groups (in-groups/out-groups) have more internal similarities than they actually do. The perception that all members of an out-group are alike ("out-group homogeneity bias") holds true of all groups, whether based on race, nationality, religion, age, or other naturally occurring group affiliations.

Cuddy et al. [41] have developed a 2 × 2 model of out-group stereotyping. The variables are cold/warm and competent/incompetent. They view Jewish stereotyping as that of "cold/competent." The competent/incompetent variable appears to have varied throughout history, with the most recent quadrant resulting in subsequent "envious prejudice." The less stability in the world, the more likely groups in this quadrant will be attacked and blamed.

Non-Jews may envy (unconsciously) Jewish accomplishments, "staying-power," etc. They may be jealous of the perceived relationship with God, including the Covenant (in-group/out-group). Götz Aly named the deadly sin of envy as the driver in his book *Why the Germans? Why the Jews? Envy, Race, Hatred, and the Prehistory of the Holocaust.*

Allport showed that face-to-face contact between members of two groups in conflict promotes positive relationships and therefore leads to prejudice reduction. The Anti-Defamation League (ADL) reports that globally, while a quarter of the world's population holds anti-Semitic views, 70% of that group have never met a Jewish person. We also know however that people who grew up personally knowing members of other groups can still hold significant prejudices.

Paluck [42] created a field intervention through a radio broadcast in a developing country that encouraged people to discuss discrimination-related topics with each other. Results showed that at the end of the study individuals in the "test" regions were actually more prejudiced and less willing to help out-group members than those from the "control" regions. This study illustrates how important it is to carry out field studies before one can claim that a particular prejudice reduction method is effective.

One does not need to have a long-established affiliation or influence from a particular group to form group-related bias. Tajfel et al. [43] in the 1970s showed that bias and discrimination could be quickly established in arbitrarily formed minimal intergroups.

So, what allows for people to submit? It is not an uncommon occurrence whereby a victim, often unconsciously and driven by a need for safety, emulates the traits of their assailant. The mechanism of "Identification with the Aggressor," incorporating a negative introject, is freeing to many young people; the previously "weak" characteristics are repressed and projected onto others, who are targeted through this new "power." Langer states in his Hitler treatise that the masses "were not only willing, but anxious, to submit to anybody who could prove to them that he was competent to fill the role." In his work, Langer implies that such followers may have come from more traditional, paternalistic families.

Augustinos has reported on research pertaining to how people disguise their prejudice (conscious or otherwise). Such discursive repertoires can include the following: (a) the denial of prejudice (i.e., "I'm the least racist person I know"), (b) grounding one's views as reflecting the external world rather than one's psychology ("It's a fact that…" "People say…"), (c) positive-self and negative-other presentation ("If they worked as hard as we have, they wouldn't be in the situation they're in…"), (d) discursive deracialization ("This isn't about race, it's about economics…,"), and (e) the use of liberal arguments for "illiberal" ends ("We need to protect the Jews from the Muslims and vice versa…").

Changing attitudes are different from changing behavior. As Jung said: "What we call civilized consciousness has steadily separated itself from the basic instincts. But these instincts have not disappeared…modern man protects himself against seeing his own split state by a system of compartments. Certain areas of outer life and of his own behavior are kept, as it were, in separate drawers and are never confronted with one another."

What Jung and many others have alluded to is that we need to (1) be aware of and (2) tolerate our discomfort—to own our feelings as our own (see mirror, not glass). We need to change the misinformation narrative.

There are numerous studies showing a "backfire effect," where dissonant-false information correction is associated with "belief polarization," a "digging in" with further divergence among opposing groups. Interestingly, often new and contrary true information may reduce self-esteem without changing belief. Cohen et al. describe one solution as coupling the affirmation of basic values with opportunities for message correction [44].

Media

As reflected in our social media, we seem addicted to outrage. Anonymity allows for communicating in ways that would never be opined in person. However, there has been more "coming out" of individuals and groups with prejudicial agendas. And, most recently there has been discussion of the use of social media in manufacturing bias for swaying not only attitudes and behaviors but also elections. Advertisers, researchers, pollsters, etc. have utilized the concept of "priming," essentially activating known or suspected biases/stereotypes. Priming has been noted in experiments of racial stereotyping [45]. Recently, Facebook, Twitter, Instagram, and other platforms have increased their surveillance and limitations on hate speech use by members. Yet-to-be discovered or utilized technologies will no doubt continue to play a role in individual and social engineering.

There have been attempts through music, the arts, and media to both enhance and reduce prejudice. Rogers and Hammerstein, both of Jewish heritage, wrote the quintessential song on the childhood development of prejudice in South Pacific's "You've Got to Be Carefully Taught." Challenges to this post-WWII musical and song by legislators who saw the production as a communist plot speak to the difficulty in addressing bias [46]. Literature, television, and more recently podcasts have been venues in which to present different cultures, lifestyles, and attitudes, with subsequent social change. In Rwanda, a controlled, yearlong field experiment revealed that a radio soap opera built around messages of reducing intergroup prejudice, violence, and survivors' trauma altered listeners' perceptions of social norms and their behavior—albeit not their beliefs—in comparison with a control group exposed to a health-focused soap opera [47]. Other groups have worked on sharing narratives and personal stories.

Leadership

While activation of certain stereotypes may be fleeting, reactivation and cumulative effects can result in prolongation. The ABCs of social psychology (affect, behavior, cognition) influence and are influenced by relationships among social groups. Particular risks occur when the individual pathology of a leader ignites the group pathology. When leaders are able to not only control a narrative (the cognitive/ belief) but also stoke the flames of emotion (affect), hate crimes (behavior) can occur. As Langer described in *A Psychoanalysis of Adolf Hitler*, "…a reciprocal relationship exists between the Fuehrer and the people and that the madness of the one stimulates and flows into the other and vice versa." Such a leader is "the expression of a state of mind existing in millions of people….in all civilized countries."

Mental Health and Prejudice

Throughout history, individuals with mental illness have been ostracized or worse. Torrey and Yolken [48] estimate that during Nazi reign, a quarter of a million people with mental illness were killed or sterilized.

While hate crimes against mentally ill individuals still occur, a more common response is that of stigmatization. Stigmatization occurs not only in the public eye but also within psychiatry [49, 50]. This appears to particularly be the case regarding patients with more severe mental illnesses. While the "schizophrenogenic mother" etiology has fallen by the wayside, when practitioners or systems can't easily treat an illness of significant complexity, the reflex is to point blame away from the provider. While there has been greater focus on cultural sensitivity/competence in the training of physicians in recent years, an anti-stigma program for medical students in the UK showed unsustained benefits in reduction of mental health stigma [51].

Self-Stigma

Earlier in the chapter, we discussed the concept of "identification with the aggressor." More commonly the internalized stigma of being part of an "out-group" results in a reduction in self-esteem and self-efficacy, particularly if there is social isolation. A stereotype about Jews is that they suffer from high levels of neuroses. A 1992 NIMH study failed to reveal a difference in anxiety disorders between religious groups [52]. A 2007 study indicated that Jews in Israel had similar rates of mood and anxiety disorders to that of Western nations [53]. A majority of the Jewish population may be more open to treatment, however. Midlarsky et al. found that Jews in New York are less stigmatizing toward therapy than other groups [54]. A survey within the last decade from NEFESH (the International Network of Orthodox Mental Health Professionals) indicated that stigma within the community had been reduced over the past 25 years and that, as a whole, individuals were "less-underserved [55]." However, "Both the chasidic and ultra-Orthodox segments of Orthodox Jewry remain particularly underserved, while the age group that needs the most attention includes children and adolescents." Jewish Family Service agencies continue to network to provide assistance for people in local federations.

Providers

Space does not allow for elaboration on the link between Judaism and the development of the fields of psychology and psychiatry. However, interestingly, a 2007 study of 1000 US physicians found that psychiatrists were more likely to be Jewish or without a religious affiliation ("spiritual but not religious"), compared to other physician groups [56].

It is well-established [57] that the majority of individuals with behavioral health issues present first to their primary care providers. Primary care clinics afford opportunities for screening, brief intervention, and referral to treatment (SBIRT) for behavioral health issues. However, when we view the spectrum of chronic diseases, identification and management of depression falls significantly behind other conditions in primary care settings [58]. Even when identified, behavioral health issues may not be referred to those with expertise. The lens through which one sees the issue will determine the approach one takes. According to Wang et al. [59], religious, non-psychiatrist physicians were more willing to refer patients to clergy and less willing to refer patients to psychiatrists. Up to a quarter of individuals seek mental health services from their religious leaders. The NEFESH survey identified that roughly "75 percent of Orthodox clinicians in New York and about 85 percent outside said that few, if any, clients are referred to their doctors by rabbis." A common fear of religious individuals considering behavioral health care is that the treatment might change their religious beliefs. A group in the UK tackled the issue of access to mental health care within the Orthodox Jewish community through a distributed leadership team with knowledge and influence, allowing for a "custom-made" service or care [60].

While the latest version of DSM includes V coding for a "religious or spiritual problem," for many individuals, mental health and religious issues are not mutually exclusive. It is incumbent upon both health-care providers and religious leaders to be culturally competent and knowledgeable.

Interventions

At the risk of overstating the obvious, the most effective interventions are those that induce a long-lasting change in attitudes and behaviors [61].

The following recommendations are based not only on analysis of research but also obviously on my opinion as a practitioner of psychiatry (intrapersonal) and population health (interpersonal):

- We need courage to self-reflect, to doubt, and to be curious. This requires risk. Who has the ego strength, the self-esteem, to tolerate this? Most people strive to do right. Haidt has described varying traits that moral people have. Some focus more on caring, some on liberty, and some on loyalty, authority, and sanctity. But most converge on the importance of fairness [62]. The Golden Rule.
- We need laws and regulations that are truly fair toward all people. Perry notes, "… the task of the criminal justice system is not only to mitigate the negative effects of hate crime for individual victims, but the communities to which they belong."
- We need to have the default position toward others as *similar*, rather than *different*. To do so we need to venture from our "in-group," which is often not a comfortable experience.
- In our dialogue with others, we should remember the elements of motivational enhancement: recalling not only the stages of change but that shame and lecturing are typically ineffective. Much of confirmation bias has to do with protecting one's identity.
- We need to acknowledge that we might not always be "right." McLean's corollary: "There are few absolutes in life. Your opinion is probably not one of them…".
- We need to foster empathy. Some countries such as New Zealand are taking strides to minimize on-line violence and increase empathy within politics, to include kindness and well-being. Related to this, we should view discrimination as a population health issue.
- We also need appropriate, scientifically valid field research on prejudice, not only of its multivariable causes but also solutions, at individual, group, and societal level. One well-known project is Harvard's Project Implicit, which studies implicit (unconscious) social cognition. The tool used is the Implicit Association Test. For those who claim to have no bias, take the test. You will likely be surprised.
- Psychiatry has been able to impact how media have reported death by suicide, in order to minimize contagion. We need media to act responsibly in their reporting of hate crimes, but we need research in order to inform best practice.

Conclusion

I had mentioned literature as a modem for teaching about prejudice. One of my favorite books as a child was *The Sneetches* by Dr. Seuss (Theodor Seuss Geisel).

> Now, the Star-Belly Sneetches Had bellies with stars. The Plain-Belly Sneetches Had none upon thars. Those stars weren't so big. They were really so small. You might think such a thing wouldn't matter at all.

According to Jonathan Cott's *Pipers at the Gates of Dawn: The Wisdom of Children's Literature,* the inspiration for the book came out of Geisel's opposition to religious intolerance. Geisel was quoted as saying, "children's literature as I write it and as I see it is satire to a great extent … there's *The Sneetches* … which was inspired by my opposition to anti-Semitism."

Geisel used the yellow star as a symbol. His was an approximation of the "yellow badge." Historically, this figure is a "sun symbol," that of an ancient "yantra" of two interpenetrating triangles. Aniela Jaffe, writing in Jung's *Man and His Symbols*, noted this Eastern meditation shape reflected the union of Shiva and Shakti (male and female divinities). Many cultures have utilized symbols, created by the union of "opposites" as representing the psyche's wholeness. It is no coincidence that the Star of David, one of the most well-recognized sun symbols, continues with prominence as mankind struggles to come to terms with intra- and interpersonal conflicts.

As we have discussed the concepts of splitting, projection, and cognitive dissonance, it is ironic that some of the most atrocious acts of violence have been done in the name of religion by groups who were all related, "split" if you will, through Abrahamic tradition. Each of those religious groups has laid claim to covenants with their Creator. Each group has unique rituals which are observed. Each religious group has factions and sects, i.e., "out-groups" within their own "in-groups." The "split" needs to be reviewed; we need not project our internal intolerance toward others. We need to see others as "whole." However, it is important to acknowledge and value differences. Trying to see the world as if there are no ethnic or racial differences is not only naïve but also, as Schofield has pointed out, counterproductive [63].

The history of the Jewish people is one of resilience; it is reflective of the human psyche: creation, exodus/exile, wandering, and finding one's sense of meaning and belonging.

The obvious take-home message is this: We all have biases, most of which we are unaware. We can all be influenced in the area of prejudice, again, often without our awareness. Throughout history, hate crimes have occurred not only individually but also via group process, at times with small "in-groups" via "groupthink" and at times to a massive national/global scale.

Much of implicit bias is learned and, as such, can be unlearned. If we do not think we have biases, or wish to find out if that is so, then change will not occur. If, as research tells us, this rigidity is part of the problem, that those who are "set" are unlikely to consider otherwise, then there is indeed a "catch-22." As we recall, this term came from a classic Joseph Heller book. In *Catch-22*, the protagonist Yossarian speaks to a young accused soldier appearing before a tribunal. "You haven't got a chance, kid," he had told him glumly. "They hate Jews." "But I'm not Jewish," answered Clevinger. "It will make no difference," Yossarian promised, and Yossarian was right. "They're after everybody."

Acknowledgments The author would like to thank Dr. Steve Wonderlich for his review and feedback. He would also like to thank Dr. Marc Basson for his input.

References

1. Allport GW. The nature of prejudice. Oxford, UK: Addison-Wesley; 1954.
2. Augustinos M, Every D. The language of "race" and prejudice (a discourse of denial, reason and Liberal-practice politics). J Lang Soc Psychol. 2007;26(2):123–41.
3. Blair IV. The malleability of automatic stereotypes and prejudice. Personal Soc Psychol Rev. 2002;6(3):242–61.
4. Duckitt J. Psychology and prejudice: a historical analysis and integrative framework. Am Psychol. 1992;47(10):1182–93.
5. Locke J, 1632–1704. A letter concerning toleration. Buffalo: Prometheus Books; 1990.
6. Pierce CM, Carew JV, Pierce-Gonzalez D, Wills D. An experiment in racism. Educ Urban Soc. 1997;10(1):61–87.
7. Sue DW, et al. Racial microaggressions in everyday life. Implications Clin Pract. 2007;62(4):271–86.
8. Nadal KL, Issa M, Griffin KE, Hamit S, Lyons OB. Religious microaggressions in the United States: Mental health implications for religious minority groups. In: Sue DW, editor. Microaggressions and marginality: Manifestation, dynamics, and impact. New York: Wiley & Sons; 2010. p. 287–310.
9. Perry B. Hate in the peaceable kingdom. In: Fleming T, O'Reilly P, editors. Violence in Canada. Whitby: de Sitter; 2015.
10. Langer WC. A psychological analysis of Adolf Hitler. Washington, DC: M.O. Branch, Office of Strategic Services; 1943.
11. Waite RGL. Adolf Hitler's guilt feelings: a problem in history and psychology. J Interdiscip Hist. 1971;1(2):229–49.
12. Jung CG. Collected works of CG Jung. (Vol. 7: two essays on analytical psychology). Princeton: Princeton University Press; 1967.
13. Blair D. Jung: a biography. Boston: Little, Brown and Co.; 2003.
14. Lewis B. Semites and Anti-Semites. An inquiry into conflict and prejudice. New York: W. W. Norton & Company; 1999.
15. Weinstein J. First amendment challenges to hate crime legislation: Where's the speech? Crim Justice Ethics. 1992;11(2):6–20.
16. Anti-Defamation League. Audit of anti-Semitic incidents: year in review 2018. https://www.adl.org/2018-audit-H.
17. Plous S. The psychology of prejudice, stereotyping, and discrimination: an overview. In: Plous S, editor. Understanding prejudice and discrimination. New York: McGraw-Hill; 2003. p. 3–48.
18. McCleary DF, Quillivan CC, Foster LN, Williams RL. Meta-analysis of correlational relationships between perspectives of truth in religion and major psychological constructs. Psychol Relig Spiritual. 2011;3(3):163–80.
19. Fein S, Spencer SJ. Prejudice as self-image maintenance: affirming the self through derogating others. J Pers Soc Psychol. 1997;73:31–44.

20. Sartre JP. Anti-Semite and Jew. New York: Schocken Books Inc.; 1944.
21. Devine PG. Stereotypes and prejudice: their automatic and controlled components. J Pers Soc Psychol. 1989;56(1):5–18.
22. Bar-Tal D. Development of social categories and stereotypes in early childhood: the case of "the Arab" concept formation, stereotype and attitudes by Jewish children in Israel. Int J Intercult Relat. 1996;20:341–70.
23. Unesco Yearbook on Peace and Conflict Studies. Greenwood; 1989.
24. Smith DL. Less than human: why we demean, enslave, and exterminate others. New York: St. Martin's Press; 2011.
25. Southern Poverty Law Center. https://www.splcenter.org/fighting-hate/extremist-files/individual/william-shockley.
26. Armstrong K. The case for god. New York: Anchor Books; 2009.
27. Pereltsvaig A, Lewis MW. The vexatious history of Indo-European studies. In: The Indo-European controversy: facts and fallacies in historical linguistics: Cambridge University Press; 2015. p. 17–52.
28. Chicago Tribune. https://www.chicagotribune.com/nation-world/ct-suspect-pittsburgh-syna-gogue-shooting-social-media-20181027-story.html.
29. Jost J, Ledgerwood A, Hardin CD. Shared reality, system justification, and the relational basis of ideological beliefs. Soc Personal Psychol Compass. 2008;2:171–86.
30. Jolley D, Douglas KM. The social consequences of conspiracism: exposure to conspiracy theories decreases the intention to engage in politics and to reduce one's carbon footprint. Br J Psychol. 2014;105:35–56.
31. Einstein KL, Glick DM. Do I think BLS data are BS? The consequences of conspiracy theories. Polit Behav. 2015;37:679–701.
32. Lewandowsky S, et al. Misinformation and its correction: continued influence and successful Debiasing. Psychol Sci Public Interest. 2012;13(3):106–31.
33. Berger J. Arousal increases social transmission of information. Psychol Sci. 2011;22:891–3.
34. Janis IL. Victims of groupthink: a psychological study of foreign-policy decisions and fias-coes. Oxford, UK: Houghton Mifflin; 1972.
35. Ellemers N, Haslam A. Social identity theory. In: Paul AM, et al., editors. Handbook of theories of social psychology, vol. Vol. 2. London: Sage; 2012.
36. Jones JT, et al. Name letter preferences are not merely mere exposure: implicit egotism as self-regulation. J Exp Soc Psychol. 2002;38:170–7.
37. Pratto F, Stewart AL. Group dominance and the half-blindness of privilege. J Soc Issues. 2012;68:28–45.
38. Sidanius J, Pratto F. Social dominance: an intergroup theory of social hierarchy and oppression. New York: Cambridge University Press; 1999.
39. Niebuhr R. Moral man and immoral society: a study in ethics and politics. New York: Charles Scribner's Sons; 1932.
40. Goldstone RL. Effects of categorization on color perception. Psychol Sci. 1995;6:298–304.
41. Cuddy A. The psychology of anti-Semitism. The New York Times https://www.nytimes.com/2018/11/03/opinion/sunday/psychology-anti-semitism.html.
42. Paluck EL. Is it better not to talk? Group polarization, extended contact, and perspective taking in Eastern Democratic Republic of Congo. Pers Soc Psychol Bull. 2010;36(9):1170–85.
43. Tajfel H, Billig MG, Bundy RP, Flament C. Social categorization and intergroup behaviour. Eur J Soc Psychol. 1971;1(2):149–78.
44. Cohen GL, et al. Bridging the partisan divide: self-affirmation reduces ideological closed-mindedness and inflexibility in negotiation. J Pers Soc Psychol. 2007;93:415–30.
45. Chen M, Bargh JA. Nonconscious behavioral confirmation processes: the self-fulfilling consequences of automatic stereotype activation. J Exp Soc Psychol. 1997;33:541–60.
46. "Georgia legislators score South Pacific; see Red philosophy in song against bias", The New York Times, March 1, 1953. https://timesmachine.nytimes.com/timesma-chine/1953/03/01/93397165.html. Subscription required.

47. Paluck EL. Reducing intergroup prejudice and conflict using the media: a field experiment in Rwanda. J Pers Soc Psychol. 2009;96(3):574–87.
48. Torrey EF, Yolken RH. Psychiatric genocide: Nazi attempts to eradicate schizophrenia. Schizophr Bull. 2010;36(1):26–32.
49. Nordt C, Rössler W, Lauber C. Attitudes of mental health professionals toward people with schizophrenia and major depression. Schizophr Bull. 2006;32:709–14.
50. Loch AA, Hengartner MP, Guarniero FB, Lawson FL, Wang YP, Gattaz WF, Rössler W. The more information, the more negative stigma towards schizophrenia: Brazilian general population and psychiatrists compared. Psychiatry Res. 2013;205:185–91.
51. Smith M. Anti-stigma campaigns: time to change. Br J Psychiatry. 2013;202:S49–50.
52. Yeung PP, Greenwald S. Jewish Americans and mental health: results of the NIMH epidemiologic catchment area study. Soc Psychiatry Psychiatr Epidemiol. 1992;27(6):292–7.
53. Levinson D, Zilber N, Lerner Y, Grinshpoon A, Levav I. Prevalence of mood and anxiety disorders in the community: results from the Israel National Health Survey. Isr J Psychiatry Relat Sci. 2007;44(2):94–103.
54. Midlarsky E, Pirutinsky S, Cohen F. Religion, ethnicity, and attitudes toward psychotherapy. J Relig Health. 2012;51:498–506.
55. Schnall E, Feinberg S, Feinberg K, Kalkstein S. Psychological disorder and stigma: A 25-year follow-up study in the Orthodox Jewish community. The 118th Annual Convention of the American Psychological Association, San Diego, CA. August, 2010.
56. Curlin FA, Odell SV, Lawrence RE, Chin MH, Lantos JD, Meador KG, Koenig HG. The relationship between psychiatry and religion among U.S. physicians. Psychiatr Serv. 2007;58(9):1193–8.
57. Kathol RG, Sargent S, Melek S. Non-traditional mental health and substance use disorder services and professionals as a core part of health in clinically integrated networks and accountable care organizations. In: Flareau BYK, Bohn JM, Konschak C, editors. Clinical integration: transforming to a system of excellence. 3rd ed. Virginia Beach: Convurgent Publishing; 2015.
58. Bishop TF, Ramsay PP, Casalino LP, Bao H, Pincus HA, Shortell SM. Care management processes used less often for depression than for other chronic conditions in US Primary Care Practices. Health Aff. 2016;35(3):394–400.
59. Wang PS, Berglund PA, Kessler RC. Patterns and correlates of contacting clergy for mental disorders in the United States. Health Serv Res. 2003;38(2):647–73.
60. McEvoy P, Williamson T, Kada R, Frazer D, Dhliwayo C, Gask L. Improving access to mental health care in an Orthodox Jewish community: a critical reflection upon the accommodation of otherness. BMC Health Serv Res. 2017;17:557.
61. Hill ME, Augustinos M. Stereotype change and prejudice reduction: short-and long-term evaluation of a cross-cultural awareness program. J Community Appl Soc Psychol. 2001;11:243–62.
62. Haidt J. The Righteous Mind: Why Good People Are Divided by Politics and Religion. New York: Pantheon Books; 2012.
63. Schofield JW. The colorblind perspective in school: causes and consequences. In: Banks JA, McGee Banks CA, editors. Multicultural education: issues and perspectives. New York: Wiley; 2009.

Countering Anti-Semitism: A Catholic Theologian's Perspective

3

Mary C. Boys

Introduction

Anti-Semitism is pernicious, an assault on the humanity of Jews. It is protean, a "Rosetta Stone that can translate animus toward one group into a universal hate for many groups" [1]. It is persistent, enduring over the course of history and in varied cultures. The complexity of anti-Semitism suggests the need to analyze it from different perspectives, such as the lenses of psychiatry that my fellow authors utilize in their chapters.

My own standpoint is that of a Catholic theologian, with particular attention to Christian manifestations of, and responsibility for, anti-Semitism. Commitment to confront and counter this odious legacy of the churches is, I believe, obligatory of Christians. As Dr. Peteet has shown in his chapter, anti-Semitism in Christianity developed in part from interpretation of New Testament texts and from a perceived need in the early church to assert its truth against Judaism—a "zero sum" claim that Christianity could only be true if Judaism were false.

In fact, certain New Testament texts provide raw materials for hostility to Jews and thus form the biblical bedrock of anti-Semitism [2]. The most prominent is the accusation that Jews were responsible for the death of Jesus; moreover, by their failure to recognize him as God's messiah, early church writers portrayed Jews as "perfidious," lacking faith and blind to God's ways—with Judas as the most traitorous of all. The Pharisees were depicted in the four canonical gospels, particularly the Gospel of Matthew, as legalistic hypocrites, as symbols of a Judaism that was mired in legalism; in the Reformation, Luther and his followers considered both Judaism and Catholicism as religions of "works righteousness." Further, most readers of the New Testament wrongly assumed that by mid-first century, Christianity had become a separate religion that superseded Judaism, from which Paul "converted" to become a Christian.

There is no question that these "raw materials" and accompanying assumptions have proven deadly to Jews and have exercised an enduring hold on many Christians over the centuries, including in the present. But contemporary scholars understand Christian origins in radically different ways. In situating texts in their social-historical and literary contexts, scholars reveal a much more complex picture of the dynamics of traditions developing in relation to one another in the Roman Empire. And just as texts can be understood in new ways—even redeemed by virtue of more nuanced readings—so too can the church's confrontation with its anti-Jewish history become a source of resolve to do justice to the Jewish people.

The question I am pursuing in this chapter is as follows: *How might we draw upon the wealth of scholarship regarding the complex relations of "Jews" and "Christians" in the early centuries of the Common Era so as to counter biblical understandings that have been fundamental to anti-Semitism?* Thus, my essay will focus principally upon contemporary scholarship on Second Temple Judaism and Christian origins that razes the biblical bedrock of anti-Semitism.

To be clear, more adequate biblical interpretations alone will not eliminate anti-Semitism in the churches, let alone in the wider culture infected by xenophobia, racism, and a resurgent white nationalism. To reinterpret troubling texts, however, allows both Jews and Christians to understand our early bonds in new ways and thereby to contribute to rebuilding a relationship.

Two Traditions Develop in Relation to One Another

Although today most Christians think of Jews and Christians as belonging to separate traditions since Pentecost, albeit with a historical linkage, shared texts, and some shared ethical foundations (e.g., Ten Commandments), religious borders were not originally so clearly demarcated. Nor were "Jews" and "Christians" distinct communities in the latter part of the first century when the gospel narratives were composed. Even if "Christian" appears in the Acts of the Apostles (11:26), it does not denote precisely what that term means today.

Two traditions—what *developed into* rabbinic Judaism and what *developed* into Christianity—grew out of Jewish life. What needs to be elucidated and emphasized is the *emergence of these two traditions in relation to one another over centuries*. As Paula Fredriksen observes, "We simply assume that 'Judaism' and 'Christianity' are two incompatible traditions because that is the way that, in large part, things worked out" [3]. How things worked out, however, obscures more complicated beginnings.

The Emergence of "Judaism": A Range of Meanings over Time

But then, precisely what makes a phenomenon "Jewish"? We now know that "Jew" had a range of meanings that changed over time. Before about 100 B.C.E., it meant a

Judean, a member of the people of the homeland, Judea; it was both a geographic and ethnic designation. Later, the Jews (*Yehudi* [Hebrew], *Ioudaioi* [Greek]) formed a political community, and membership could be extended even to those outside of Judea. Then, a third meaning emerged: a Jew was someone who believed in certain tenets (e.g., worship of the one God who made heaven and earth and gave Israel the Torah) and observed certain practices (e.g. Sabbath, circumcision, dietary and purity norms, sacrifices in the Temple in Jerusalem, and annual contribution of ½ shekel donations for its upkeep). In this third usage, "Jew" suggests a way of life and a culture rather than ethnic/geographic origin. The first use of the term "Judaism" (*Ioudaismos*) occurs in 2 Maccabees (e.g., 2:21 and 14:37–44). Shaye J. D. Cohen, among others, argues this translation is too narrow because it does not yet designate a religion but rather "Judaeanness," the opposite of those who adopt foreign ways ("paganness") and who adopt "Greek" ways (*Hellenismos*) [4].

Moreover, we must take care not to present "Judaism/Judeanness" as monolithic. While distinctive tenets and practices generally characterized Jewish life at the dawn of the Common Era, differences in how Torah was understood and how practices were observed were evident. We can presume a spectrum of intensity with regard to precisely how Shabbat was observed, the extent to which the dietary laws were uniformly followed, and the function of the Temple for those in Galilee and in the Diaspora. In Fredriksen's metaphor: "We have a better sense of how things worked if we imagine the Torah as widely dispersed sheet music: the notes were the notes, but Jews played a lot of improv" [5].

In about the second century B.C.E., voluntary groups formed; we know a few by name (e.g., Pharisees, Sadducees, Essenes). Likely around the late 20s and early 30s of the first century C.E., the first disciples of Jesus of Nazareth also formed one such voluntary group, thus forming the first generation of "Jesus's Movement" or the Followers of the "Way"; this latter term is from the Acts of the Apostles (9:2, 18:26, 19:9,23; 22:4, 24:22).

The Emergence of "Christianity": Key Phases

In the initial phase of what eventually would become Christianity, the Jewish teacher Jesus of Nazareth taught and preached about God's kingdom throughout Galilee and Judea. We know about this period, however, only through the lens of the post-resurrection community. Jesus' disciples are Jews who seem to have limited interaction with Gentiles. In the year 33 of the Common Era, the Roman governor of Judea, Pontius Pilate, executed Jesus by crucifixion. Then "Jesus's Movement" took a distinctive turn, as some among his disciples experienced him alive, claiming that God had raised Jesus from the dead. For his followers the resurrection was *the* decisive event, leading to an outpouring of the Spirit of God upon the community. Now the teaching and preaching were not only about the imminent coming of God's kingdom but also about Jesus as God's divine "agent" or messiah ("Christ").

Two other related developments contributed to the reshaping of the Followers of the Way. Paul and his colleagues spread the word about Jesus to Gentiles throughout the Mediterranean. As considerable scholarship has revealed, Paul considered himself still an "Israelite," but one who followed Jesus; his was not so much a "conversion" as a "call" to be the Apostle to the Gentiles. Krister Stendahl was the first to argue:

> Paul's message was related not to some conversion from the hopeless works righteousness of Judaism into a happy justified status as a Christian. Rather, the center of gravity in Paul's theological work is related to the fact that he knew himself to be called to be the Apostle to the Gentiles, an Apostle of the one God who is Creator of both Jews and Gentiles [6].

Thus, by the end of the first century of the C.E., the "Followers of the Way" included large numbers of Gentiles, thereby intensifying questions about identity, including to what extent Gentile "followers" of Jesus should follow Jewish practices, particularly boundary markers such as the dietary laws and circumcision.

It was during this period, roughly from the 70s to the early 100s of the second century C.E., that rivalry between the other Jewish groups and the "Followers of the Way" (now a mixed Jewish/Gentile group) intensified. At its core was an argument about who was more faithful to God: those who follow the Way of Torah or those who follow the Way of Jesus? This was also the timeframe for the composition of the four canonical gospels (Matthew, Mark, Luke, and John). We can see some of the tensions reflected in certain gospel passages and then developed in literature from early church writers, for whom apologetics of the "nascent" movement was a primary task.

A key question revolved around religious leadership. After the destruction of the Temple in 70 C.E. and forced exile from Jerusalem, it is likely that Jews shaped by Pharisaic thought and practice exercised more influence than did other voluntary groups; they became the predecessors for rabbinic Judaism. The conflicts of the later first and early second centuries found their way into New Testament texts ostensibly *about Jesus' ministry in the 30s C.E.* Matthew, for example, likely regarded Pharisees as rivals in his time (ca. 85 CE), so he criticized them by depicting Jesus—whose teachings had broad similarity to those of the Pharisees—as their harsh critic some 50 years earlier:

> Then Jesus said to the crowds and to his disciples, 'The scribes and the Pharisees sit on Moses' seat; therefore, do whatever they teach you and follow it; but do not do as they do, for they do not practice what they teach. They tie up heavy burdens, hard to bear, and lay them on the shoulders of others; but they themselves are unwilling to lift a finger to move them. They do all their deeds to be seen by others; for they make their phylacteries broad and their fringes long. They love to have the place of honor at banquets and the best seats in the synagogues, and to be greeted with respect in the market-places, and to have people call them rabbi. But you are not to be called rabbi, for you have one teacher, and you are all students'. (Matthew 23: 1–8)

The disparagement of the Pharisees evident in Matthew but also in Mark and Luke pales in comparison to the Johannine rhetoric of binary opposition. Among the numerous examples are as follows:

- "He came to what was his own, and his own people did not accept him" (John 1:11).
- "Abide in me as I abide in you. Just as the branch cannot bear fruit by itself unless it abides in the vine, neither can you unless you abide in me. I am the vine,

you are the branches. Those who abide in me and I in them bear much fruit, because apart from me you can do nothing. Whoever does not abide in me is thrown away like a branch and withers; such branches are gathered, thrown into the fire, and burned" (John 15: 4–6).

- "Then Pilate took Jesus and had him flogged. And the soldiers wove a crown of thorns and put it on his head, and they dressed him in a purple robe. They kept coming up to him, saying, 'Hail, King of the Jews!' and striking him on the face. Pilate went out again and said to them, 'Look, I am bringing him out to you to let you know that I find no case against him.' So Jesus came out, wearing the crown of thorns and the purple robe. Pilate said to them, 'Here is the man!' When the chief priests and the police saw him, they shouted, 'Crucify him! Crucify him!' Pilate said to them, 'Take him yourselves and crucify him; I find no case against him.' The Jews answered him, 'We have a law, and according to that law he ought to die because he has claimed to be the Son of God'" (John 19:1–7).
- "But you have been anointed by the Holy One, and all of you have knowledge. I write to you, not because you do not know the truth, but because you know it, and you know that no lie comes from the truth. Who is the liar but the one who denies that Jesus is the Christ? This is the antichrist, the one who denies the Father and the Son" (1 John 20–22).
- "Many deceivers have gone out into the world, those who do not confess that Jesus Christ has come in the flesh; any such person is the deceiver and the antichrist!" (2 John 7).

A considerable body of commentary by both Jewish and Christian scholars on the Johannine writings has developed in recent years, with scholars mindful of the dangers of the language of binary opposition. "Jews" in the Fourth Gospel seem to be a group the evangelist fiercely opposed, but whoever they were, they do not appear to be identical with Jews as a people. Consider, for example, this text from John 20:19: "When it was evening on that day, the first day of the week, and the doors of the house where the disciples had met were locked for fear of the Jews, Jesus came and stood among them and said, 'Peace be with you'." The disciples (and Jesus, of course) were all Jews. So whom did John have in mind when he wrote that the [Jewish] disciples were fearful of the "Jews"?

The Philosophical and Literary Context

The gospels were not alone in antiquity to use heightened language against the other, whether a philosophical school or a religious movement. Varying interpretations about how Torah was to be lived among Jewish groups gave rise to tension and hostility among them. Moreover, in the world of antiquity, arguments against other schools of thought could sometimes include vilifying one's opponents. The heightened language drew upon the rhetorical conventions of the literary elite of antiquity. The Dead Sea Scrolls (DSS) provide some vivid examples, such as railing against the "wicked priests" and viewing themselves as the "Sons of the Light" in contrast to the "Sons of Darkness." We see in the DSS (as well as in ancient philosophical literature of the time more generally) two tendencies that made their way into the NT: binaries (good/evil, with evil projected on to those who practiced or believed differently) and disparagement; disparagement on occasion morphed into demonization.

The rhetoric of disparagement and, in some cases, demonization in the gospel accounts was part and parcel of the rhetoric philosophers and religious groups employed in the Greco-Roman period to argue against each other, as Luke Timothy Johnson has argued [7]. When, however, these texts circulated in the next centuries, their intra-familial tone was lost. It was no longer a bitter family argument *within* Jewish life, but rather a debate about Christianity against Judaism. Thus, some of the harsh passages were now read as polemics against Jews. As Krister Stendahl phrased this problem: "Words like that grow legs and walk out of their context" [8].

Two developments compounded the problem. Considerable works by the literary elite of the early church elaborated on the polemical template in the gospels. John Chrysostom (347–407), who has the dubious honor of being the most vituperative and vindictive of this literary elite, preached eight "Homilies Against the Judaizers," who were most likely the common folk of Antioch, attending both the synagogue for its feasts and the church for *its* feasts: "Finally, if the ceremonies of the Jews move you to admiration, what do you have in common with us? If the Jewish ceremonies are venerable and great, ours are lies. But if ours are true, as they *are* true, theirs are filled with deceit" (*Discourse* I.6.5).

Despite the fact that in many places Jews and Christians interacted peacefully, Christian texts, both in the New Testament and in early church writings, "engraved" binary opposition and disparagement onto Christian identity—a problem exacerbated when the late fourth-century Theodosius I (379–395) declared Christianity as the official religion of the Roman Empire. Christian political power added to the rhetoric of binary opposition and disparagement of the other had tragic consequences for Jews—and impugned the moral integrity of Christianity.

Social History

Numerous scholars have recently taken issue with the very notion of *the* partings of the ways between "Judaism" and "Christianity" in the late first century or early second century. The ways, of course, did eventually part, but at different times, under different circumstances, and in different locations—and never completely, since Jews and Christians have interacted continuously over the centuries. Perhaps the fourth century C.E. was *a* decisive turning point (e.g., the Council of Nicaea in 325), but, given the many variant forms of Judaism and Christianity, no single, definitive turning point can be accurately identified.

In brief, the complex process by which Jews and Christians came to define themselves in mutually exclusive terms developed over the course of several centuries. In this period, church leaders tended to speak the language of odious contrast, whereas the boundary lines for many of the more "ordinary" followers of Jesus were more fluid. John Chrysostom's diatribes against the "Judaizers" who participated in the worship of both church and synagogue exemplify the tensions between the literary elite and ordinary people.

Over the centuries, the New Testament texts that depicted Jesus as against Jewish leaders (e.g., Matthew 23) and placed the blame for the crucifixion on "the Jews" (e.g., John 19: 4–7) became fundamental components of anti-Jewish rhetoric. In the early church, an entire literature developed among the literary elite that a later age categorized as *Adversus Judaeos*. In this rhetorical realm, certain themes formed a constellation of charges. The North Star of the constellation was the claim that the Jews as a people are Christ killers; surrounding this were accusations of their faithlessness, blindness, carnality, and legalism. These claims resonated through theological commentary, pastoral exhortation, and popular culture. They have not entirely disappeared, though they are cited less often now, especially in the churches of the West that have sought to repair relations with Jews. But the texts are still there—and words matter.

Despite the negative depiction in key New Testament texts, in fact, "Jews" and "Christians" in the first three centuries in many places lived as neighbors. Some, particularly some church leaders who gained ascendancy, understood following the Way of Christ as a path separate from and superior to Judaism. Their supersessionist views dominated the extant literature from that period. For many others, however, the boundary was less fixed. In their perspective, the Way of Christ did not preclude connection to Jewish beliefs and practices.

Eventually, however, supersessionist theologies and negative depictions of Jews and Judaism dominated Christian Europe, as was manifest in the Crusades beginning in the eleventh century. In the High Middle Ages, the language of invective against Jews intensified, with accusations of ritual murder and blood libel; Jews became scapegoats for the Plague (1347–1351). While in many respects the Reformation benefitted Jews, the malevolent views of Martin Luther, especially his 1543 essay "On the Jews and Their Lies," excoriated Jews and recommended treating them violently. The Venetian Republic's creation of a Jewish ghetto in Venice in 1516 and the Vatican's similar move in 1555 in Rome symbolized the contempt for Jews that had developed. In the case of the Roman ghetto, Pope Paul IV made it clear that his purpose was to make conditions so dire for Jews that they would be compelled to convert; the ghetto lasted until 1870. During the Enlightenment, philosophers, always suspicious of Jewish loyalties, debated the "Jewish Question." The rise of National Socialism in the 1930s and 1940s made Jews pariahs for whom the "final solution" was genocide. Hitler had Christianity's centuries-long disparagement of Judaism on which to build his virulent hatred of Jews:

> Though the [Catholic] Church rejected the National Socialism racist form of antisemitism that preached a 'struggle against the Jewish race' and made blood the sole determining factor of Jewish identity, it nevertheless, almost since its foundation, continued to promote a religious-based antisemitism, often referred to as anti-Judaism, by blaming Jews for Jesus' crucifixion. Regardless of the theological logic underlying antisemitism, the negative portrayal of Jews facilitated discrimination and persecution. Even when Catholics tried to distance themselves from antisemitism or at least demonstrate moral sympathy toward Jews, it was very difficult to show any theological sympathy [9].

I am not suggesting a straight line between accusations that the Jews were responsible for the death of Jesus and the Nazi death camps. Drawing a trajectory from the New Testament's depiction of Jews to Auschwitz ignores social context and function, distorts historical complexity, and conflates the teaching of contempt with state-sanctioned genocide. Nevertheless, Christians have an ethical responsibility to examine the effects Christian teaching had on Jews—and on their own tradition. The legacy of *Adversus Judaeos* weighs heavily on Christians.

A Church Confronts Its History

The Second Vatican Council and Its Precedents

In this second section, I will focus on developments in Catholicism that reveal not only a reckoning with its legacy of anti-Jewish teaching but also its increasing sophistication in the interpretation of problematic biblical texts. Other Christian churches have also issued significant documents and engaged in actions to counter anti-Semitism. In view of the limitations of space, however, it will suffice to call attention to advances in my own tradition.

It is well known that the Second Vatican Council (1962–1965) inaugurated a revolution in the teaching of the Catholic Church with regard to Jews and Judaism, particularly in its decree *Nostra Aetate*, issued on October 28, 1965. Most famously, it declared in §4 Sect 4: "True, the Jewish authorities and those who followed their lead pressed for the death of Christ; still, what happened in His passion cannot be charged against all the Jews, without distinction, then alive, nor against the Jews of today" [10].

Of course, this dramatic change of the church's posture had precedents, as some groups in the church had been pressing for rethinking traditional understandings of Judaism. *Amici Israel*, founded in 1926 in Rome, promoted reconciliation between Jews and Catholics. They challenged the notion that Jews were "Christ killers" and advocated speaking about God's love for the Jewish people. The association also sought to eliminate negative references to Jews in liturgy and preaching. In 1928, they appealed to Pope Pius XI to reform the Good Friday prayer for the Jews, which then read:

Let us pray also for the perfidious Jews [*perfidis Judaeis*]: that Almighty God may remove the veil from their hearts; so that they too may acknowledge Jesus Christ our Lord. Almighty and eternal God, who dost not exclude from thy mercy even Jewish faithlessness [*Judicam perfidiam*]: hear our prayers, which we offer for the blindness of that people; that acknowledging the light of thy Truth, which is Christ, they may be delivered from their darkness. Through the same our Lord Jesus Christ, who lives and reigns with thee in the unity of the Holy Spirit, God, for ever and ever. Amen [11].

In particular, *Amici Israel* proposed removing the terms *perfidis* and *perfidiam*, which referred to unbelief. Their petition, favorably received by an expert in liturgy, met with opposition from high-ranking Vatican officials. Pope Pius XI issued a statement on March 25, 1928, that included the first official condemnation of anti-Semitism in the church's history, but its negative depiction of Jews—"the people formerly chosen by God"—reveals the typical understanding of Jews and Judaism in Catholic life before Vatican II [12]. Moreover, the pope censured *Amici Israel* and suppressed the association because of what he regarded as its erroneous initiatives. It is ironical that the pope condemned anti-Semitism while dissolving the very group that had sought to counter it. In August 1947, a group of Protestants and Catholics, along with some Jews (including French historian, Jules Isaac), convened the International Emergency Conference on Anti-Semitism in Seelisberg, Switzerland. Christian members issued a document advocating ten points that the churches should teach as a way of countering anti-Semitism. Among them were three that bear similarity to what *Nostra Aetate* §4 decreed in 1965:

- Avoid distorting or misrepresenting biblical or post-biblical Judaism with the object of extolling Christianity.
- Avoid using the word *Jews* in the exclusive sense of the enemies of Jesus and *The Enemies of Jesus* to designate the whole Jewish people.
- Avoid presenting the Passion in such a way as to bring the odium of the killing of Jesus upon all Jews or upon Jews alone [13].

Among the Catholic participants at Seelisberg was Gertrud Luckner, whose courageous work on behalf of German Jews had resulted in her imprisonment in the concentration camp at Ravensbrück. She became a leading member of the so-called Freiburg Circle, a postwar group of Catholics who sought to awaken consciousness of their duties and responsibilities toward Jews. Luckner founded the *Freiburger Rundbrief* (a circular letter) in 1948 to keep memory of the Holocaust alive, to advocate dialogue with Jews, and to advocate for economic restitution.

Karl Thieme (1902–1963), whom Luckner had recruited as theological adviser to the *Freiburger Rundbrief*, underwent a remarkable evolution in his own thought that later exercised profound influence on those who drafted NA. While in a 1945 book he had spoken of Jews as "enemies of the Christian name," a few years afterward, he declared he had undergone a "conversion," due in large measure to the opportunity in the postwar years to engage Jews such as Martin Buber in conversation. These conversations enabled him to realize after Auschwitz just how offensive it was to missionize Jews. In August 1950 he announced in a public letter his "conviction that a Jewish person, not only as an individual person, but also in a certain sense precisely as 'Jew' can be pleasing to God …. one can assume that even in distance from Christ the Jewish people enjoys special guidance and special grace" [14]. Thieme was the first major Catholic thinker to grasp Paul's claim in Romans that Jews remained God's "beloved" people (Romans 11:28).

The most passionately debated issue at the Council was whether or not *Nostra Aetate* should include language about converting Jews. Thieme's influence is apparent in the final wording of NA: "In company with the Prophets and the same Apostle [Paul], the Church awaits the day, known to God alone, when all people will call on the Lord with a single voice and 'serve him with one accord'" [10]. In other words, the decree portrays Jews and Christians as before God at the end of time—thus, implying no mission to convert Jews.

Post-conciliar Developments

Tracing the effects of *Nostra Aetate* necessitates situating them in the wider horizon of the totality of the documents of Vatican II and the voluminous commentary on the Council. Even at nearly 60 years, this modest document is still being interpreted, as is Vatican II itself. NA's effects may be seen most notably in the interrelated areas of liturgy and Scripture. Less visible but crucial is the church's confrontation with its history vis-à-vis Jews, particularly the *Shoah* (Holocaust).

In 1970, a new lectionary replaced the 1570 Tridentine Roman Missal, providing a far more extensive selection of biblical texts, including a reading nearly every Sunday from the Old Testament/Hebrew Bible, which had virtually been ignored in the earlier missal. Given the typical lack of familiarity with the Old Testament, this inclusion of texts in turn spurred many Catholics to engage in study of the Bible. It also exposed Catholics to sacred texts shared with Jews.

Also appearing in 1970 was a revised prayer for Jews on Good Friday—the revision that *Amici Israel* had sought in 1926. The contrast with the formulation of 1570 is stark:

> Let us pray for the Jewish people, the first to hear the word of God, that they may continue to grow in the love of his name and in faithfulness to his covenant. Almighty and eternal God, long ago you gave your promise to Abraham and his posterity. Listen to your Church as we pray that the people you first made your own may arrive at the fullness of redemption. We ask this through Christ our Lord. Amen [15].

In December 1974, the newly created Vatican Commission on Religious Relations with Jews issued the first of its instructions, "Guidelines and Suggestions for Implementing the Conciliar Declaration *Nostra Aetate*" (n. 4). The Commission urged that attention be paid to passages that could be interpreted to show Jews in an unfavorable light. Further, it recommended that the "Old Testament and the Jewish tradition founded upon it must not be set against the New Testament in such a way that the former seems to constitute a religion of only justice, fear and legalism, with no appeal to the love of God and neighbor (cf. *Deut* 6:5, *Lev* 19:18, *Matt* 22:34–40)" [16].

The Commission returned to this theme a decade later in its "Notes on the Correct Way to Present Jews and Judaism" (1985). While Catholic tradition has accentuated the unity of the Scriptures and presented the New Testament as a fulfillment of the Old, the Jewish tradition reads their Scriptures through the lenses of rabbinic commentary. The Catholic interpretation, in the Commission's view, differed in emphasis, but should not be read as implying that God's promises to the Jewish people have been abrogated. To the contrary: In the 1982 formulation of Pope John Paul that is cited in the "Notes," Jews are "the people of God of the Old Covenant, which has never been revoked" [17].

What was far too subtly expressed in NA has now been more candidly addressed in subsequent documents on biblical study. For example, in 2001 the Pontifical Biblical Commission [PBC], an international group of about 20 leading Catholic biblical scholars, issued a lengthy study, *The Jewish People and Their Sacred Scripture in the Christian Bible*. They clarified that in using the nomenclature "Old" Testament, the church has "no wish to suggest that the Jewish Scriptures are outdated or surpassed. Christianity's appropriation of the "Old" Testament is a rereading, a "retrospective perception"—a theological interpretation of texts Christians share with Jews. Thus, it differs from Jewish readings, which are nonetheless "possible": "Both readings are bound up with the vision of their respective faiths, of which the readings are the result and expression. Consequently, both are irreducible" [18].

This 2001 document is of particular importance in providing a more cogent explanation about alleged Jewish culpability for the death of Jesus, as well as laying out more nuanced interpretive principles. Historically, "only a minority of Jews contemporaneous with Jesus were hostile to him… a smaller number were responsible for handing him over to the Roman authorities… fewer still wanted him killed, undoubtedly for religious reasons that seemed important to them." Note also the admission that blaming Jews for Jesus' death "has had disastrous consequences throughout history" [19]. Cardinal Edward Irdis Cassidy, then President of the Commission on Religious Relations with the Jews, had been even more forthright when he confessed in May 1998 that the "Church-ordered ghetto was the antechamber to the Nazi death camps" [20].

In addition to developments in biblical interpretation, Catholic historians, including Edward Flannery [21], Donald Dietrich [22], Michael Phayer [23], Robert Krieg [24], John Connelly [14], and Kevin Spicer [9], were writing major books about anti-Semitism and the Shoah. Theologians such as Gregory Baum [25], Eugene Fisher [26], and John Pawlikowski [27] raised ethical questions and challenged aspects of traditional church teaching. Chairs in Jewish Studies and Centers for Jewish-Christian Relations were established in Catholic colleges and universities. In early May 2019 the Pontifical Biblical Institute in Rome sponsored a conference on "Jesus and the Pharisees" to celebrate its 110th anniversary, with papers given (and available on video) by distinguished Jewish and Christian scholars [28].

Profound friendships have developed between scholars, whether in the ecumenical Christian Scholars Group on Jewish-Christian Relations or in interreligious organizations such as the International Council of Christians and Jews (ICCJ).

Conclusion

My own profession involves the classroom, not a therapeutic, psychoanalytic, or spiritual-care setting. Nonetheless, deep emotions often arise in teaching, particularly when Jews and Christians study history together. In spring 2018, Professor Shuly Rubin Schwartz (Jewish Theological Seminary of America) and I (Union Theological Seminary) co-taught "Studies in Jewish-Christian Relations" for students from both our institutions. Most of the JTS students were familiar with the historical material, but had never studied it in the presence of Christians. At times their anger was palpable, although they seemed unsure how to express it in the presence of the UTS students, who were largely paralyzed with shame in facing a history that they had not previously encountered, let alone in the presence of Jews. From a pedagogical perspective, this meant doing our own emotional homework, allowing uncomfortable silences, being available for conversations after class, structuring discussion in small groups, and requiring joint projects. As personal relationships developed among members of the course, the emotional atmosphere changed. Anger and shame had not disappeared but were ameliorated in large part by mutual respect, openness, and appreciation for learning in the presence of the other.

What might our classroom experience imply for mental health practitioners? Because Christians typically have little awareness of the shadow side of their own history vis-à-vis Jews, they need encouragement and accompaniment to step out of their comfort zone to face the wounds inflicted by their own tradition. For the most part, Christians have learned about Judaism only from what they've been taught by their own Christian teachers, so opportunities to understand Judaism through experiences, such as an invitation to a Seder or Shabbat dinner, may prompt questions that lead to deeper understandings. Jews often view Christianity as fundamentally anti-Semitic. Understanding the complexity of Christian identity formation in the matrix of Second Temple Judaism provides essential context, as does knowledge of the many efforts in Christian churches to repair relationships with Jews and Judaism.

Among the most important contributions mental health practitioners might make is to encourage engagement with those who are "other" and to foster development of empathy. Helping persons to deal with their fears of those who differ from them in a significant way is vital in this time when the strident rhetoric of some political leaders stokes fires of racial hatred, demeans the humanity of certain groups, and promotes ethnonationalism. The ability to empathize with the pain of the other is crucial to the health of society. To gather in common witness when a terrorist act has violated a synagogue or a church is a moving experience that deepens one's compassion. Standing in solidarity with the religious other to protest inhumane conditions and working together to counter racism and intolerance are acts of what René Girard terms "disruptive empathy" that will not only enhance relations between Jews and Christians but also contribute to the healing our polarized society [29].

A final note. On June 29, 2019, I arrived in Lund, Sweden, for the ICCJ's annual conference meeting this year on the theme "Transformations Within and Between: How Does Our New Relationship Affect Jewish and Christian Self-Understanding?" En route by taxi from Lund's central train station to the conference, I noted a few neo-Nazis gathering for what later arrivals confirmed was a small demonstration—a stark reminder as I gathered with Jews and Christians from 23 nations that anti-Semitism remains pernicious, protean, and persistent. Thus, our efforts to counter it must be shrewd, sagacious, and strategic.

References

1. Green E. Why the Charlottesville marchers were obsessed with Jews. https://www.theatlantic.com/politics/archive/2017/08/nazis-racism-charlottesville/536928/.
2. Boys MC. Redeeming our sacred story: the death of Jesus and relations between Jews and Christians. New York: Paulist; 2013.
3. Fredriksen P. When Christians were Jews: the first generation. New Haven: Yale University Press; 2018. p. 186.
4. Cohen SJD. The beginnings of Jewishness. Berkeley: University of California Press; 1999.
5. Fredriksen P. When Christians were Jews: the first generation. New Haven: Yale University Press; 2018. p. 185.
6. Stendahl K. Paul among Jews and gentiles. Philadelphia: Fortress; 1976.
7. Johnson LT. The New Testament's anti-Jewish slander and the conventions of ancient polemic. J Biblic Lit. 1989;108(3):419–41.
8. Stendahl K. "From God's perspective we are all minorities; http://www.jcrelations.net/From+God%E2%80%99s+Perspective+we+are+all+Minorities.2224.0.html?L=3.
9. Spicer K. Hitler's priests: catholic clergy and the national socialism. DeKalb: Northern Illinois University Press; 2008. p. 229–30.
10. https://www.ccjr.us/dialogika-resources/documents-and-statements/roman-catholic/second-vatican-council/nostra-aetate.
11. In Boys MC. Has God only one blessing? Judaism as a source of Christian self-understanding. New York: Paulist; 2000. p. 203.
12. Acta Apostolicae Sedis 1928;20:103–4. www.vatican.va/archive/aas/index_en.htm.
13. https://www.ajcf.fr/IMG/pdf/Seelisberg.pdf.
14. Connelly J. From enemy to brother: the revolution in Catholic teaching on the Jews, 1933–1965. Cambridge: Harvard University Press; 2012. p. 204–5.
15. In Boys, M. Has God only one blessing?; p. 203.
16. https://www.ccjr.us/dialogika-resources/documents-and-statements/roman-catholic/vatican-curia/guidelines.
17. https://www.ccjr.us/dialogika-resources/documents-and-statements/roman-catholic/vatican-curia/notes.
18. http://www.vatican.va/roman_curia/congregations/cfaith/pcb_documents/rc_con_cfaith_doc_20020212_popolo-ebraico_en.html.
19. Ibid.
20. Carroll J. Constantine's sword: the Church and the Jews, vol. 376. Boston: Houghton Mifflin; 2001.
21. Flannery E. The anguish of the Jews. New York: Paulist Press; 1985.
22. Dietrich D. God and humanity in Auschwitz: Jewish-Christian relations and sanctioned murder. New Brunswick: Transaction Publishers; 1995.
23. Phayer M. The Catholic Church and the Holocaust, 1930–1965. Bloomington: Indiana University Press; 2000.
24. Krieg R. Catholic theologians in Nazi Germany. New York: Continuum; 2004.
25. Baum G. Is the new testament anti-Semitic? A reexamination of the new testament. Paulist: Glen Rock; 1965.
26. Fisher EJ. Faith without prejudice: rebuilding Christian attitudes toward Judaism. New York: Paulist Press; 1977.
27. Pawlikowski JT. The challenge of the holocaust for Christian theology. New York: Center for Studies of the Holocaust; 1978.
28. https://www.jesusandthepharisees.org/.
29. Barnett VJ. Bystanders: conscience and complicity during the Holocaust. Westport: Praeger; 1999. p. 150–7.

Some Neuro-Biologic Determinants of Intergroup Bias That Affect the Development of Anti-Semitism

Madeline W. Harford

Anti-Semitism Is a Cultural Phenomenon Rooted in the Biology of Out-Group Dynamics

Human beings are social creatures biologically predisposed to group living [1, 2]. At the same time, they exhibit a consistent capacity to organize their social structures into in-groups and out-groups. In humans, groupings can be stable or they can quickly change. Treatment of the out-group has been noted to be much less favorable than the treatment of the in-group. This tendency is apparent in human children as young as 5 [3]. It has been observed in every culture studied [4].

A surprising finding has been the observation that primate relatives of humans, rhesus macaques, show the capacity to identify an "other." They can identify a member of another troop of macaques consistently and instantaneously, even when the other member was born in the in-group but migrated to another troop in adolescence. Though the face might have been familiar, the face was identified with the new troop that was joined [5].

The fact that us and them groupings occur in all primates suggests that there are ancient phylogenetic roots to the perception of out-groups. In-groups provide belonging, safety, and identity. Out-groups are viewed with apprehension and vigilance. Out-groups can also be viewed with disgust, fear, envy, and dehumanization. Some out-groups, such as children or the elderly, can be viewed with warmth [6]. Much of the time out-group treatment is biased and destructive.

Anti-Semitism is an example of out-group mistreatment and conflict. It is also a very complex social phenomenon. It cannot be explained simply by neuro-biology. But neuro-biology tells us that the tendency for humans to create these groups is innate and a means of organizing the world to maximize an individual's chance of

M. W. Harford (✉)
Private Practice, Dallas, TX, USA

University of Texas Southwestern Medical School, Dallas, TX, USA
e-mail: madeline.harford@gmail.com

© Springer Nature Switzerland AG 2020
H. S. Moffic et al. (eds.), *Anti-Semitism and Psychiatry*,
https://doi.org/10.1007/978-3-030-37745-8_4

survival and success. Neuro-biology also tells you that group formation is fluid, highly dependent on social context, and influenced by hierarchy, the presence or absence of empathy, and the capacity to dehumanize or objectify another.

I have focused my attention on the research that has been done in identifying how the basic concepts of "us" and "them" are represented in the brain. Furthermore, I have been curious how these concepts affect the processing of fear, anxiety, and aggression. The thousands of years of anti-Semitism in many parts of the world call for an understanding of these processes at all levels. It has not always been explicitly acknowledged that the biology of electrical charges and neurotransmitters and automatic brain circuits influence behavior in predictable ways. At times in history, Jews have had an esteemed place in local society, but in a few short years, that place can be destroyed and anti-Semitism can erupt with massacres or genocide. In the United States today, Jews have been able to advance and thrive for more than 50 years. But the recent re-emergence of overt anti-Semitism with the deaths of innocent Jews in their synagogues should remind us of the tenuous nature of group status.

Specific areas of the brain contain neurons that are dedicated to specific functions: modulation of fear, the acquisition of memory, empathy, the identification of the other, and the identification of a human being as opposed to a thing. Neuronal circuits, pathways that are activated repeatedly under specific circumstances between areas, can be defined postmortem but also in vivo with new imaging equipment. While controversies remain, there is much to be learned from the current data that can inform our study of anti-Semitism. The neuro-biology that is active in the identification of the other, of hierarchy, of empathy, of dislike, and of dehumanization acts automatically and below conscious awareness and can be documented in fMRI studies. The belief that we are fully rational beings and think through problems in logical ways is not supported by the data. In fact, automaticity and conflation of pathways, basic body needs, and higher-order thinking occur often in ways that are surprising and shocking.

Research done over the past 20 years has shown that automatic reactions, outside of conscious awareness, often dictate our assessments and behavior. A study performed on people either holding a cold or warm drink in their hand while meeting someone new revealed the following: if they are holding the warm drink, they are more likely to describe the new person as a warm person; the opposite is true when holding a cold drink [7]. Another study asked whether Australian courtroom judges rendered similar decisions before or after lunch.

The finding that for the same crime, judges would deny parole more often before lunch than after lunch suggests that the judges' physiologic state of hunger affected their capacity for assessing and interpreting the law. The fragility of our higher-order goals comes to the fore when we consider that automatic and non-conscious activity of the brain holds so much sway in our internal worlds [8]. Correctives for some of these findings seem obvious. If you are a judge, make sure you do not allow yourself to get too hungry or at least keep in mind that you are a different judge when you are hungry. When treating patients, psychiatry residents are taught to monitor their own state of mind. Counter-transference and other feelings can interfere with effective therapy. Understanding more of our unconscious patterns continues to be a crucial part of the education of a psychiatrist.

Our constructed sense of self, our capacity for empathy, and our relationships with others are all influenced by areas of the brain that process information outside of conscious awareness. Human memory and brain function is so malleable that we can construct facts (a real memory) that are based on information we are given, even if the information has no basis in reality. Elizabeth Loftus at the University of California, Irvine, performed an amazing study that documented the process of "implanting" memory in adult subjects [9]. Fully one-fourth of her subjects accepted a fantasy story of their own childhood as real and, on later visits, even embellished this story with details that had not been provided by the researchers. That capacity to create story as if it were a factual experience can lead to all sorts of beliefs capable of affecting behavior.

The simple act of repeating a lie can make it seem like truth. Temple University psychologist Lynn Hasher and colleagues showed in a pioneering study published in 1977 that people will rate statements as true, whether true or not, when the statements are repeated three or more times [10]. If pictures are included as was done in a 2012 study, published in the *Psychonomic Bulletin and Review*, people are more likely to believe the statements, whether true or not [11]. And adding vivid language helps spread lies more quickly [12]. The tendency to believe what we are told, rather than to use critical thinking skills, is a shortcut in our information processing and has played a role in the thousands of years of anti-Semitism. The blood libel story, the false accusation that Jews kill Christian children to use for Passover rituals, has been traced to a village in twelfth-century England.

The story was fabricated when a young man went missing. E.M. Rose describes the trajectory of this false belief in his book, *The Murder of William of Norwich* [13].

Brain areas that are pertinent to my discussion include the amygdala, the hippocampus, the prefrontal cortex, the fusiform gyrus, the insula, the mesolimbic dopamine system, the anterior cingulate cortex, and the nucleus accumbens.

Neuro-biologists emphasize that these areas of the brain function as components of circuits or neurological matrices. They are not centers that act independently, but, rather, act in concert with other parts of the brain to create specific circuits. Defining these circuits has allowed us to think about a "pain matrix" in the brain that helps to explain phenomena such as phantom limb pain; the "reward circuit" helps understand addiction.

The limbic system (especially the amygdala and the hippocampus) is the area that plays a central role in processing emotions in humans. The amygdala is a center of 13 nuclei innervated from the thalamus, the hippocampus, and the prefrontal cortex. These nuclei send projections to the hypothalamus and brain stem. The amygdala plays a major role in processing information and regulating autonomic responses associated with fear, arousal, emotional responses, hormonal secretions, and memory. The amygdala appears to influence what memories are stored and where they are stored. Scientists have identified specific locations of neurons in the amygdala that are responsible for fear conditioning, an associative learning process by which we learn, through experience, to fear. Through hearing stories told by people we trust, we learn who the enemy is. There are also areas of the amygdala that can change what we have learned [14].

The hippocampus is associated with memory, episodic memory, long-term memory, and spatial navigation. Damage to the hippocampus affects the ability to inhibit behavioral responses that have been previously learned. Loss of the hippocampi prevents humans from learning and storing new information [15].

The prefrontal cortex (PFC) coordinates and adjusts complex behaviors. It helps regulate impulses and organizes emotional reactions. It works to direct attention and focus and to ignore external distractions. Complex planning, prioritizing competitive and simultaneous information, and personality are major functions of the PFC [16]. Activation of critical thinking skills, which can play a role in diminishing automatic reactions, requires time and effort. A study by Hughes et al. showed that learning to trust in-group members was a much faster process than learning to trust out-group members. The latter requires more input from the prefrontal cortex [17].

The fusiform gyrus is associated with face recognition (damage to the area causes prosopagnosia or inability to recognize faces). It is also associated with high-level visual processing, color processing, body recognition, word recognition, and the ability to distinguish between a real human face and a facsimile of a face. This area is active in determining in-group versus out-group membership [18].

The insular cortex works to facilitate assessment of decisions when there is risk to the individual. It activates when there is anticipation of negative stimuli. Lesions of the insula increase risky decisions. It also plays a role in moral decision making, anxiety, bodily awareness of pain, warmth, and stomach distension. It receives inputs from the thalamus and amygdala and sends projections to the primary and secondary sensory cortices. It is also activated by olfactory and gustatory sensations associated with disgust, including moral disgust [19].

The mesolimbic dopamine system originates in the ventral tegmental area and projects toward the forebrain through the nucleus accumbens. This pathway integrates the amygdala and the hippocampus and informs the individual of how rewarding a behavior might be and how salient a given incentive might be. Many think that the mesolimbic pathway is involved in conditions such as addiction and depression. It is also active during the experience of emotional pain caused by social exclusion.

The nucleus accumbens (NA), part of the basal ganglia, functions in creating motivation. Based on the activation of the mesolimbic pathway, the NA coordinates motivation with motor action. The NA is activated by pleasant food intake, sex, drugs of abuse, and alcohol and is associated with the release of dopamine [20] in the amygdala and "the other."

Social psychologists, primatologists, and other scientists have studied the development of the concept of "the other." It appears to be a fluid process. Psychologist Terri Apter notes that the "fundamental basis of grouping – what makes someone different from someone else – is often constructed. Group identity can be defined by the team you support, the religion you adhere to, the work you do, your country of origin. The importance of that identify fluctuates with context."

On the other hand, there appears to be a biologic basis for the perception of "the other." As most would intuit, survival of any individual requires brain function that apprehends and processes threat.

Scientific study of the last century and a half has identified the limbic system and its circuits as the center of emotional and behavioral expression. In particular, the amygdala has been noted to activate whenever fear or threat is being processed.

The limbic system has also been tied to identifying "the other" and identifying threat. In particular, the amygdala has been an intense focus of study because of the data that implicates a central role for its activation in fear and aggressive behavior.

In imaging studies, when an animal is being aggressive, the amygdala consistently lights up. If you lesion the amygdala in an animal, aggression declines [21]. If you show human subjects pictures that provoke anger, neuro-imaging studies show intense activation of the amygdala [22].

Joseph E. LeDoux has a theory that the amygdala is activated whenever humans are exposed to fear, even when the threat is subliminal. Along with neural activity in the amygdala, body responses associated with fear such as sweating and increased heart rate also occur.

LeDoux posits that the main action of the amygdala is to activate brain areas that increase the secretion of chemicals throughout the brain (norepinephrine, acetylcholine, dopamine, and serotonin) and hormones such as adrenalin and cortisol. These chemicals alert the organism that something important is happening. As a result, attention systems in the neocortex guide the perceptual searching of the environment for an explanation for the highly aroused state. LeDoux suggests that there is activation of cognitive systems in the neocortex that runs parallel to the circuit output of the amygdala. The meaning of the environmental stimuli present is aided by the retrieval of memories. If the stimuli are known sources of danger, "fear" schema is retrieved. LeDoux also suggests that a "feeling" of fear is an outcome of multiple processes (attention, perception, memory, and arousal) that coalesce into conscious awareness [22]. Since many people tell stories about the dangers posed by Jews, it appears likely that a frequent schema that is aroused under conditions of threat relates to memories of such stories.

The amygdala helps mediate both innate and learned fears. Innate fears are those that occur without any prior experience with the threat and are thought to be encoded in the brain. Examples include automatic reactions to seeing spiders or to experience falling. Hoehl et al. at the Max Planck Institute for Human Cognitive and Brain Sciences in Leipzig, Germany, studied infants 6 months old, who were exposed to images of spiders or flowers and images of snakes and fish. The infants were held on their parent's laps under constant light conditions. When the infants were exposed to spiders, their pupils dilated to a significantly larger degree than when visualizing flowers. The results were less impressive with the distinction between fish and snakes, but were also present [23]. These results support the theory that there is an evolved preparedness for fears of these ancestral threats.

Studies of brain reactions to sensory cues show that the human brain is exquisitely attuned to the color of someone's face. Depending on the color, the amygdala activates quicker (as shown with neuro-imaging) when the perception of the color of the face one sees is different from one's own. The fusiform area of the brain plays a major role in identifying faces as human. There is less activation of this area when the face seen is different from faces one is familiar with. People who look "different" are more difficult to identify and are more easily grouped together and stereotyped [24].

Learned fears are processed via conditioning. Humans are predisposed to enhance their own survival by identifying dangerous environmental stimuli quickly and marshalling their resources to enhance their own survival and to avoid harm. There is a genetic continuum to harm avoidance, with some people having extremely high aversion to harm [25].

I am emphasizing the study of fear circuits as they play a central role in the dynamics of bigotry and scapegoating. It is not always consciously expressed, but if you study history, the competition for resources, for power, and for dominance plays a major role in the rise of bigotry and violence.

Such fear circuits can be constructed by innate fears or extrinsic social teaching or individually constructed as a way to explain danger and stay safe.

I have also been heartened by studies that show that automatic brain circuits can be modified by activity from the PFC. Research in humans suggests that the anterior cingulate gyrus and the PFC contribute to regulation of fear behavior. Imaging studies of adults who have a subliminal exposure to faces of people considered as "other" activate the amygdala. But if the exposure continues for 500 milliseconds, the PFC and the anterior cingulate gyrus are also activated and can dampen the amygdala activation [26]. In some animal studies that are suggestive for application in human brains, a group in Korea has shown that reducing input from the anterior cingulate cortex to the basolateral nuclei of the amygdala increases innate fear responses to fox urine [27].

People have been shown to be partial to their in-group when there is intergroup conflict [28]. In fact, empathy and fair treatment are also affected by the definition of in-group and out-group status. Baumgartner et al., in a study published in 2013, look at the role of the dorsomedial PFC. They found that people who were more likely to be impartial in the punishment of in-group and out-group members had larger and thicker gray matter volume of their dorsomedial PFC [29].

Empathy

Empathy can be defined as the capacity to feel distress when you witness someone else experiencing pain. It is a complex emotion that is highly variable. In order to empathize, people must first categorize the "other" as a human rather than an object, then appreciate that the "other" has a mind, and finally view the "other" through trait dimensions of warmth and competence [30]. Social neuroscience reliably implicates activation of regions of medial prefrontal cortex in mind perception [31].

People do not ascribe minds to others in any consistent way. In fact, when study participants in Susan Fiske's study viewed homeless people or drug addicts, their medial prefrontal cortex failed to activate. Instead the insula, which activates with disgust, was more active. Fiske also showed that study participants failed to use intent verbs in describing the target's typical day, a finding that has been related to discounting a mind. Empathy is different for in-group pain than it is for out-group pain. Studies of imaging empathy circuits, which involve the coupling of limbic structures, the ventral motor prefrontal cortex, and the insula, show that there is less activation of these circuits when the subject in pain is considered a member of the out-group than if it is part of the in-group. In order to empathize with the "other," it is necessary to override a habitual behavior and involve the frontal cortex in a higher cognitive load activity [32].

Hierarchy, Conformity, and Obedience to Self-Identified Group

In Hannah Arendt's book, *Eichmann in Jerusalem*, she describes a dynamic process that she calls the banality of evil. She covered Adolf Eichmann's trial in Jerusalem in 1961. His explanation for his actions to the court during the trial casts a picture of the ordinary person who becomes convinced that a leader must be right if that leader has successfully climbed the hierarchy and managed to obtain great power. In his memoirs, he wrote, "Hitler may have been wrong all down the line, but one thing is beyond dispute: the man was able to work his way up from lance corporal in the German Army to Fuhrer of a people of almost 80 million.

His success alone proved to me that I should subordinate myself to this man." Eichmann claimed he believed in an orderly society; and in Germany at the time, he had to follow the Fuhrer and the laws that his leader imposed. What do we know about humans and hierarchies and the brain?

Robin Dunbar has shown that the bigger the average size of the social group of a species, the bigger the brain, relative to body size, and the larger the size of the neocortex relative to the size of the brain. He proposes that increases in social complexity and the evolutionary expansion of the neocortex are linked. A neuro-imaging study of captive macaque monkeys seems to add credence to this theory. The monkeys were housed in groups of different sizes. The larger the group size, the thicker the size of the prefrontal cortex and the superior temporal gyrus. In humans, there appears to be a similar pattern; the larger the size of someone's social network, the larger the ventromedial prefrontal cortex, orbital prefrontal cortex, and amygdala. This is correlated to the person's skills in getting along with others [33].

There is much evidence that social learning skills, which are honed in the context of your group, are a marker for successful adaption in the world. We seek to master our environment and ensure our safety and success. A significant way to do that is to have a group and to conform to its teachings, whether the teaching is "correct" or not. A study performed with vervet monkeys in 2013 by Andrew Whitten of the University of Saint Andrews shows this type of learning and its social transmission. The vervet monkeys were given two different containers of maize, one dyed pink and the other dyed blue. One color had a bitter additive. The monkeys learned to avoid the container of the maize that tasted bitter. The bitter additive was removed from the maize, but the monkeys continued to eat only from the color that was previously identified as tasty. As infants were born or new members migrated into the troop, they all continued to pick only from the one color bin, even though both bins were now being filled with the same maize [34].

Animal studies are only suggestive of what happens with humans, but there is documented evidence that humans conform to social teaching without having evidence or data for the teaching and subsequent behavior.

The Cagots were a minority in France, who were persecuted by their neighbors for seven centuries. There was no clear understanding of why they were persecuted as they looked like everyone around them. It was only during the French Revolution that the Cagots were able to burn their birth certificates in government offices to change their status [35].

Detecting rank is another automatic brain activity; it takes 40 milliseconds to distinguish between a dominant face (with direct gaze) and a subordinate one (with averted eyes and lowered eyebrows) [35]. But an irony of detecting rank is that there is often no relationship between rank and capability. Take for an example the alpha male of the African Savanna baboon. Primatologists used to believe that they led their troop in daily foraging for food. In actual fact, Dr. Sapolsky has documented that the troop follows the old females, who have the most experience in identifying spots for eating. This helps maintain the troop's success, but the females do not have the same rank or privileges that the alpha male has. Yet rank and hierarchy continue to exist in communities of primates. Imaging studies related to submitting to others suggest that the amygdala and insular cortex light up when you think that you are out of step with others. There is also activation of the vmPFC, the anterior cingulate cortex, and the nucleus accumbens. This is a network mobilized during reinforcement learning. Being submissive to the leader appears to be related, at least in part, to the basic biology of fear of not being included in your group and being left out [35].

Dehumanizing

Fear of the other, obedience to hierarchy, and empathy play a role in stigmatizing others. But the process of dehumanizing, which is a predictor of aggressive outcomes, such as support for torture, armed conflict, and reluctance to provide aid to victims of violence, appears to be a brain circuit that operates with a different pattern [36]. Emile Bruneau and his colleagues at the Peace and Conflict Neuroscience Lab have performed studies with people who espouse ideas that entire groups of people are no better than pigs or pests.

Dr. Bruneau was surprised that there were many people who expressed these ideas without much hesitation. He had expected some reticence from most, but instead found that a significant proportion of the people he interviewed from around the world were comfortable sharing with him and his team the idea that the entire population of Muslims, Africans, Jews, and Mexicans or a number of others were not fully human. Dr. Bruneau and his team used fMRI to identify the areas of the brain that were activated when his study subjects rated different groups of people: Americans, Europeans, surgeons, Muslims, Roma, and the homeless. He also included animals like puppies and rats.

He measured the degree of dislike that they had for these groups and also the degree that these groups were viewed less than human by their ranking on the "Ascent of Man" scale. He found that dislike was correlated with brain patterns that were distinct from the brain patterns of dehumanization. Regions in the left inferior parietal cortex and the left inferior frontal cortex were selectively parametrically modulated [37].

Hughes et al. looked at the brain circuits when people were engaged in activities involving trust of in-group members. They found dissociable mechanisms in the brain in those situations. When trusting in-group members, the striatum and the ventromedial PFC were highly active. When trusting out-group members, the dorsal anterior cingulate gyrus and the dorsal and the ventromedial PFC were active. It appeared that there was much higher involvement of neural control of the PFC in order to trust the out-group [38].

Conclusion

Anti-Semitism is a form of out-group derogation that has waxed and waned for over 2000 years of history. Jews are seen by many as being different (misinformation has often been used to stoke the differences), and they are often treated as an out-group, though this varies with social context.

There have been many periods of peaceful co-existence and just as many times of pogroms, slaughter, expulsions, and genocide throughout history. Non-Jews have feared and dehumanized Jews, and Jews of course have also feared and dehumanized non-Jews. Brain processes that prompt human beings to guard against the threat of "otherness" operate in everyone.

The task of humans, if we are to mitigate senseless intergroup conflict, requires understanding of our automatic biases and having the will to overcome them. Many organizations have taken on this mission. The Anti-Defamation League, the Southern Poverty Law Center, and Doctors Without Borders are all examples of efforts to increase group empathy, trust, and cooperation across human barriers. Schools can also teach empathy for out-groups. A famous example is that of the elementary school teacher who divided her classroom into in-groups and out-groups by eye color. The in-group was able to exclude the out-group at recess and had special privileges. The next day she switched the groups. Interviews many years later with these students, now adults, showed what a powerful exercise this was in helping the students recognize their innate capacity to depreciate the other [39].

Psychiatrists spend much of their clinical time dealing with individual patients who need to be more mindful of their internal world and how this affects themselves and others. Perhaps in order to do more primary prevention, we could facilitate the dissemination of the very significant insights that social scientist and neuroscientist have provided into the very sophisticated but potentially harmful automatic workings of fear, empathy, and obedience to hierarchy that exist in the human mind. Some of these insights have become common knowledge. Continued discussion and highlighting of how these processes affect intergroup conflict will hopefully gradually erode discrimination and bias toward minorities.

References

1. Caporeal R. The evolution of truly social cognition; the core configuration model. Personal Soc Psychol Rev. 1997;1(4):276–98.
2. Dunbar RIM. The social brain hypothesis. Evol Anthropol. 1998; https://doi.org/10.1002/(SICJ)1520-6505(1998)6:5<178::AID-EVANS>3.0.CO;2-8.
3. Dunham Y, Baron AS, Carey S. Consequences of "Minimal" Group Affiliations in children. Child Dev. March 2011;82(3):793–811.
4. Brown DE. Human universals. New York: McGraw-Hill Humanities; 1991.
5. Mahayan N, Martinez MA, Gutierrez NL, Diesendruck G, Banaji MR, Santos LR. The evolution of intergroup Bias: perceptions and attitudes in rhesus macaques. Attitudes and Social Cognition. J Pers Soc Psychol. 2011;100(3):387–405.
6. Fiske ST. Stereotype content: "warmth and competence endure". Curr Dir Psychol Sci. 2018;27(2):67–73.
7. Williams LE, Bargh JA. Experiencing physical warmth promotes interpersonal warmth. Science. 2008;322(5901):606–7.
8. Danziger S, Levav J, Aunaim–Perso L. Extraneous factors in judicial decisions. Proc Natl Acad Sci U S A. 2011;108(17):6889–92.
9. Loftis EF, Hoffman HG. Misinformation and memory: the creation of memory. J Exp Psychol Gen. 1989;118:100–4.
10. Kapur N, Cole J, Manly T, Viskontas I, Nintoman A, Hasher L, Pascual–Leone A. Positive clinical neuroscience: explorations in positive neurology. Neuroscientist: Rev J Bringing Neurobiol Neurol Psychiatry. 2013;19:354–69.
11. Polage D. Making up history: false memories of fake news stories. Eur J Psychol. 2012;8(2):245–50. https://doi.org/10.5964/ejop.8i2.456.
12. Brady WJ, Willis JA, Jost JT, Tucker JA, Van Bavel JJ. Emotion shapes the diffusion of moralized content in social networks. Proc Natl Acad Sci U S A. 2017;114(28):7313–8.
13. Rose EM. The Murder of William of Norwich. The origins of the Blood Libel in Midieval Europe. New York: Oxford University Press; 2015.
14. Sah P, Faver E, Lopez De Armentia L, Power J. The Amygdaloid Complex: anatomy and Physiology. Physiol Rev. 2003;83(3):803–34.
15. Chan RW, Leong ATL, Ho LC, Gao PP, Wong EC, Dong CM, Wang X, He J, Chan YS, Lim LW, Wu EX. Low-frequency hippocampal-cortical activity drives brain-wide resting state functional MRI connectivity. Proc Natl Acad Sci U S A. 2017;114(33):E6972–81.
16. PFC – U.S. Department of Health and Human Services. http://www.hhs.gov/opa/familylife/techassistance/etraining/adolescentbrain/development/prefrontalcortex.
17. Hughes BL, Ambady N, Zaki J. Trusting out-group, but not in-group members, requires control: neural and behavioral evidence. Soc Cogn Affect Neurosci. 2017;12(3):372–81.
18. Weiner KS, Zilles K. The anatomical and functional specialization of the fusiform gyrus. Neuropsychologia. 2016;83:48–62.
19. Namkung H, Kim SH, Sawa A. The insula: an underestimated brain area in clinical neuroscience, psychiatry, and neurology. Trends Neurosci. 2017;40(4):200–7.
20. Stott SRW, Ang S–L. Patterning and cell type specification in the developing CNS and PNS. Amsterdam, The Netherlands: Elsevier; 2013. p. 435–53.
21. Nelson R, Trainer B. Neural mechanisms of aggression. Nat Rev Neurosci. 2007;8:536.

22. Le Doux J. The emotional brain: the mysterious underpinning of emotional life. New York: Simon and Schuster; 1998.
23. Hoehl S, Hellmer K, Johansson M, Gredsback G, et al. Front Psychol. 2017;8:1710.
24. Brosch T, Bar-David E, Phelps EA. Implicit race bias decreases the similarity of neural representations of black and white falls. Psychol Sci. 2013;24:160–6. Abstract. PDF.
25. Cloninger CR, Svarkic DM, Przybeck TR. A psychosociologic model of temperament and character. Arch Gen Psychiatry. 1993;50:975–90.
26. Cunningham W, et al. Separable neural components of the processing of black and white faces. Psychol Sci. 2004;15:806.
27. Jhang J, et al. Anterior cingulate cortex. 2018; https://doi.org/10.1038/S41467-018-05090-Y.
28. Hobson NM, Inzlicht M. The mere presence of an out –group member disrupts the brain's feedback – monitoring system. Soc Cogn Affect Neurosci. 2016;11(11):1698–706.
29. Baumgartner T, Schiller B, Hill C, Knoch D. Impartiality in human is predicted by brain structure of dorsomedial prefrontal cortex. Social and affective Neuroscience, Department of Psychology, University of Basel, Broomansgasse 8, CH-4055 Basil, Switzerland. Neuroimage. 2013;81:317–24.
30. Fiske ST, Cuddy AJC, Glick P, Xu J. A model of (often mixed) stereotype content: competence and warmth respectively follow from perceived status and competition. J Pers Soc Psychol. 2002;82(6):878–902.
31. Gray HM, Wegner GK. Dimensions of mind perception. Science. 2007;315(5812):619.
32. Lamm C, et al. The neural substrate of human empathy: effects of perspective taking and cognitive appraisal. J Neurosci. 2007;19:42.
33. Dunbar RIM. Coevolution of neocortical size, group size, and language in humans. Behav Brain Sizes. 1993;16(4):681–735.
34. Van de Waal E, Borgeaud C, Whiten A. Potent social learning and conformity shape the wild primate's foraging decisions. Science. 2013;340:483–5.
35. Thomas S. The last untouchable in Europe. The Independent News. 2008.
36. Rule NO, et al. Perceptions of dominance following glimpses of faces and bodies. Perception. 2012;41:687.
37. Bruneau E, Ner J, Nour K, Saxe R. Denying humanity: the distinct neural correlates of blatant dehumanization. J Exp Psychol. 2018;147(7):1078–93.
38. Hughes BL, Ambody N, Zakin J. Trusting out-group, but not in-group members, requires control: neural and behavioral evidence. Soc Cogn Affect Neurosci. 2017;12(3):372–81.
39. Bland K. The Republic/AZ Central.com CDT. 2015.

Barry Marcus

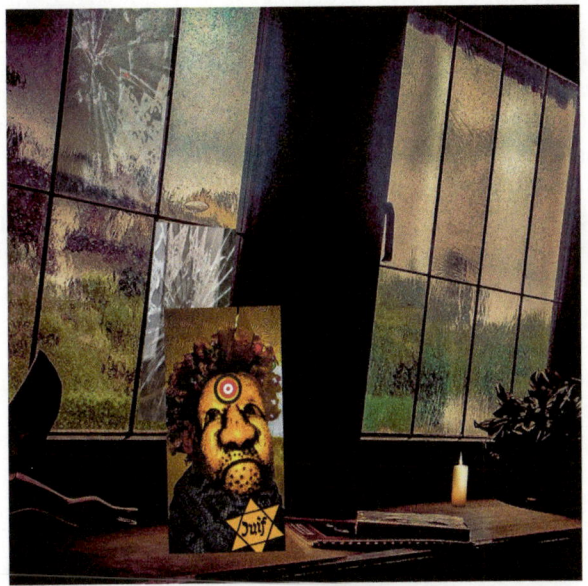

Introduction

Kristallnacht of the Soul – by Barry Marcus (2019)

A portrait becomes a target. A person becomes an object to be used or discarded at will. Beginning outside the window, inside the mind. The window in the image was my German window, inside my German home. Shattered glass shows that the invasion of anti-Semitism into my sheltered life has begun.

B. Marcus (✉)
Bainbridge Island, WA, USA
e-mail: Barmar46@icloud.com

It is November 9 and Kristallnacht has begun! It is coming for me, I fear. I can hear shouts and screams emanating from the street outside my German home. The sounds of marching boots and shattering glass pierce the peace to which I have grown accustomed in our quiet neighborhood. The disturbance continues to escalate, growing louder outside my window and within my head and heart.

I know what will come next. There will be an insistent knock upon my door. As they have come for others, they have come for me. A man in a black uniform will profer a question to which he already knows the answer: "Sind sie Juden?" Am I Jewish? That is a question I often ask myself. But in this circumstance there is not a shred of doubt lingering in the air. As I stand shaking in fear and uncertainty, he will speak in the affirmative: "Sie sind Juden!"In his demanding intrusion, I cannot deny that I am inescapably Jewish. What comes next is already predetermined. Soon I will be placed on a train headed to Auschwitz, Dachau, or Bergen-Belsen, wearing the black and gray striped uniform of death. A small yellow badge will designate my identity, past, present, and future. The star that is the symbol of my faith turned against me, the "Jude." Such is art used as a weapon.

I sit in my chair confused. Frozen to my seat. All I need to do is get up and go to the window. One look will confirm what I already know. But my attention is transfixed on a contemplation of contradictions. The sounds are definitely reverberating within me. But how can they really be coming from outside? Yes, I am certain that today is November 9, a date associated with the beginning of Holocaust. But I also know that Kristallnacht is but history. The outburst of anti-Semitism that began on the evening of November 9, 1931. My experience, right here and now, seems identical, but transposed to the year 2012.

Is this a reoccurrence? A memory or hallucination? Perhaps it is an expression of a Hawkingesque bending of space/time feeding back through a black hole. More than likely, it is the timeless and visceral impact of anti-Semitism on a Jewish man who unavoidably finds himself living in a land that lit the flame of the Final Solution!

At last I gain the composure and courage to look outside my window. There I see the street looking back at me. Innocent of the crimes still ringing in my ears.

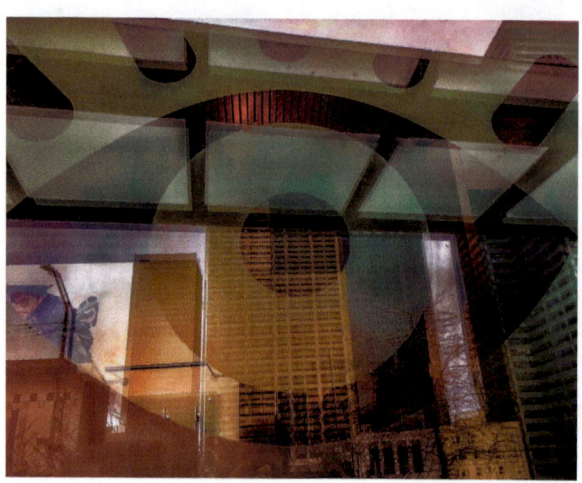

The Watchful Eye of God – by Barry Marcus (2018)

God is omniscient, omnipotent, and omnipresent. This is quite a pressure for a child who senses his own father possesses these same powers. The large eye of God is juxtaposed over a concrete urban setting of my childhood. Eyes peering out from the transformed angel on the left. Always on watch.This image also represents the scrutiny of Jews and their feeling of anti-Semitism lurking in a watchful eye.

I grew up having little knowledge of the biblical foundations of anti-Semitism. That my Jewish ancestors had been deemed guilty of the crime of "deicide," the act of killing Jesus and thus God himself (according to Christian theology). Early gospels placed responsibility on their Jewish contemporaries as well as on all Jews for generations to come. Thus, knowingly or not, I was a criminal, a murderer, and a monster to many who had made up their minds without my acquaintance.

I was sheltered, however, from the notion that I was in any real danger of anti-Semitic prejudice or violence. Unlike some of my friends, I knew of no relatives who had been victims of the Holocaust. I was neither fearful of Gentiles nor particularly anchored in my own Jewish identity. For, although I came from a Jewish family living in a Jewish neighborhood, there were few visible signs of Judaism in our home. We didn't light candles on Friday nights or go to temple the following morning. There were no Jewish pictures, books, or symbols in our house. I don't remember talking about what it meant to be Jewish or how to observe and practice Judaism. I heard little mention of the Holocaust as an event or of the lessons learned.

What my parents made constant reference to was money. The little money that my father made as a salesman and the comparative Jewish wealth he saw around him. He spent most waking hours either at work as a furniture salesman or occupied with repair and replenish projects around the house. We could not afford to seek paid labor and, besides, no one could live up to my father's standards but my father. I believe he resented what he perceived as the unattainable Jewish expectations to achieve wealth. And as such, that he was mirroring what he saw around him and internalizing a personal anti-Semitic shadow as well.

My paternal grandmother, Rose, resided in our home. Although she had immigrated from Romania to the United States after the turn of the century, she never talked about what circumstances led her to take the long and perilous journey across the sea. I suspect she was one of the many Jews who were fleeing anti-Semitic oppression at that time. Although I may have had some limited notion of that growing up, it has presented itself in a new light in the telling of this story.

On occasion I would walk a few blocks from my house to visit my friend David. I always felt anxiety upon entering his home. Once he opened the door, I could not help but see the intimidating painting at the end of the hallway. It was a portrait of an old man wearing a prayer shawl over his shoulders and a "yamulka" upon his head. His right arm was bound in strange serpentine black leather that wound all the way up his arm. It ended in a pair of square black blocks, resting on the center of his forehead. The man in this strange garb was a fearful sight. Almost as threatening to me as the paintings of Jesus I saw on occasion.

When I entered David's home, I walked right up to the painting and stood before it. I was committed to carry on a silent staring contest with this old man. A self-identified ritual I had to perform in order to be qualified to pass on through the hallway and on out to the family room. I did not linger too long. I respected the power this strange man had over me, but only at a distance. I now recognize that my reaction to this menacing figure was, in part, a way of creating a separation from both the painting and myself. Rather than own my discomfort with a Judaism that was threatening to my fragile self-identity, I projected that shadow onto the painting. Onto Judaism itself. I could find no comfortable reference to all that appeared before me. I was enveloped in a kind of dizzy distrust. Here I was, an ambivalent Jew, rejecting an unrealized part of myself. Was this perhaps the very seed that, if nurtured, could grow into a living expression of self-hating anti-Semitism?

Although I was intimidated by the portrait hanging in David's home, I am sure that his parents had no knowledge of my frightened reaction. For them, the portrait was a source of Jewish pride. It hung in honor of Jewish faith and tradition. This prayerful man of God was an idealized Jew. A standard bearer for the chosen people. He was an ever-present mirror of dignity reflecting back upon the Jewish viewer.

My fear of the intimidating Jewish man pictured in the painting on David's wall also extended to God Himself. I knew of His Old Testament reputation. Of His wrath and the punishing consequences He administered for violating His rules and commands. I heard the stories. I saw the pictures of this other stern old man pointing His accusatory finger at me. One had no choice but to follow His directions and yield to His demands. Thou shalt do this! Thou shalt do that! And the whole list of what thou shalt not do. This God had thunder and lightning at His disposal. His voice, my father's voice, becoming my own voice from within. There was no escape. Where would one even go? God was omniscient, omnipotent, and omnipresent! And there I was, just a frightened child with braces on his teeth shaking in fear of the darkness. I was no match for the powers that be.

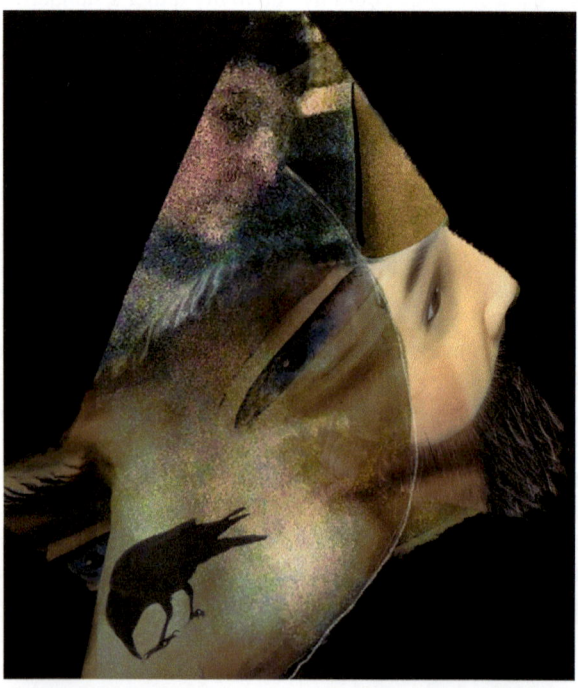

Anti-Semitism: My Introduction

How They See Us – by Barry Marcus (2019)

The origin of this image is artistic portrayals of anti-Semitism beginning in the European Middle Ages. The depictions of Jews evolved from embellishments of clothing and inserted symbols of usury, greed, and deceit into embodied distinctions and associations with magic, sorcery, and the devil. This assemblage is in reference to the origins of anti-Semitic art. The pointed hat and large nose became enduring symbols of the vile and inferior Jew. The crow, as a thief of bright shiny objects, symbolized the view of Jews consumed by the material and obsessed with money and wealth that they obtained at the expense of others.

The Crawford Country Club was just a few blocks down from our house, directly across the street from the Red Owl grocery store. I used to take my younger sister, Leslie, to Red Owl as a special treat, pulling her little red Radio Flyer wagon behind me as she sat inside. As we got closer to our destination, I always felt a heightened sense of anxiety and confusion. I would glance in the direction of the Club, but never hold that gaze. As if we would be turned to salt if I looked too closely. Not that there was much to see from our distanced vantage point. Just a hedge covered wrought iron fence wrapping completely around the block. The tall foreboding locked gate stood as a firm reminder that my sister and I were forbidden to enter. I had heard whispers among my friends that Jews were not allowed to be members. Although I did not understand the gravity and full implications of such a puzzling exclusion, I dared not cross the street and peer into the gated entrance.

Years later, as a teenager, I was always eager to find a well-paying summer job after school let out. One highly sought-after job was to serve as a caddy at one of the public or private golf clubs in the area. The most elite and lucrative place to caddy was the Crawford Country Club. Although no Jew was accepted as a member, Jewish boys were allowed to shoulder the weight of a heavy bag of iron and required to hand over the proper club as requested by the golfers, their "masters." Jewish caddies knew that there were other unstated requirements as well. They had to withstand the subtle and not so subtle remarks directed their way: "You're not bad for a "kike." "Hold on to your tip, I know you Jews are good at that." On occasion, a member would reject a caddy outright. In his eyes, a Jew was not even worthy of carrying the bag of a righteous Christian member. I did not have the gumption or the fortitude to endure such slights. I stuck close to home, mowing neighbors' lawns within a safe vicinity of my home.

I had heard other whispers of anti-Semitism in stories that circulated around our neighborhood. A mix of references to a generalized form of prejudice and specific stories of the Holocaust. I knew that some of my friends' parents had been survivors of the death camps. A few friends told me that they had lost multiple relatives among the 6 million Jews slaughtered by the Nazis.

I was made all too aware of the shadow of a Holocaust survivor when I visited my friend Marty. I literally prayed that his strange and scary mother would not answer the door. When she did, it was always an awkward encounter. Unlike the parents of other friends, she did not greet me with a smile and a "good to see you" acknowledgment. She seemed frightened and frail, confused and shaken, not sure whether to let me in the house or push me away. Each time that I approached her door, I was, once again, a stranger and potential danger. Sometimes, as I waited for Marty at the door (I don't recall if I ever actually entered the house), I saw the pattern of indelible blue numbers scrawled across her slight wrist. I was shocked by their physical appearance, the way the brutal marks were etched into her unwilling skin. Sometimes she caught me lingering a bit too long, staring at the signs of her violation. When she caught me, she would immediately pull her long sleeve back over her wrist thereby breaking the unintentional revelation of the source of her broken soul. That action brought us both a kind of relief. I was fine with the cover up for fear that the horror of her branded wrist might touch me as well.

My father too had warned me about the impact of anti-Semitism. He told me of his experience as a young tenor banjo player as a member of a prominent local band traveling the Midwestern states. The group played in bars and clubs, often greeted by a foreboding that was sign posted inside: "No Dogs or Jews Allowed." If my father shared his own reaction to such menace or any other details about these occurrences, I do not recall hearing it. It seems to me that he would always stop right at that sign and go no further.

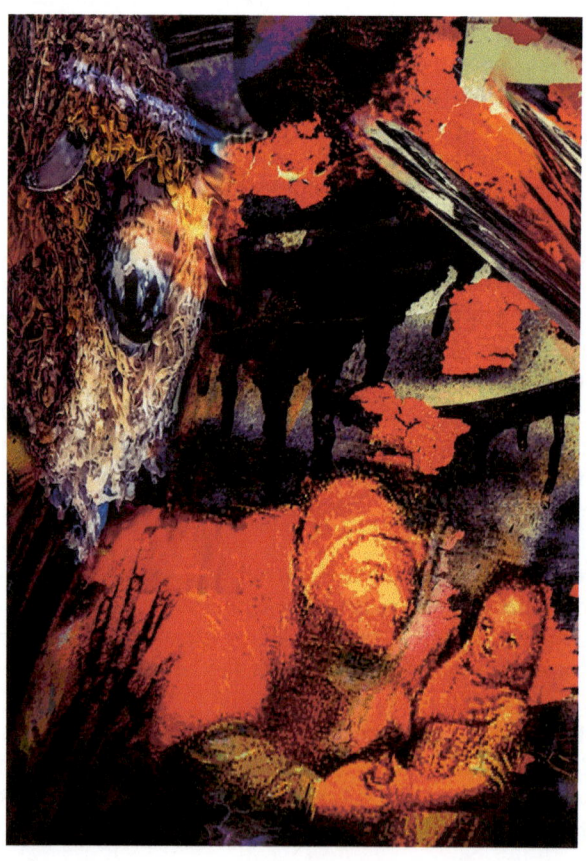

Anti-Semitism: In the Flesh

Drawn in Blood: A Danger to Their Children – by Barry Marcus (2019)

This image is reference to the burgeoning anti-Semitism of the Middle Ages and its expression through art. The figurative element is derived from a Fresco painting of blood libel by Adam Swach, a seventeenth-century Franciscan monk (in the public domain). Blood libel was an accusation and myth that Jewish women kidnapped and murdered Christian children in order to use their blood in preparation of the Passover "matzo," as an element of a secret and demonic dark ritual. Within the context of my story, the bloody saturation of the entire image symbolizes the raw flesh served up in an anti-Semitic incident that I describe further in the text. I inserted a stylized sheep to indicate the ignorant followers of the blood libel mythology.

Every Christmas my family and I would drive through Kennelworth, the Gentile neighborhood not too far from our own little Jewish middle class "ghetto." Kennelworth was considered a place of great opulence where the residents displayed their wealth by decorating their homes in resplendent signs of Christmas. This extravagance was in the spirit of implicit competition among neighbors wanting to flaunt their wealth and claim the status of Christmas supremacy. These contests worked out well for us folk who found great joy and entertainment in circling around the streets of Kennelworth. The bright flashing lights and animated figures delighted me. As a child, this was the closest I was ever going to get to Disneyland.

Eventually I learned that there was a darker side to Kennelworth. One that was not advertised in the colorful light of Christmas celebration. The word out on the streets of our Jewish neighborhood was that Kennelworth was yet another place close by that did not like Jews.

As I grew up, I discovered that, despite the shadows of anti-Jewish sentiment, Kennelworth had an attraction that could not be denied. Steak and onion rings at the Kennelworth Inn. I could count on the steaks to be large and juicy, cooked to my specifications. Rare, if you please! The onion rings were always plump, crisp, and generous in number. When I was served them on a shiny silver platter, then smothered with Heinz ketchup (had to be Heinz), all my thoughts of anti-anything seemed to fade behind the positivity of a delectable meal.

I went to Kennelworth Inn with a group of my friends to enjoy such a meal a number of weekend evenings. Because of the warnings about the community's prejudice, we always entered the restaurant tentatively. A bit on guard. Staff were very polite. A little too much so. Their typically polished "Welcome to the Kennelworth Inn" always seemed formal, stiff, and generic. Disingenuous. There was nothing in that sterile greeting that implied any kind of personal recognition or connection. The tone was superficial and passively withholding. Neutral at best. We probably should have taken the not so subtle "hint" and walked back to our cars. But, oh those onion rings!

One Friday evening we gathered at the restaurant for a birthday celebration. After we completed the ritualized greeting, we sat down at a large rectangular table.

It appeared to be the largest table in the room. When the waiter arrived, he was proper and poised, offering a slight undertone of patronizing graciousness. We expected his attentiveness. He had to know a big tip awaited him from us "regulars."

"And what will you be ordering, sir," the waiter inquired of me? "I'll have a steak and an order of onion rings for the table," I replied. "And how would you like your steak cooked, sir?" I answered the same as I always had: "Rare and juicy!"

It seemed that we waited for hours before our food was brought to the table. It was probably no more than 45 minutes or so, but longer than it should have been. When he finally arrived with our food, the waiter put my plated steak on the table before me, pausing just long enough to look me in the eye as if to say that he was complicit in what was about to follow. There on that plate was definitely a steak, but it was not pink and rare as I had ordered. No, this steak was black and burnt to a crisp. In retrospect, I cannot help but think of all the Jews who were shoved one by one into Nazi ovens. They too became blackened and burned. Was that the chef's intention? To remind me of those atrocities and imply my fate as well? Likely not, but the reference is impossible for me now to ignore completely.

I stared down at my plate startled and confused. There could be no mistake. This was not a case of accident or miscommunication. It was clearly intentional. "Send it back," came spontaneous calls from my friends around the table. Of course I would do so. I was not shy or hesitant to assert myself when necessary. "Excuse me, waiter, this steak is not cooked the way I ordered it," I stated with just a slight edge of outrage. "Would you like me to take it back and bring you another, sir?" he said in a monotone. There was no apology expressed or implied. "Yes," I said, "and please make sure that this one comes back rare. Just as I had ordered it." "Most certainly, sir" the waiter said with a smile that had a tinge of self-satisfaction.

To my amazement, this time the waiter returned in less than 5 minutes. He placed the plate before me and said: "One rare steak, as you like it, sir!" The entire table went silent but for few whispered gasps. This steak was not rare, it was cold and raw. At this point I was numb. The message was clear. Written in the flesh and blood that was on my plate. Written even deeper onto my own flesh and blood and that of my ancestors. There was nothing subtle about this flagrant display!

My friend, Mickey, received the message too. He would not remain silent. Mickey stood up abruptly and gestured and gesticulated fervently as if he was in the midst of some kind of seizure. He amplified his outrage by shouting a diatribe of obscenities for everyone to hear. Next he picked up my slaughtered steak and waved it around over his head for everyone to see. Then he threw it across the room aimed at our still smiling waiter. "We're getting the hell out of here," he announced with a rebel yell. And that was that. We were gone, never to return. Still, I wondered, what was it they saw in my Jewishness that provoked such aggression? How was I the enemy? For the first time in my life, the impact of anti-Semitism was deeply personal.

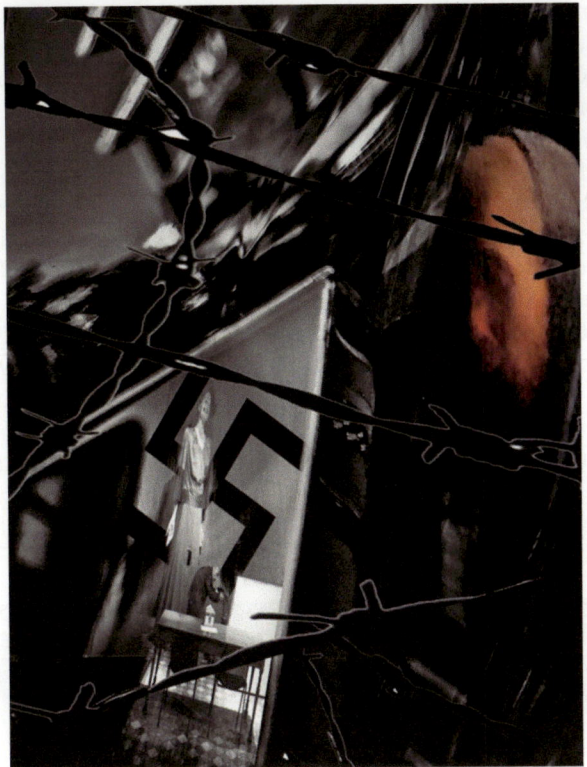

Anti-Semitism: German Immersion

Hell Realm – by Barry Marcus (2019)

> Living in Germany for 5 years provided me with many opportunities to visit and view the instruments and impact of the Holocaust. The death camp of Dachau and the Holocaust Museum in Berlin were but two examples of my immersion into that horror. The message of this image, I believe, is self-evident in both its suffocating darkness and in the vivid flesh of the hopelessly resigned Jewish victim moving into the inevitable. The embedded black and white figurative image on the left is also a reference to the looming destiny of the old and feeble Jewish man about to disappear into oblivion.

In moving to Germany many years later, I found myself to be in a situation antithetical to my mostly sheltered experience as a member of God's chosen people. Here, too, Jews had been chosen: chosen for extermination. It was as if the Holocaust from the past was ever present and ever possible here and now and in the future.

Although I made good friends and lived relatively free from direct expressions of bigotry and hate, I felt very vulnerable and constantly on guard. As if ghosts of the

Gestapo loomed over my shoulders, posing a threat all around me. As if spirits from the concentration camps hovered above me in horror. Could the seeds and ashes of genocide find new life there before me? The instruction to "never forget" was unnecessary in the midst of reminders all around.

A visit to Dachau shook my soul. I saw the ovens, real ovens, close at hand. Their sole purpose had been to dispose of real human beings. One after the other. Were the fires still lit as I stood there in intense gaze? I was sure I saw the burning flames and inhaled the smoldering flesh! There were the train tracks. Winding their way into the camp and then coming to an abrupt end at the final destination. Unfathomable! Unforgettable!

The Holocaust Museum too was overwhelming. The building itself was both minimalist and stark, yet still elegant in its beauty. The interior wound around as it moved the visitor up along multiple exhibits of impossibility. All in a grand scale. But its most visceral impact came through the way it told tragic individual human stories through short narratives, photographs, and personal effects. As I encountered these remnants of lives lost, I wept. From start to finish. As I moved out the door, I was still weeping. Clearly there was no escape. I was one of them.

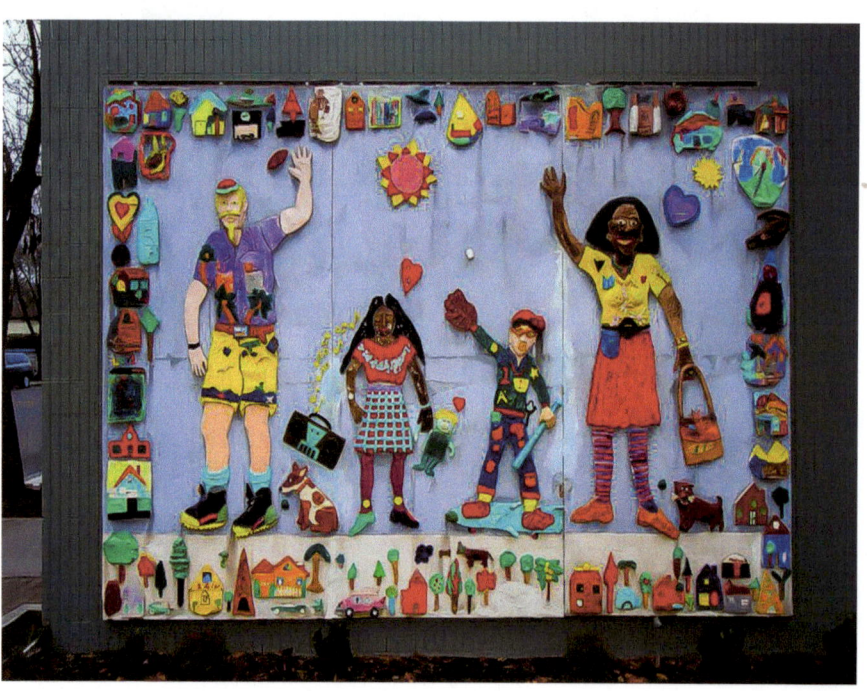

Art in Response to Trauma

The Davis Family Mural – created by the children of Families First Residential Program, Davis, California

> Each of four residential houses collaborated with an established ceramic artist to create one member of an idealized multicultural nuclear family, pets inclusive. Every child was provided an opportunity to create his own version of a house imagined as appearing along the borders of the mural. The children learned that while each on his own made an important contribution, it took the house as a whole to create a single family member and only all together as a community could a nurturing family be born.

In the shadow of Germany, the Holocaust, and the ever-present threats of anti-Semitism, I continue to recognize the pattern and enduring effects of trauma. As a mental health director and practitioner for over 25 years, I have treated children and adults suffering from deep wounds, self-inflicted and otherwise.

Over the course of my career, I have found that art offers a container for chaos. That individuals suffering from trauma turned within or without can find refuge in the creative process and result. That the resistance and turmoil of directly re-experiencing and confronting traumatic events can be mitigated by channeling these forces onto a page, across a canvas, or into a song. By focusing attention outside oneself and engaging in the task at hand, an individual can create a safe distance from self-reference and the external object of attention. This tangible creation can be viewed with pride and satisfaction or be seen as something to be disposed of or discarded. In some instances, the act of destruction, itself, can be a cathartic physical expression of pent-up frustration and rage. Thus the art maker has control of what is made and how it is used in contrast to the overwhelming out of control nature of trauma.

There has been an increasing emphasis on the use of expressive art therapies in treating severe trauma and for increasing individual resiliency. These practices are informed by contemporary research in trauma intervention, neurodevelopment, and related fields. Given that many of the adaptive survival methods in which survivors engage are primitive and associated with lower brain activity, expressive arts have demonstrated positive results in building neural plasticity. By releasing into the flow of the creative process, those struggling in hypervigilant protective behaviors can find respite and relief from the concerted effort to control everything in and around them. In the process, they can access alternate parts of the brain and build new pathways of resiliency. This work has direct application in working with individuals and communities that have been the targets of anti-Semitism. Sadly, given the now all too common attacks on places of worship, there will be ample opportunity to explore this topic now and in the future.

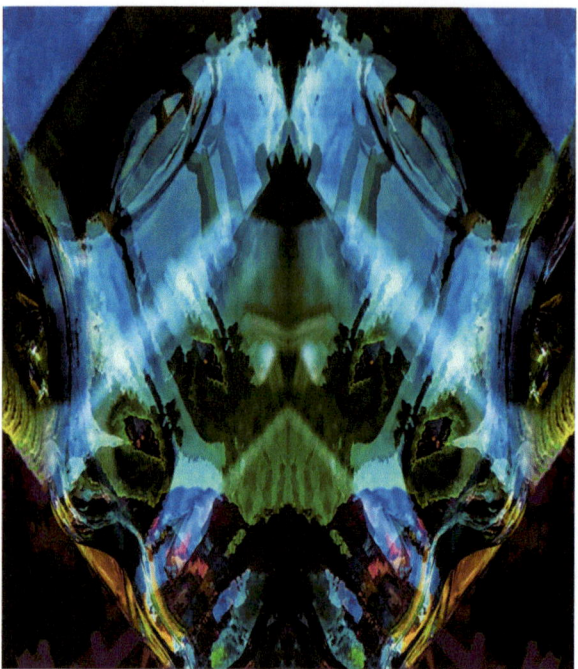

Conclusion

Look Out Your Window – by Barry Marcus (2019)

> According to the esteemed Jewish mystic and philosopher, Martin Buber, a relationship with God requires a letting go of ego and the restrictions that separate I from other. In the "I-you" encounter, which Buber refers to as "love," there is no boundary or separation. "I" relates as if the entire universe existed through "you." The process is transformational for both participants. Love and transformation. A reminder the enduring forces that run counter to anti-Semitism.

I live on an island now. Bainbridge Island. Surrounded by the vital waters of the Puget Sound just a 30-minute ferry ride from Seattle.

This is a far cry from the claustrophobic confines of my Jewish worries in Germany.

As I sit and contemplate the ways I might bring closure to this chapter, I am mesmerized by the natural beauty I see moving just outside my window. Sometimes sea lions. On occasion orcas. Always big ships bringing their cargos to and from port. This flow of nature is ever changing. Calm waters turning into choppy seas. Waves crashing up upon the shore and then receding to reveal the rocky beach beneath. Muscular clouds rolling in and out, bringing wind and rain in overcast only to withdraw and reveal the sunshine that was previously obscured. It all unfolds in the moment as I bear witness. If I pay attention and let go of my own expectations, revelation abounds.

These waters mark time yet also transcend it. I imagine a past where there were no signs of human life, just the percolating presence of cellular activity evolving into forms of higher life. I envision a future that is uncertain. Will the human touch bring healing to these troubled waters or continue on the destructive path of ignorance and exploitation?

The history of the Jewish people has been subject to the same kinds of ebb and flow. Temporary and timeless. Through almost 6000 years of persecution and perseverance, Jews have endured destructive upheavals and tumultuous seas of change. Steeped in a culture rich in creativity and tradition, Jews possess a living calendar that is in sync with the seasons and history. Through their ability to adapt to challenge and uncertainty, they continue to find ways to be resourceful and resilient. To overcome the ongoing spread of anti-Semitic hatred and violence. Despite threats to their very existence, Jewish waters always run deep and unrestrained.

Like the life I see outside my window, I too am subject to the forces of change and impermanence. While I look out through the glass that appears to separate me from the flow of life outside, I recognize that there is no separation at all. It is just the appearance of separation. I am not merely a witness to the flow of life I view, I am one with it. A descendant of generations of ancestors. Within me in spirit and substance. Rippling through me like waves through the waters of time.

All is not flow. This chapter included. What I have created here, in fact, is not the chapter I intended to write nor what I envisioned as I proceeded. Many may think that a personal narrative would be a product of recall, a recounting through a process of self-dictation. My story, however, has unfolded with far more mystery and uncertainty. It is, essentially, a weaving of what I thought I knew with threads of what I surprisingly discovered in facing the blank page. A journey of inspired direction, false starts, and dead ends. This is the power of art. Of trusting in the process without pressing a predetermined outcome. As I began this chapter, I felt burdened and ashamed by my ambivalent sense of Jewish identity. I started out with the assumption that I was not a "legitimate" Jew. That by failing to adhere to what I had determined were the basic requirements of Jewish authenticity, I was an imposter pretending to be a Jew in good standing. Neither learned nor observant in the formal customs of Jewish practice, I judged myself harshly. Channeling the criticism of the stern rabbi of my youth. The wrathful eye of the ever-watching God of the Old Testament. By allowing the story to unfold and the images to reveal themselves to me, I have experienced revelation and healing. The whole of this creation is greater than the sum of its parts. This gestalt has infused me with a sense of dignity and pride. It exists as a mirror reflecting the darkness and the light that gives shape to a newfound self-acceptance.

Art is both a mirror and a window. It is a process of tempering intention with attention. Allowing the raw nature of experience to make itself known on the spot.

When I enter into a relationship with the art process, I feel a sense of heightened awareness as well as a note of cautionary hesitation. Will I get it right? Can I step away from the constraints of my hungry ego and open up to the unknown?

As an artist I feel I am a steward of spirit. Exploring the source at its origin, following its winding path out to deeper waters. Seeking to be in the flow of inspiration. Suddenly a moment arises. An opening where I lose all sense of time and space. There I find an embodied fullness that knows no bounds! Will anybody like the object of my expression? I hope so. But, that is really not my chief concern. I am neither interested in decoration nor in ornamentation nor in making things "pretty." The vivid, energetic rawness of life, that is what I serve. And always I am but an apprentice.

Art, too, can serve a purpose. It can promote a specific agenda or point of view. In this way, art can exert a power all its own, functioning as a deliberate call to action! Such has been the nature of anti-Semitism through the ages. Such is the possibility for an equal and opposite reaction!

It is my intention that, as art, this chapter will engage the viewing participant in mystery and reflection. That it will be experienced viscerally and inspire empathy through its depiction of anti-Semitism. Through the power of the pen and the impact of the image, it is my goal to motivate creative and effective action as a force to counter anti- Semitic hate speech and violence. Art as a healer and a sword. Good work to inspire good works, lighting a spark of co-creation in the Jewish tradition of Tikkun Olam: the imperative to heal the world!

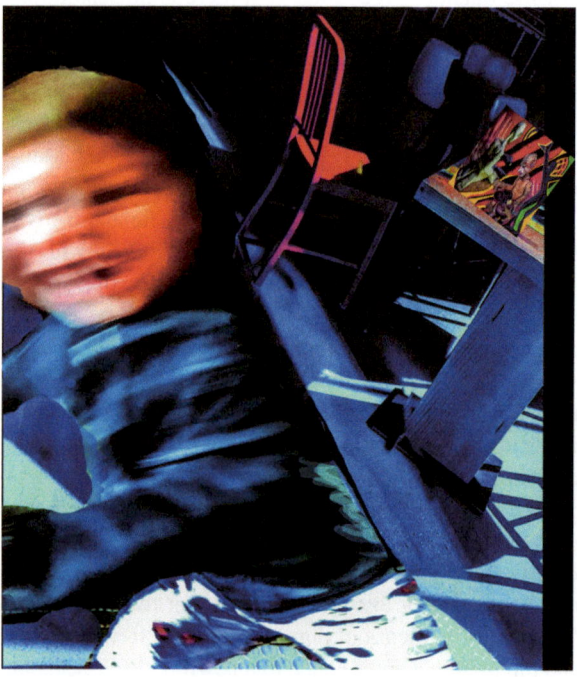

The Artist's Free Spirit – by Barry Marcus (2019)

There is work to be done as an artist. Skills to be honed, methods to apply. It takes patience and persistence. There are details to articulate through diligence and routine. Sometimes the stuff of the mundane. Sitting down in my chair before my table is where it appears I make my art. That is true to some extent. The viewer can see such evidence in the completed image on display atop the table. It is the very same image that introduced this chapter. But there is the artist in me that does not take a seat. He takes leave on his own exuberant exploration. In the form of unlimited engagement with possibility. Like an enthusiastic child. Like my grandson in this picture. He, an expression of generations of Jews to come!

A Social Psychiatrist Looks at Antisemitism and Jewish Identity

6

Stanley J. J. Freeman

The human animal is very much a social animal – like wolves, not like bears – and like many other social animals, we use the group to protect us and to facilitate most aspects of our lives. Beyond our tribal affiliation, we belong to a wide variety of other social units: our religion as a whole, a particular branch of our religion, our immediate family, our extended family, a political party, our nation, our city, our province, fellow supporters of a sports team, graduates of our university, and on and on. Our attachment to some of the groups can be sporadic depending on circumstances and on the need for some of the benefits available from that group at a particular time. For example, some groups can be the source of a significant proportion of our self-esteem. When one of our groups achieves honor or power, we act and feel as though it is we, ourselves, who have earned the accolades. If the Blue Jays were to win the World Series, it would be as though I had won and I would proclaim my affiliation to that group by wearing a Blue Jays sweater and cap. Often, humans deride or hate or even, sometimes, kill those who are not in their group. Any threat or imagined threat by, or serious competition with, another group, usually serves to increase the strength of the bonding within each of the contending groups. Group leaders often use this phenomenon politically to consolidate their power or to distract their constituents from their current problems. "It's not we who have failed. It's the international conspiracy by the crafty Jews that has done it to us," or "The welfare money given to the useless blacks has caused our colossal deficit," or "To make our group great again, I'm going to build a high wall to keep out the foreign rapists."

The drive to group formation appears to be firmly embedded in our DNA. The bonding may become even more powerful when there is poverty or famine, or any other kind of threat to our safety or stability. But, if the threat appears beyond control, the group may disintegrate leaving its former members to seek new groups through avenues such as migration or criminal activity or terrorism. In the case of

S. J. J. Freeman (✉)
Professor Emeritus, Department of Psychiatry, University of Toronto, Toronto, ON, Canada
e-mail: nastanfreeman@gmail.com

© Springer Nature Switzerland AG 2020
H. S. Moffic et al. (eds.), *Anti-Semitism and Psychiatry*,
https://doi.org/10.1007/978-3-030-37745-8_6

the Jews, however, the unbelievably destructive antisemitism during the Holocaust did not cause disintegration of the group. Only a small number of survivors rejected their Jewish identity; the majority retained it. Probably, it takes the experience of centuries of recurrent persecution to develop the belief that, if you wait long enough, the present pain will end.

There seems to be a startling relationship between the degree of antisemitism and its effect on Jewish identity. If we characterize the antisemitism as mild, intermediate, and very strong, we find that intermediate antisemitism, like that in pre-Hitler Europe and in North America during most of the twentieth century, has often promoted stronger Jewish bonding and, with it, all manner of social, scientific, and artistic creativity. Minimal criteria of intermediate antisemitism would appear to be rule of law and no specific anti-Jewish legislation at any level of government. Mild antisemitism may be said to exist when there are actual laws against prejudicial behavior toward Jews and, above all, a widespread public acceptance of their value and rights as fellow citizens. Such conditions existed in the United States from at least 1975 to 2015, contributing largely to a decrease in Jewish identity as evidenced by the marriage of over 50% of young Jews to non-Jews [1]. In contrast, the very strong antisemitism of the Holocaust failed to diminish the sense of Jewish identity in its survivors!

With the present multiplicity of growing crises in our world – the deterioration of the environment, income inequality, the replacement of jobs by artificial intelligence and globalism, and the resultant huge population movements – it is hard to imagine a decrease in nationalism or other major forms of grouping in the near future. Indeed, the reverse is true. There are presently more independent nations in the world than there were in the late 1940s and religious fervor and strife are on the rise. And so is antisemitism. As worldwide stress increases, we can expect both old and new national or religious groupings to consolidate by seeking scapegoats. Prejudice against any group of people arises from a variety of geographical, political, economic, and sociological factors, almost all of which were, and are, in operation against the Jewish people.

What Do We Mean by Jewish Identity?

To an Orthodox Jew the answer to this question is simple. You are a Jew if your mother was Jewish, if you believe in the Abrahamic definition of God, and if you observe the myriad commandments, festivals, and customs that are traditional with your particular subgroup of Jews, such as East European Jews or those of Spanish descent. Indeed, many scholars believe that the Jewish sages introduced this complex array of observance in order to keep the Jews occupied with being Jewish and to separate them from the Gentile population. Nevertheless, for the past two centuries, Jewish identity has begun to include an increasing number of cultural attributes that are more or less unrelated to religion. This is even true of formal synagogue practice, an example of which originated in the nineteenth century with German Reform Jews who averred, "We are Germans of the Jewish faith," a faith which they observed by a markedly watered-down set of religious rituals. At one point, they even deleted the usual Saturday services, celebrating the Sabbath by services on Friday evening and Sunday morning – and without the traditional head covering. Today, a large number of American Jews who are synagogue members are not there primarily for religious reasons. The synagogue for them has become not so much the *religious center* but the *central location* for their version of Jewish identity: the celebration of certain holidays, festivals, and life milestones like Bar Mitzvahs, weddings, and funerals. Concerts, film festivals, lectures, and the like take place in the synagogue as well. In this way, Jewish identity has expanded its parameters beyond worship and the study of scripture.

Jewish identity has had all kinds of other claims made on it. The *Yiddishists* of the late nineteenth century and into the middle of the twentieth century noted that you could speak a common language to perfect strangers as you travelled from Russia to Poland to Lithuania to England to America to Argentina. Their mantra became "Yiddish will save the Jewish people. It will preserve our identity." They supported what grew into an excellent body of Yiddish literature and founded the Jewish Scientific Institute (YIVO) which formalized the language, produced excellent research on its development, and gave rise to dictionaries and other linguistic publications.

Zionism increasingly became another major factor in the definition of Jewish identity from the time of Theodor Herzl in the late nineteenth century right up to very recent years when a split between Western Jews, especially in the United States, and Israeli Jews began to appear. This concerned mainly what the Western Jews believed to be the undemocratic, imperialistic behavior of the current Israeli government toward the Palestinian population. But the Western Jews were objecting as Jews to Jews and it was probable that there was little diminution in the proportion of Jewish identity they derived from the existence of the State of Israel. In a recent conversation with a Canadian world traveller, he told me that, in the absence of any other common language, he was able to communicate in Hebrew and get much-needed help from strangers in three different countries – Hebrew replacing Yiddish as the lingua franca of the Jewish people, thanks to Zionism.

It appears, then, that Jewish identity now consists of a variable blend of religious, cultural, and nationalistic components, some or all of which are subscribed to by people all over the world who call themselves Jews. But there is another extremely important force that holds this group together. On several occasions in my lifetime, I have been accused of not being a Jew– but only by Jews who felt I did not live up to the demands of their definition of the group (usually the religious demands). But I cannot remember a single instance where my being Jewish was denied by a Gentile. This simple fact illustrates the point that one of the crucial forces that promotes and preserves Jewish identity is the attitude toward Jews, whether positive or negative, held by non-Jews. As the Jews of fifteenth-century Spain or twentieth-century Germany found out, no matter who or what they thought they were, their identity as Jews was forced on them by external antisemitic forces. Even generations after the end of the Spanish Inquisition, the descendants of Spanish Jews, who converted to Catholicism to save their lives, were labelled and often punished as

"Conversos" ostensibly loyal, albeit secretly, to their Jewish heritage. It appears very clear, therefore, that one of the most powerful determinants of Jewish identity comes from outside, from the fact that the outside world insists that the Jewish people are a distinct group.

As has always been the case, diminution of prejudice and of persecution increases the rate of assimilation of any minority group in any society with a resultant loss or blurring of ethnic identity. In turn, increased assimilation hastens the diminution of prejudice and persecution because the "strangers within our gates" become less strange. They begin to talk, dress, and behave like "us." They begin to have similar tastes and similar goals. Some differences are, however, permissible and even desirable, such as those that allow the majority group to compliment itself on having a "multicultural society" within which various minority groups celebrate their holidays by wearing colorful costumes and performing their "ethnic dances." It feels good, even adventurous, for most non-Jews to be invited to a Passover Seder or for members of the majority group to watch a Chinese New Year's Festival – as long as these new entrants into our society abide by "our" laws (not *Talmudic laws* or *Sharia*) and increasingly live their daily lives as "we" do.

Is It Important to Preserve Jewish Identity?

Before talking about how to preserve Jewish identity, we must ask the difficult question, "Why should we try to preserve it?" For me, as for many modern, Western Jews, a large part of the reason is very personal. I love the beautiful, positive aspects of Jewish culture, especially that of East Europe: the Yiddish language, the humor, the music, and all of those things in which my Jewish childhood was nestled. Most people who grew up with major affiliations to any other group would probably give similar answers. But, the answer that has more general importance is that historical factors have brought about the formation of a unique group whose values and creative forces have been of great value to the world scientifically and artistically and in the refinement and development of desirable moral, political, and cultural institutions like the improved status of women or the legal system.

How Has Jewish Identity Been Preserved in the Past?

The Jews and the Romani are two examples of people who, without a geographic homeland, managed to survive over the centuries without a degree of assimilation that would spell the end of their identity and culture. In both instances they maintained marked differences in most aspects of communal and family life from the peoples among whom they lived and who usually reviled and persecuted them. Through much of classical antiquity and medieval times and up to the *Haskallah* (the time of Jewish Enlightenment in the late eighteenth century), the Jews practiced a form of religion that was complex and intense in its daily demands. Blessings had to be said many times a day before and after food; phylacteries had to be worn for certain prayers; one had to kiss the *mezuza* on every door post as one passed through; certain times of the day required prayer with a *minyan* composed of at least ten men; special clothing was prescribed; festivals and fasts were frequent. It is generally understood that these customs were introduced by the rabbis who redefined Judaism after the exodus from Israel. Their intention was to preserve Jewish identity by keeping the Jews busy being Jews and by making them different in appearance and lifestyle from the majority group around them. Again, for both the Romani and the Jews, prejudice against them was significantly fueled by these marked differences in life style, while conformity to the differences was reinforced, in turn, by the prejudice. It is noteworthy, however, that the Jews almost always managed to reach much more successful levels of economic and intellectually creative success. This came about because of a number of cultural characteristics which evolved over the centuries, particularly a love and respect for learning along with many commandments about the importance of charity and *tikkun olam* (the repair of the world).

To a considerable degree, these cultural characteristics enabled persecuted, ghettoized Jews to create highly organized sub-communities quite separate from those of the host communities in which they lived. This usually took place in enforced ghettos but sometimes, as in Montreal in the first half of the twentieth century, they were simply areas in which Jews chose to live comfortably close to each other. Here they could organize charities, synagogues, schools, festivals, and most of the attributes of ordinary urban or village life. Montreal Jews often had only a rudimentary knowledge of French, and although their English was much better, many of them communicated almost entirely in Yiddish. My mother-in-law, who came to Canada as a young child, was intelligent and well-read in English literature, and yet her excellent English was spoken with a pronounced Yiddish accent. This was undoubtedly because she was able to carry out most of the functions necessary for daily living within the vibrant, Yiddish-speaking sub-community in Montreal. Who needed assimilation?

Another factor contributing to Jewish survival has been a persistent sense of being in the right, which probably originated in the belief that they were the Chosen People. Social anthropologists have long noted that a sense of "chosenness," of being a member of a special or superior group, often correlates with the preservation and unity of that group, for example, the Rastafarians of Ethiopia. When the Jews were reviled by their neighbors, they refused to believe that they were inferior or dirty or avaricious. They believed they were actually quite special and it has long been known that self-esteem correlates with resilience in the face of stress as well as with ambition and performance. "If you won't let us own land, we'll invent banking!"

A more contentious reason for survival bases it on genetic factors. Recently, several geneticists (believe it or not, *not* Jewish geneticists) have hypothesized that the survival of the Jews as a people (not to mention the plethora of Nobel Prizes won by them) in the face of incredible and continuous stress is, to a significant degree, a function of their IQ. The claim is that, for Jews, the mode of the normal distribution curve for intelligence is shifted to the right [2]. This is attributed to the fact that only the fittest survived persecution in the past two, or even three, millennia. Others have theorized that literacy and learning were demanded by Jewish tradition and those who could not meet the standard stood less of a chance of finding a mate. Another hypothesis suggests that when the Jews were forced out of ancient Israel to Babylon, only the most highly skilled artisans were taken and that it was their descendants who returned and reconstituted the Jewish people. Presumably, high IQ allows for greater creativity in meeting the stress of antisemitism. Whether or not these genetic theories have any validity remains to be seen but the next point is much more solidly explanatory.

Jews are often called "The People of the Book." From very early times, they have always written down their history, their philosophy, their religion, and their liturgy. In the last two centuries especially, they have added a huge body of scientific, musical, artistic, and literary creations. These accomplishments have been the outcome of an almost relentless pursuit of education and achievement.

Unfortunately, many of these highly adaptive mechanisms are prone to diminish sharply as assimilation progresses. As children of minimally assimilated, Jewish immigrants, my generation of high school and university students won a disproportionate number of the available scholarships. But our place has been taken by the children of similar minimally assimilated Chinese and South Asian immigrants. Apparently it is not just a cultural tradition of learning that matters. It is also the fact that for new immigrants or those suffering prejudice for any other reason, "you have to be ten times as good to have one-tenth the chance." Therefore, their children are inculcated with a drive to succeed academically and vocationally. Nevertheless, with successful assimilation, there is a decrease in desperation and, rather than an intense focus on achieving excellence, it becomes acceptable, for example, to learn to play the guitar instead of the violin – even a guitar equipped with a capo! It appears then that in an accepting environment that facilitates assimilation, it is not only religious observance that decreases but other factors that promote cultural identity also tend to lose their potency, all of this within a mere two or three generations.

There are two conclusions to be drawn from the foregoing. The first is that it is important to preserve Jewish identity because the centuries of persecution, in combination with the biblical and rabbinic laws of the Jews, have produced a people with a unique blend of social responsibility and respect for intellectual achievement. They have an ongoing record of artistic, scientific, and political creativity which the world needs, especially in a time of increasingly acute global problems. Obviously there are notable exceptions, usually short-lived, to this assertion, for example, the way the current Israeli government is handling the West Bank situation. But, as mentioned above, the vociferous objection to this by the American Jewish community indicates that the attribute of social responsibility remains strong enough to override chauvinistic loyalties.

The second conclusion is that a large part of Jewish identity is maintained by antisemitism – usually intermediate antisemitism as defined above – and that a reduction of antisemitism to the level of mild antisemitism leads to increasing assimilation and a weakening of Jewish identity.

Can Jewish Identity Be Preserved in the Absence of Antisemitism?

What Won't Work

Both the lifestyle and the fecundity of the Ultra-Orthodox seem to be effective at present in prolonging Jewish identity. Their number worldwide is increasing. But the great majority of modern Jews would not dream of separating themselves from the world around them and from most connections to art, literature, and science. Besides, in a time of all-pervasive technology and addictive social media, it is doubtful that it will be possible for the Ultra-Orthodox to isolate their children indefinitely from the surrounding culture.

Would "Modern Orthodoxy" be more successful? Many Orthodox but less enthusiastically observant Jews are today active in the workplace, artistic life, and educational institutions of the dominant culture. This is only possible where anti-semitism is muted enough to tolerate this degree of participation by observant Jews. The majority of the Jews who came from Eastern Europe to North America between 1880 and 1910 were observant, but this did not stop the inexorable progress of assimilation even at a time when antisemitism was more openly expressed than it is today. Three or four generations later, most of their grandchildren and great-grandchildren live much like the majority of the people in the surrounding culture. To the degree that their Jewish identity remains intact, it is being maintained by cultural factors other than religion.

What Might Work

It is obvious that the existence of a national homeland strongly defines the identity of a people, even for those who do not actually live there, for example, the Irish of the United States or the Ukrainians of Canada. Will the existence of the State of Israel function in the same way? There are, unfortunately, some caveats here. Will Israel survive, given that an increasing part of the world is opposed to it? Will it remain a democratic, just society that Western Jews can identify with? There are currently some disquieting signs that it might not. Many erstwhile Zionists are bemoaning the disappearance of the ardent idealism that characterized the Jewish populations of Palestine and Israel only two or three generations ago [3]. The establishment of a Jewish state was driven by idealism and socialistic definitions of democratic liberalism. This has gone the way it usually does when a new state becomes successful. Idealism has been superseded by strivings for political power as it did in the Soviet Union after the Revolution. At the same time, the usual materialistic aspirations of ordinary families have come to the fore, "Can I get a job that will enable me to buy a car?" Is this the beginning of a schism between being Jewish and being Israeli? Despite these negative portents, the existence of a national homeland where there is pride in the history, ethics, and creativity of the Jews may well become of major importance for the preservation of Jewish identity.

Since the majority of Jews will continue to live in the Diaspora, it is obvious that Jewish education and organized Jewish communal activities will be crucial to the preservation of Jewish identity. So far, most Jewish communities remain highly organized with regard to charity, Jewish education, and political (especially Zionist) advocacy. These functions are often mediated through synagogues and community centers, but big-budget facilities like day schools are dependent on organized community charities. Lately however, and perhaps inevitably, there is a tendency for the leadership of these community charities to be taken over by successful young businessmen who, too often, are more concerned with providing good workout facilities than good, affordable Jewish schools.

To Sum Up

It appears that religious observance will not be effective in preserving Jewish identity for the great majority of modern Jews. The existence of an ethical and creative State of Israel coupled with thoroughgoing Jewish education and communal activities in the Diaspora might work – especially if Jews continue to be told that they are Jews by the majority populations among whom they live.

Assimilation is the major agent that weakens Jewish identity.

Antisemitism, in turn, is the major agent that weakens assimilation.

Therefore, we must conclude with this outrageous contradiction:

The most antisemitic thing they can do to us is to do away with antisemitism.

References

1. Smith GA, Cooperman A. What happens when Jews intermarry?. Pew Research Center. 2013. https://www.pewresearch.org/fact-tank/2013/11/12/what-happens-when-jews-intermarry/. Accessed on January 2020.
2. Cochran G, Harpending H. The 10,000 year explosion. New York: Basic Books; 2009.
3. Shavit A. My promised land – the triumph and tragedy of Israel. New York: Spiegel and Grau; 2013.

How Anti-Semitism and the Shoah Helped Shape Twentieth-Century Psychiatry

7

Sharon Packer

Introduction

Anti-Semitism in general and the Holocaust (Shoah) in particular helped shape the course of twentieth-century American psychiatry, although anti-Semitic attitudes toward Jewish physicians date to medieval times, long before the Reich's arrival.

When Freud started psychoanalysis as the nineteenth century ended, he boasted that only a "G-dless Jew" could have invented psychoanalysis [1]. Fearful that his embryonic psychoanalytic movement would be dismissed as a "Jewish national affair" because he and most movement members were Jewish, Freud welcomed Carl Gustav Jung into his circle, hoping that this son of a Protestant minister would ease psychoanalysis' acceptance by Gentiles. Jung had devised important word association tests and personality theories about introverts and extroverts.

Freud's relationship with Jung bore bitter fruit. They later parted ways [2]. Jung was welcomed into the Gentile world—and the Nazi regime. Psychologist M.H. Goering, cousin of Nazi Field Marshall Goering, appointed Jung as chair of the German Medical Committee for Psychotherapy after the Nazis ousted the Jewish chair and members [3]. Debates about Jung's alleged anti-Semitism, and his motivations for accepting this position, have raged for decades, as noted in Aryeh Maidenbaum's essay on "Jung and the Specter of Anti-Semiticism" [4].

While many Freudian ideas have lost their place of importance in American psychiatry, Freud's fear that psychoanalysis would be dubbed a "Jewish science" was eerily accurate, for that is how the Nazis described psychoanalysis before banning it altogether and burning Freud's books (and other supposedly subversive books). Bonfires were lit in 33 German towns and cities. Freud's ironic reaction to the book burning was also on-target, albeit not wholly correct. He wrote to Ernest Jones, "What progress we are making. In the Middle Ages, they would have burned me.

S. Packer (✉)
Mount Sinai Beth Israel, New York City, NY, USA
e-mail: drpacker@hotmail.com

© Springer Nature Switzerland AG 2020
H. S. Moffic et al. (eds.), *Anti-Semitism and Psychiatry*,
https://doi.org/10.1007/978-3-030-37745-8_7

Now they are content with burning my books." Freud did not know that three of his four sisters would be gassed and probably incinerated in concentration camps, although their exact fate is not fully known. A fourth sister reportedly died of disease en route to another camp. None were able to access funds Freud left for their escape from Europe [5].

Freud himself was reluctant to leave Austria, even though most psychoanalysts had already fled by the time the Nazis interrogated his daughter Anna in 1938, which finally prompted his departure for England. Many psychiatrists and psychoanalysts did not fare so well and perished in the Holocaust, or were interred in concentration camps, but some future psychiatrists and their families took flight in response to the impending Nazi terror. A few hundred analysts, some with international reputations, arrived as refugees in America, where they established or fortified analytic institutes, trained new analysts, and chaired prestigious American psychiatry departments, to the point that psychoanalytic ideas prevailed in American psychiatry for a full 40 years, until being displaced by biopsychiatry in the mid-1980s.

This essay will trace anti-Semitic attitudes toward Jewish physicians before Freud, followed by a brief account of the Reich's restrictions on Jewish doctors, psychoanalysts, and scientists, propelling many analysts (and even an anti-psychiatrist) to resettle in the Americas. We will add anecdotes about some émigré analysts and also acknowledge displaced medicinal chemists whose discoveries impacted American psychiatry. We will assess the help—or harm—from this mid-century influx of analysts and speculate about the trajectory that American psychiatry might have taken, had the Reich's anti-Semitism not forced analysts to flee and to find safe haven in America (and, sadly, to leave so many millions more behind).

Anti-Semitic Attitudes Toward Jewish Doctors in Europe Before Freud

Christian Europe viewed Jewish doctors as "different" from other healers long before Freud [6]. In medieval times, Church authorities forbade Christians from consulting Jewish healers, who were considered not only heretics but who also charged fees for services that were otherwise offered free via Christian charity at healing shrines. In spite of formal injunctions and added costs, Christians often called on Jewish doctors clandestinely, partly because they attributed special, even supernatural, abilities to Jewish doctors and partly because Jews did not link mental or medical illness to the Christian concept of Satan.

Folkloric ideas aside, Christian patients could expect more from medieval Jewish doctors because Jews could access several systems of medicine, even though all but a few Christian-European institutions (as opposed to Muslim-European institutions) banned Jews from studying at medicine institutions until Italian institutions admitted them in the 1700s.

Medieval Jewish physicians studied Hebrew translations of Greek and Islamic medical texts at a time when medical theories of Hippocrates and Galen, considered pagan, were forbidden to Christians. Although outdated, those sources were far superior to the supernatural texts permitted by the Church. Some Jewish doctors, notably Maimonides, who was born in Spain but worked in North Africa, were educated at Muslim medical schools. Others transmitted medical knowledge informally from father to son and, occasionally, to daughters. During the Enlightenment (1637–1800), Jewish doctors acquired medicinal herbs from the East via Jewish traders [7].

The Renaissance: Paracelsus the Alchemist and Jewish Alchemists

By the early Renaissance, sufficient numbers of Jews practiced medicine to provoke Paracelsus to undermine his competitors by claiming that Jews were not unique in their proficiency at medicine. Born in 1493, the contentious and coarse-mannered alchemist laid the foundations for modern medicine by introducing specific treatments for specific ailments.

European Jews in Christian countries (in contrast to Muslim-dominated regions) were rumored to dabble in the mystical and possibly demonic *Kabbalah*. That school of thought had long simmered beneath the surface of rabbinical Judaism but came to the fore in various locations at various times [8]. Writing about *The Jewish Alchemists*, Israeli-born anthropologist Raphael Patai notes that many late medieval and Renaissance alchemists were Jewish and many Jewish alchemists were practicing physicians. This association between occultism and alchemy, between Jews and occultism, and between Jewish physicians and *Kabbalah* cemented beliefs among the general public that Jewish physicians accessed esoteric information.

Sir Walter Scott saluted the connection between medieval Jewish magic, mysticism, and medicine in his nineteenth-century novel, *Ivanhoe* (1820), stating that "But the Jews, both male and female, possessed and practiced the medical science in all its branches, and the monarchs and powerful barons of the time frequently committed themselves to the charge of some experienced sage among the despised people, when wounded or in sickness. The aid of the Jewish physicians was not less eagerly sought after, though a general belief prevailed among the Christians, that the Jewish rabbis were deeply acquainted with the occult sciences, and particularly with the cabalistical art which had its name and origin in the studies of the sages of Israel" [9]. A female Jewish physician named Rebecca is cast in the role of heroine in *Ivanhoe*.

Freud's "Jewish National Affair" in Austria

Early on, Freud studied under the French neurologist Charcot in Paris and encountered Charcot's anti-Jewish ideas about Jewish tendencies toward "degeneration." In Catholic Vienna, Freud portrayed himself as an "outsider" [10] in spite of the social support from his local B'nai B'rith chapter (and from many Jewish Viennese doctors). Although half of Austrian medical professors were Jewish when Freud sought an academic appointment, he felt stymied by the religiously intolerant, politically regressive, Catholic-controlled Austria, especially since rudimentary "quotas" on Jews made it more difficult—but not impossible—to succeed.

Freud's concerns were not unrealistic, given that Vienna was the first European city to elect an overtly anti-Semitic government. When Karl Lueger became mayor in 1895, Lueger served as a prototype of anti-Semitic success for a still striving (but artistically unsuccessful) Austrian art student named Adolf Hitler. Hitler coined his most anti-Semitic stereotypes during his Viennese studies [11]. As a result, the failed artist succeeded in orchestrating the worst man-made catastrophe that the world has witnessed.

Freud and Other Physicians in Pre-Holocaust Germany and Austria

In 1933, when Americans were suffering through in the Great Depression, standing in breadlines, sometimes living in make-shift tent cities called "Hoovervilles" (named for then-President Herbert Hoover), the Germans voted for Hitler. In 1933, half of Germany's practicing physicians were Jewish or had hidden Jewish origins. Up to 40% of female German medical students were Jewish, for Jewish women flocked to medical schools once Germany admitted them [6, p. 235]. Austria had even more Jewish physicians than Germany. Then, in 1933, Jewish doctors were expelled from the German medical insurance program that subsidized medical care. With their economic opportunities severely restricted, many emigrated elsewhere, often to England.

Conditions progressively worsened for Jews. The 1933 boycotts of Jewish doctors, shops, lawyers, and stores were soon followed by the "Law for the Restoration of the Professional Civil Service," which banned Jews from government jobs. Books by Freud and Jewish anthropologist Franz Boas were set aflame in 1933.

After President Paul von Hindenburg's death in mid-1934, the powers of the Chancellor and President were combined, granting Hitler complete control. The 1935 Nuremberg Laws outlawed marriage between Jew and non-Jew. The "Reich Citizenship Law" stripped all Jews, even quarter- and half-Jews, of citizenship. Barred from voting, Jews could not officially oppose even harsher anti-Jewish laws that were being planned.

For instance, no new medical licenses were granted to Jews. In response, a substantial number of newly minted doctors committed suicide, knowing that they could not earn a living. In 1936, Jews were banned from all professional jobs. By the fall of 1938, only "Aryan" doctors could treat "Aryan" patients. Later in 1938, German laws prohibited Jewish doctors from practicing medicine altogether. The few hundred remaining Jewish doctors were demoted and all Jewish hospitals, save for one Jewish hospital in Berlin, were closed and their staff transported to ghettos or concentration camps [6, p. 264].

Since psychoanalysis initially attracted neurologists (as opposed to psychiatrists), those doctors faced the same restrictions as all other physicians, but most physicians had left before the worst restrictions on medical practice evolved. The psychoanalysts (who were not necessarily physicians) were among the first intellectuals to leave Europe, since they had been barred from practicing or teaching psychoanalysis as early as 1933 because the Nazis viewed psychoanalysis as a system of thought as much as a medical specialty [12]. A few left far earlier at Freud's bidding, intending to seed psychoanalytic societies elsewhere.

America's Introduction to Psychoanalysis

In the United States, Adolf Meyer was the most prominent American psychiatrist of his day. Meyer was Professor of Psychiatry at Johns Hopkins between 1910 and 1941. Originally a Kraepelinian who emphasized nosology, Meyer embraced nearly even new trend, from psychoanalysis to Dr. Cotton's peculiar concepts of "autointoxication" as a cause of psychosis.

America had been introduced to psychoanalysis through A.A. Brill's 1907 English translations of Freud's writings and via Freud's 1909 visit (with Jung and Ferenczi) to the United States. The psychoanalytic field gained a far firmer footing in America as émigré analysts arrived in major cities and established or reinvigorated psychoanalytic institutes. Many had international reputations before emigrating. Psychoanalysts such as Lawrence Kubie, M.D. (and many more), promised financial support for refugee analysts and secured hospital positions for the physicians, to comply with stringent immigration demands. Their presence familiarized hospital staff with psychoanalytic ideas. The Menninger Clinic in Topeka, Kansas, welcomed many displaced Jewish analysts, including Otto Kernberg, for Karl Menninger had studied with Freud. As practicing Protestants, they were well-poised to promote this exotic European import [13].

Psychoanalytic ideas infiltrated America through another less expected, non-academic route. Many Hollywood luminaries entered psychoanalysis via the reinvigorated Los Angeles Institute and Society for Psychoanalytic Studies. Major studios made movies that lionized psychoanalysts' miraculous, but hyperbolic, couch cures. A prime player at the L.A. Institute was an émigré psychoanalyst named Ernst Simmel, who made a name for himself for successfully treating World War I shell-shocked soldiers with a short course of hypnosis combined with psychoanalytic insights—even before he formally trained in psychoanalysis.

Analysts Who Survived the Camps (or Claimed They Did)

While many psychiatrists and psychoanalysts perished in the Holocaust, some future psychiatrists and their families took flight in response to the impending Nazi terror. A young Thomas Szasz, later known for his so-called (but incorrectly called) anti-psychiatry manifesto on *The Myth of Mental Illness* (1961), left Europe before his native Hungary was overrun by the Reich. Szasz's writings were enshrined by anti-psychiatry activists and self-described psychiatric survivors [14]. He transmuted his antipathy to fascism and the Nazified Europe he witnessed in his youth into his iconoclastic anti-psychiatry attitudes against the psychiatric diagnostic canon. Szasz continues to intrigue (and infuriate) psychiatrists to this day, having inspired Knoll's 2019 collection of essays, after impugning the morality of psychiatric treatment protocols [15]. Szasz opposed state-mandated treatments of mental illness, such as involuntary incarceration and forced medication, basing his ideas on ideology rather than direct clinical experience or up-to-date scientific data.

Szasz was so opposed to involuntary hospitalization that he refused to complete a psychiatry residency that mandated rotations in locked wards and instead trained at a program that treated only persons who were not psychotic enough to merit involuntary admission. He became a psychoanalyst who offered office-based treatment to patients. He maintained a professorship and mentored residents, even though he condemned the concept of mental illness, which young psychiatrists were training to treat. In yet another paradox, Szasz distanced himself from left of center "anti-psychiatrists" of the 1960s, reminding readers that he himself was a conservative libertarian and a registered Republican.

Viktor Frankl, M.D., a Viennese psychoanalyst who founded existential analysis (logotherapy) and authored the best-selling *Man's Search for Meaning* (1946) (and other books), did not escape the Nazis, but instead was incarcerated in concentration camps where he was forced to function as a physician. Frankl's book recounts his experiences as a camp doctor charged with treating typhus patients who died at the end of each day. He details the deaths of camp inmates who shriveled up and succumbed after they lost their wills to live. Paradoxically, he explains how his superficially meaningless work that did not change his patients' prognoses gave meaning to his own daily existence. Frankl's impact on contemporary psychiatry is limited, possibly because logotherapy is headquartered in Austin, Texas, far from New York City or other major cities with influential analytic institutes. Still, his authority as a psychiatric self-help author persists for the general public [16].

Bruno Bettelheim, Ph.D., was another self-described concentration camp survivor, but his concentration camp accounts have been disputed. He swayed psychiatry, psychology, and the public, having held a professorship in psychology and a high-ranking administrative post at the University of Chicago's Orthogenic School for Autistic Children. He was acclaimed (by some) as a child psychologist, even though he was not trained as a psychiatrist and there are no records of training as a psychologist. He claimed that his European psychology education records were lost during the war years. His credentials as a psychoanalyst are not disputed.

With a Ph.D. in aesthetics, Bettelheim was well-equipped to write a well-received book about the psychological symbolism of fairy tales, *The Uses of Enchantment* (1976). Bettelheim chronicled his own (probably factitious) concentration camp experiences in a widely cited 1943 paper on "Individual and Mass Behavior in Extreme Situations." That paper made him a de facto spokesman about human adaptability to the stresses of concentration camps. He was criticized for attributing ghetto-dwelling Jews' conscription into camps to their own passive attitudes. His pronouncements about children of the kibbutz, reared by the collective rather than by biological parents, found a receptive audience, although he based his conclusions in *Children of the Dream* (1967) on time-limited observations without an experimental design [17].

Perhaps most importantly, Bettelheim promoted now-debunked and much-maligned yet highly persuasive theories implicating "refrigerator mothers" for their children's autism. *The Empty Fortress* (1967), his book about autism, established him as an expert on what we now call ASD. However, most students did not meet criteria for ASD, either then or now.

Bettelheim's generation-shaping claims caused immeasurable suffering to mothers who were blamed for their children's neurologically based disorders. After his death by suicide, he stood accused of abusing children at the Orthogenic School. Many medical journals subsequently denounced his studies on autism.

The Exit of Analysts from Europe and Their Export to America

As stated earlier, some analysts left Europe early enough to emigrate to safer shores. Many—but not all—eschewed their Jewish identities or renounced their religious roots, possibly to react against the Nazi-imposed Jewish identities symbolized by the yellow star, possibly because they were already assimilated or simply not religious before the start of the war, and possibly in support of Freud's anti-religion attitude as articulated in *The Future of an Illusion* (1929). For a few, Zionism, Socialism, or Communism substituted for religion.

Franz Alexander had already relocated to Chicago in response to Freud's request. Alexander, a psychoanalyst and later an historian of psychiatry, founded the field of psychosomatic medicine. He was joined by analyst Therese Benedek, another proponent of psychosomatic medicine. Karen Horney, who countered Freud's emphasis on penis envy and founded feminist psychoanalysis in the process, accepted Franz Alexander's invitation to assist him in Chicago. Even though she was not Jewish, she was concerned about the rise of Nazism in Germany—and about her falling out with Freud. She left Germany in 1932, before Hitler's ascension, and opened the Horney Institute in her adopted American homeland.

Alfred Adler, also an Austrian and the founder of "individual psychology," had hoped to spread socialism via psychoanalysis. Adler was a colleague of Freud rather than a disciple. Burdened by bone deformities from childhood rickets, Adler emphasized the "inferiority complex" as the driver of personality and the propeller of achievement. Alder was born Jewish but converted to Christianity. Still, the Nazis closed his 22 child guidance clinics because he belonged to the "Jewish race" (which overshadowed religion). Without professional opportunities in Austria, Adler accepted a professorship at the Long Island College of Medicine, but died in 1937, before Kristallnacht. Adler lectured widely and attracted sincere followers as well as cultlike devotees, some of whom developed very unusual practices.

Erik Erikson was the son of a Jewish mother and an unnamed Danish man. Erikson lacked formal education in psychology but earned a diploma in psychoanalysis in Vienna. He introduced the term "identity crisis," identified eight stages of psychosocial development, and established his own brand of "Eriksonian psychology" that emphasized adolescence. After leading a peripatetic artist's life, he ultimately earned a Pulitzer Prize. At school in Denmark, due to his Nordic appearance, Erikson was teased by Jews but was bullied by Nordics because of his Jewish heritage. Erikson headed to America early on and taught at Harvard for decades.

Other psychoanalysts who moved to America included Otto Rank, Sandor Ferenczi, Felix and Helen Deutsch, Rene Spitz, Heinz Hartmann, Fritz Redl, Erich Fromm, Wilhelm Reich, Frieda Fromm-Reichmann, Margaret Mahler, Heinz Kohut, David Rapaport, Edith Weigert, Otto Fenichel, Theodor Reik, Siegfried Bernfeld, Hans Sachs (an attorney by training), Sandor Rado (who was instrumental in forming the Columbia University Center for Psychoanalytic Training and Research), Ernst Kris (an art historian whose attempts to enter medical school were thwarted by Nazi law), and Kurt Eissler (a devoted Freudian and Goethe scholar who maintained the Freud Archives). Psychoanalyst and pediatrician Hilde Bruch, famed for her early studies of eating disorders, initially emigrated to England, where she practiced pediatrics before accepting a professorship in the United States.

Virtually the entire staff of the Berlin Psychoanalytic Institute relocated to New York, thanks to the intervention of the New York Psychoanalytic Society. Other analysts made their way to Chicago, Boston, Los Angeles, or Buenos Aires. In Vienna, the Psychoanalytic Society shriveled from 69 members in 1935 to 3 in 1945. Laura Fermi estimated that 190 European psychoanalysts emigrated to the United States in response to Hitler, whereas historian of psychiatry Edward Shorter identified about 250 analysts. When the war ended, the United States had more psychoanalysts than the rest of the world combined.

Several analysts mentioned above deserve extra discussion because they wielded disproportionate influence on psychiatric theory or practice or on the public's perception of psychiatry. Theodor Reik was a lay analyst whose 50-plus books and articles covered literary and musical figures, masochism, and Christian martyrs, plus several Jewish-specific topics, including "Kol Nidrei" and "The Shofar," *Jewish Wit* (1962), and *Pagan Rites in Judaism* (1964).

Otto Rank, Ph.D., did not hold an M.D. but was a high-ranking member of Freud's inner circle. Rank left Europe after the passage of the Nuremberg Laws but died in 1939, before the death camps came into being. Rank's name is often linked to his 1929 theories about "birth trauma," but his most enduring impact stemmed from his *The Myth of the Birth of the Hero: A Psychological Exploration of Myth* (1909) and, secondarily, through *Art and Artist* (1932). Rank's research on hero myths was co-opted by Joseph Campbell, who credited Rank in a barely visible footnote on the first page of Campbell's multi-volume *The Hero with a Thousand Faces* (1948). Campbell received recognition for Rank's pioneering research after appearing in a 1988 PBS television documentary about myth.

The legacy of Wilhelm Reich, M.D., revolved around his controversial claims about his "orgone machine" as well as "political psychiatry." Reich's book on *The Mass Psychology of Fascism* (1938) [18] references his European experiences. It inspired 1960s' student radicals who threw books at the Parisian police. Reich invented the term "sexual revolution" but his persistent marketing of his "orgone box," which he claimed could transfer biological energy that others called "God," led to fraud charges and incarceration. His practice of massaging undressed patients invited the ire of the medical, psychoanalytic, and judicial establishments. He lost his license to practice and his personal freedom, but he left his mark on the turbulent 1960s before dying in prison. Discussants at Weill Cornell History of Psychiatry seminars attributed his erratic and sexually preoccupied behavior to undiagnosed and untreated bipolar disorder (S. Packer, personal account from History of Psychiatry seminars).

Social psychologist, philosopher, and psychoanalyst Erich Fromm was born into an Orthodox Jewish family, descendants of a long line of rabbis. His tome on *Escape from Freedom* (1941) attempted to explain why the authoritarian personality epitomized by Hitler appealed to otherwise rational people. This study emphasizes his reactions to the Nazi regime, although World War I, rather than World War II, powerfully impacted his point of view. Fromm's book about *The Art of Loving* (1956) brought fame, while his social and political psychology studies won academicians' admiration. *You Shall Be as Gods: A Radical Interpretation of the Old Testament and Its Tradition* (1966) looks back to his Jewish background, while his collaborative books about *Zen Buddhism and Psychoanalysis* (1960) foreshadowed Americans' infatuation with Eastern meditation techniques. Frieda Reichmann, another refugee from the Reich, introduced him to psychoanalysis. Eleven years his senior, she had been his psychoanalyst and subsequently became his wife (and then his ex-wife).

Frieda Fromm-Reichmann, M.D., left a semi-permanent mark on American psychiatry by introducing the concept of the schizophrenogenic mother. Her friend Gershom Scholem, the German-born librarian-turned-academician who single-handedly turned Jewish mysticism into a subject of serious study, praised Reichmann's Heidelberg-based "Torah-peutics" which combined Torah teachings with psychotherapy sessions. Her then-husband Erich Fromm collaborated, but both eventually abandoned orthodoxy and embraced socialism instead [19].

She also appears in a highly romanticized, autobiographical account of a young woman's lengthy stay at Chestnut Lodge, a onetime psychoanalytic stronghold which has since closed. *I Never Promised You a Rose Garden* (1964) was the creation of the pseudonymous author Hannah Green, who later revealed her name as Joanne Greenberg. After the memoir landed in high school and college curricula, the book became a best-seller and then a film. Greenberg/Green later enjoyed a successful career as a children's book author.

Greenberg's story-telling skills convinced the book-buying public that talk therapy alone could cure the florid hallucinations and delusions of schizophrenia, although many have questioned whether the author suffered from what is today considered as schizophrenia. Greenberg's book arrived around the same time as the emerging anti-psychiatry movement. "Dr. Fried," portrayed as an ever-patient analyst who valorized every word spoken by her distraught patient, reified the era's *zeitgeist* [20].

Helene Deutsch, M.D., a Polish-Jewish psychoanalyst, coined the concept of the "as if" borderline personality. Her 1944 publication fortified sexist ideas of the

1950s but clashed with the ethos of feminist movement that emerged in the late 1960s. Deutsch's *The Psychology of Women* was hailed as the first analytic study devoted to women, but later denounced by Susan Brownmiller, author of the 1975 feminist treatise, *Against Our Will: Men, Women and Rape*. Reacting to Deutsch's claim that masochism, narcissism, and passivity permeate the female character, Brownmiller called Deutsch both a "pioneer" and a "traitor" [21].

Empirically based discoveries of displaced Austrian-Jewish psychoanalyst and child psychiatrist, Rene Spitz, M.D., endure. In the 1940s, Dr. Spitz identified "marasmus" and "anaclitic depression" in hospitalized infants deprived of their mothers. He linked their early deaths to social isolation and lack of stimulation. Interest in infant development in per-term infants and the emotional impact of children's protracted hospitalization soared in response to his studies.

The Hungarian-Jewish Margaret Mahler, M.D., was another luminary in the field of child development. A relatively late refugee who left after the Anschluss in 1938, Mahler forged the term "separation-individuation." Never an observant Jew, Mahler's Jewish identity was shaped by her mother's death during the Holocaust and by the anti-Semitism experienced during her youth. According to the Jewish Women's Archives (www.jwa.org), Dr. Mahler's last wish "was that her ashes … be interred in the Jewish cemetery in Sopron [Hungary]…".

Experiences of Otto Kernberg, M.D., in Nazi-controlled Austria, with first-hand views of Kristallnacht, shaped his views of ego psychology and the fragmentation of the self, as displayed in borderline personality disorder. In interviews with Emily Kuriloff, Kernberg imputes his psychoanalytic theories to his out-of-the-way training in Chile and his Midwestern "exile" at the Menninger Institute in Kansas, where he was free to create his own concepts, undeterred by psychoanalytic hard-liners who dominated major North American institutes [22].

As an analyst with interests in personality disorders, like Kernberg, Heinz Kohut, M.D. recognizes the influences of his pre- and post-Reich life on his concepts of "self-psychology," stating that "I've led two totally different, perhaps unbridgeable lives," leading him to identify the "fragmented self" in borderline personalities [22, p. 2]. In contrast to Kernberg, who celebrates his Jewish heritage, Kohut's historian-son confirmed that Kohut concealed his Jewish background and that their German-born family worshiped *Werther* and German Kultur.

A contemporary psychiatrist, E. Fuller Torrey, M.D., who is well-known as a passionate advocate for the seriously mentally ill, recounts the travels and travails of displaced analysts in his book about *Freudian Fraud: The Malignant Effect of Freud's Theory on American Thought and Culture* (1992). The book's subtitle sums up his opposition to Freudian ideas that distanced psychiatry from biological basics. Torrey blames both East Coast intellectuals and Hollywood moguls for spreading the false "Freudian faith" across America and diverting attention from the seriously mentally ill and the biological basis of their distress. He attributes psychoanalysis' overblown status in America to the flood of refugee analysts from Nazi-run Europe but credits the film industry for public perceptions of the "couch cure."

Influence of the Holocaust on Biological Psychiatry

Without disputing Torrey's assertion that Nazified Europe (and the Shoah and anti-Semitism, by implication) led to an exodus of psychoanalysts coming to America, who in turn influenced American psychiatry and society overall and prioritized office-based private practices that treated "problems" rather than "symptoms," in lieu of for the sometimes hospitalized seriously mentally ill, we should also note that some European Jewish émigrés paved new paths in the study of child development, apart from strict psychoanalytic theory.

Moreover, anti-Semitism and the Shoah influenced biological psychiatry's trajectory. Medicinal chemist Leo Sternbach developed the best-selling benzodiazepines, Librium and Valium, but transferred patent rights to his employer, pharmaceutical giant, Hoffman-La Roche, which in turn transferred Sternbach to America, far from Nazified Europe, where his life was threatened. The benzodiazepines have been both revered and reviled. They remain essential to detoxification regimens and are used for conscious sedation during surgical procedures, quelling acute psychotic agitation, or as rescue treatments for panic disorder.

A year earlier, a displaced physician and researcher named Frank Berger, M.D., inadvertently developed meprobamate, marketed as Miltown or Equanil, which became the most sought-after medication of its day. Psychiatrist and neurophysiologist Manfred Sakel, M.D., similarly fled the Nazis in 1936, after presenting his findings on insulin coma therapy (ICT) for treating schizophrenia. Dr. Sakel continued his research at Harlem Valley State Hospital. Sakel's ICT was eventually eclipsed by comparatively safer ECT and finally by phenothiazines, which were introduced to America in 1954, but his ICT treatment remained popular through the 1950s and is featured in *A Beautiful Mind* (2001), a film about a brilliant (but anti-Semitic) mathematician named John Nash, who suffered from schizophrenia.

A more tangential by-product of European anti-Semitism is the case of chemist Raphael Mechoulam, Ph.D., who isolated endogenous cannabinoids and phytocannabinoids while at Israel's Weizmann Institute of Science. The role of exogenous cannabis in the induction of psychosis (and in the possible relief of symptoms of autism, serious neurological disorders, or pain syndromes) is being studied and is gaining interest in America, where cannabis is marketed as medical marijuana. Born to a Bulgarian physician who was temporarily interred in a concentration camp, Raphael Mechoulam and family found safe haven in Israel, where he learned laboratory and research skills during mandated service in the Israeli army (IDF).

Franz Josef Kallmann, M.D., the German-born psychiatrist whose otherwise exemplary twin studies on the inheritability of mental illness were used to promote Nazi-era racial hygiene policies, also immigrated to the United States in response to the Nazis—for different reasons. Kallmann was not reared in the Jewish religion—his Jewish-born father had converted to Christianity—but he was removed from his academic position because the Reich viewed Jews as a "race."

Perhaps the most impressive example of Holocaust-stimulated neuropsychiatry discoveries is Nobel Laureate Eric Kandel, M.D. The Viennese-born Dr. Kandel dates his interest in memory's role in PTSD to his personal recollections of Kristallnacht, the "Night of Broken Glass," which marks, for some, the start of the Holocaust. Unlike many Jewish-born psychoanalysts who renounced their Jewish identities or distanced themselves from their Jewish religion, Dr. Kandel emphasizes his Yeshiva education in Brooklyn and his Jewish roots in Vienna. In his Nobel Prize acceptance speech, Dr. Kandel notes that "Even prior to the Anschluss in 1938, anti-Semitism was a chronic feature of Viennese life." "This viciousness … culminated in the horrors of Kristallnacht…." "… the experiences of my last year in Vienna helped to determine my later interests in the mind, in how people behave, the unpredictability of motivation, and the persistence of memory" [23].

Pendulum Swings After World War II and into 1980s America

Aside from the popularity of tranquilizers such as Librium and Valium, Equanil, or Miltown, America's appreciation of neurogenetics and biological psychiatry was upended partly because the Shoah made concepts of the inheritability of mental illness and intergenerational transmission of "degeneration" unpalatable to Americans and partly because of respected muck-raking journalists such as Albert Deutsch, who wrote *The Shame of the States* (1947) (and earlier versions). Deutsch toured the "shameful" state hospitals, comparing them to concentration camps and Dante's Inferno. Memoirists such as Mary Jane Ward, whose book about *The Snake Pit* became an iconic film in 1948, also swayed public opinion. *Suddenly, Last Summer* (1959), loosely based on Tennessee Williams' sister's lobotomy, added to a turn toward psychological explanations of mental illnesses as it reminded Americans of needless lobotomies in the 1950s America. The Nuremberg Trials, broadcast on TV, showcased the horrors of the Holocaust, and Stanley Kramer's Academy Award-winning, all-star film, *Judgment at Nuremberg* (1961), pushed American sentiment even further away from anything related to Nazis' emphasis on racial purity, eugenics, and "degeneration" [24].

Historian Edward Shorter's subchapter on "Psychoanalysis and the American Jews" suggests that psychoanalysis acquired nearly totemic meaning to Jews after the war, so that Jewish doctors who had previously opposed psychoanalysis (and there were many) withheld their critiques, out of respect for the suffering of their co-religionists and to avoid inflicting further misery [25]. Undeterred by those detractors, psychoanalysis supplanted neuropsychiatry and neurogenetics.

In the mid-1980s, a paradigm shift occurred, largely in response to a landmark lawsuit against Chestnut Lodge, the fabled psychoanalytic bastion featured in *I Never Promised You a Rose Garden*. Biological psychiatry had been simmering beneath the surface and was still available via electro- or insulin shock, psychosurgery, or the once-miraculous but later maligned "neuroleptics," as well as side effect-ridden (and occasionally lethal) early antidepressants. Then a depressed nephrologist named Raphael Osheroff successfully sued the Lodge for failing to prescribe appropriate psychopharmacological treatment and continuing to treat him, unsuccessfully, for months on end, with psychoanalytically oriented therapy [26].

After his mother arranged his transfer to another facility, Dr. Osheroff received antidepressant medications that relieved his symptoms within weeks. In the interim, Dr. Osheroff had lost his medical practice, his many dialysis centers, and contact with his sons, which reportedly pained him more than anything else. The two sides settled, and a precedent was set. The pendulum began to sway. Experimental results (scientific evidence) overruled opinions of theorists.

As the century ended, and the new millennium began, psychoanalyst-turned-neuroscience researcher Eric Kandel shared the 2000 Nobel Prize in Physiology or Medicine for discoveries about ways that neurons encode memories. Kandel's personal transition from psychoanalysis to laboratory science mirrors the shift in psychiatric sentiments. A year earlier, Dr. Kandel had summarized his personal sentiments in his paper about "Biology and the Future of Psychoanalysis," published by the *American Journal of Psychiatry* in 1999 [27]. Dr. Kandel reminds us that Freud himself predicted that "all of [our] provisional ideas in psychology will presumably one day be based on an organic substructure," so that biopsychiatry will supplant psychoanalysis.

Dr. Kandel proceeds to recommend ways to revitalize psychoanalysis through the introduction of contemporary scientific methodology, complete with experimental designs that confirm (or refute) analytic theories and treatments. Even more boldly, he suggests the equivalent of a "Flexner Report for the Psychoanalytic Institutes," to evaluate extant training institutes with the same rigor applied by physician Abraham Flexner, who scrutinized American medical schools for his Flexner Report. That 1910 report led to the closure of many inadequate institutions—and to the establishment of medical education and practice standards.

Conclusion

Activist-psychiatrist E. Fuller Torrey attributes American acceptance of psychoanalysis to the forced emigration of analysts out of Europe and into America. That conclusion is largely correct, in this author's opinion, save for the few caveats mentioned above. Indeed, the "psychoanalytic reign" in mid-century America and until the last quarter for the twentieth century directed attention onto relatively healthy persons with "problems of living," rather than the most seriously mentally ill. In fact, sometimes psychoanalytic treatments were used for psychosis, with little impact, just as Freud predicted. Concepts such as "refrigerator mothers" (accused of inducing autism) or schizophrenogenic mothers (blamed for schizophrenia), introduced by analysts, harmed both patients and parents and distracted researchers away from biological contributors to (or better cures for) such illnesses. We can only wonder how many opportunities to advance the treatment or understand the origins of serious mentally illness were missed because of this misplaced emphasis on orthodox psychoanalysis.

Admittedly, discoveries such as Prozac, which popularized psychopharmacology in the later 1980s, largely targeted the not-so-seriously ill (as was true for psychoanalysis) and offered little benefit to persons struggling with schizophrenia or autistic spectrum disorder.

While contemporary America's approach to serious mental illness is far removed from the Nazi's horrific Operation T-4, which murdered 200,000 mentally and physically challenged persons until the Nazis suspended their project in response to protests by Protestant clergy (and subsequently re-appropriated those gas chambers for their "final solution" to annihilate Jews and Gypsies), much remains to be done for the persons who need the most. Delays in identifying the causes, and advancing the care, of the most seriously mentally ill can be construed as yet another casualty, albeit a circuitous one, of anti-Semitism and the Shoah.

References

1. Gay P. A godless Jew: Freud, atheism, and the making of psychoanalysis. New Haven: Yale University Press; 1989.
2. McGuire W (ed.). Freud-Jung letters: the correspondence between Sigmund Freud and C.G. Jung. Princeton: Princeton University Press, 1974.
3. Maidenbaum A. Carl Jung and the specter of anti-Semitism. In: Anti-Semitism & psychiatry, in production; Maidenbaum A, editor. Jung and the shadow of anti-Semitism. Boston: Shambala Publications; 1991.
4. Cocks G. Psychotherapy in the Third Reich. New York: Oxford University Press; 1985.
5. Freud S. Letter to Ernest Jones (1933), as quoted in The Columbia dictionary of quotations by Robert Andrews; 1993. p. 779.
6. Efron J. Medicine and the German Jews: a history. New Haven: Yale University Press; 2001.
7. Ruderman D. Jewish thought and scientific discovery in early modern Europe. New Haven: Yale University Press; 1995.
8. Packer S. Jewish mystical movements and the European ergot epidemics. Isr J Psychiatr. 1998;35:3.
9. Scott W. Ivanhoe. New York: Pocket Library; 1959, as quoted in Efron J. Medicine and the German Jews: a history. New Haven: Yale University Press; 2001.
10. Richards AD. The Jewish world of Sigmund Freud. Essays on the cultural roots and the problem of religious identity. McFarland: Jefferson; 2010.
11. Beller S. Vienna and the Jews 1867–1938: a cultural history. Cambridge: Cambridge University Press; 1989.
12. Kurtzweil E. Freud's reception in the United States. In: Roth MS, editor. Freud: conflict and culture. New York: Vintage Books; 1998. p. 127–39.
13. Friedman LJ. Menninger: the family and the clinic. Topeka: University of Kansas; 1992.
14. Whitaker R. Mad in America: bad science, bad medicine, and the enduring mistreatment of the mentally ill. New York: Perseus Books Group; 2001; Mad in America: science, psychiatry and social justice. www.madinamerica.com. Accessed 7 July 2019.
15. Knoll JL, Haldipur CV, Luft VC. Thomas Szasz: an appraisal of his legacy. Oxford: Oxford University Press; 2019.
16. Batthyany A, editor. Logotherapy and existential analysis: proceedings of the Viktor Frankl Institute, vol. I. Cham: Springer International AG; 2016.
17. Packer S. Book Review: *Bettelheim* by Nina Sutton. Jewish Book Review, 1996; Sutton N. Bettelheim: a life and a legacy. New York: Basic Books; 1996.
18. Reich W. The mass psychology of fascism. Trans. Vincent R. Carfango. New York: Farrar, Strauss & Giroux; 1970.
19. Hornstein GA. To redeem one person is to redeem the world: the life of Frieda Fromm-Reichmann. New York: The Free Press; 2000.

20. Green DB. This day in Jewish history 1957: real-life basis for "Rose Garden" psychiatrist dies. Haaretz, April 27, 2016. https://www.haaretz.com/amp/jewish/.premium-1957-real-life-basis-for-rose-garden-psychiatrist-dies-1.5376578. Accessed 25 July 2019.
21. Brownmiller S. Against our will: men, women and rape. New York: Simon & Schuster; 1975, requoted in Jewish Women's Archive, jwi.org.
22. Kuriloff EA. Contemporary psychoanalysis and the legacy of the Third Reich: history, memory, tradition. New Jersey: Routledge; 2013. p. 63–6.
23. www.nobelprize.org.
24. Packer S. Cinema's sinister psychiatrists. McFarland: Jefferson; 2012.
25. Shorter E. A history of psychiatry. New York: Wiley; 1997. p. 181–9.
26. Packer S. Raphael Osheroff, MD: a belated obituary. Psychiatric Times, June 28, 2013. http://www.psychiatrictimes.com/blogs/couch-crisis/belated-obituary-raphael-j-osheroff-md.
27. Kandel E. Biology and the future of psychoanalysis: a new intellectual framework for psychiatry revisited. Am J Psychiatr. 1999;156:505–24.

Part II

Psychiatric Implications of Anti-semitism

Internalized Anti-Semitism: A Painful Consequence of Assimilation

My Personal Story of a Jewish Identity Lost and Found

John S. Tamerin

When Steve Moffic invited me to contribute a chapter to this book, I had just experienced my one and only episode of overt anti-Semitism in 50 years of clinical practice. It came in the form of a vitriolic email from a man who attended a single meeting of a pro bono support group I had facilitated for 20 years for people with depression and/or bipolar disorder. Fifty years ago, when I was 30, I might have felt threatened or embarrassed and perhaps would have even taken his comments personally since my identity as a Jew at that time was ambivalent and insecure. In contrast, now at 81, I was not disturbed but merely experienced his ugly anti-Semitism as a manifestation of the helpless rage of a deeply disturbed individual. What follows is a narrative of my journey as a Jew from an identity once lost to one rediscovered.

I was born on September 16, 1937, at the Park East Hospital on the Upper East Side of Manhattan. I came to my first home on Riverside Drive and 78th Street, a lovely apartment overlooking Riverside Park and the Hudson River.

My grandparents had come to the United States from Russia as children and ultimately settled in Hudson, New York, where both of my parents were born. None of my grandparents attended college. My mother's father started a small department store and moved gradually into the middle class. My father's father had a modest store selling stoves but devoted most of his time to studying the Torah.

Both of my parents went on to college as the first members of their families to go beyond high school. My mother went to the New Jersey College for Women later named Douglass College in honor of its founder and dean, Mabel Smith Douglass. It subsequently became part of Rutgers University.

For the purposes of this essay which is an exploration of anti-Semitism and my personal Jewish odyssey, I believe it is essential to relate a story which occurred to my mother a couple of years after she arrived at college. Her name was Gertrude Rabinowitz. She was a small woman with a large personality and considerable

J. S. Tamerin (✉)
Weill Cornell School of Medicine, New York, NY, USA
e-mail: jtamerin@optonline.net

© Springer Nature Switzerland AG 2020

H. S. Moffic et al. (eds.), *Anti-Semitism and Psychiatry*,
https://doi.org/10.1007/978-3-030-37745-8_8

101

musical talent and was receiving a good deal of attention on campus. As a young girl she had played the piano at silent movies in the Hudson movie theater to earn extra money. As my mother related the story to me, she was in late adolescence – perhaps 18–19 years old having skipped a year or two in high school – and she was summoned to the dean's office one day where she was chastised by Dean Douglass with the following words: "We don't want anyone with a name like Rabinowitz being so visible on our campus." Quite a shock for a young girl from Hudson, New York.

This experience was indelibly etched into my mother's psyche and ultimately into mine. I guess the message to her and then from her to me was that being too visibly Jewish could be dangerous not to one's life (as had become evident in Europe) but rather as to how one was perceived and perception became all important to my parents and then ultimately to me.

I should add that these memories will never disappear though so many other events, activities, and interactions that happened to my parents and/or to me have been easily forgotten.

My father, who came from a very modest home, graduated from high school two years early and at barely 16 came by himself to New York City to attend New York University. Needing to support himself, he tutored boys for their Bar Mitzvahs. He was an outstanding student and, rather amazingly, was accepted into Cornell Medical School, well-known at that time for its anti-Semitic bias. He graduated near the top of his class and was a member of Alpha Omega Alpha, the medical honor society for distinguished graduates.

My father's last name at that time was Tamarin. It was a Russian name and the accent was on the second *a*. My father decided to "smooth" it out and Aryanize his last name by changing it to Tamerin. Both of my parents died in their early 60s almost 50 years ago and are buried in Hudson, New York, next to their parents and my grandparents. It is somewhat amusing, yet revealing, to see all the other relatives named Tamarin (including my father's brother) buried next to my father whose name had become Joseph Arthur Tamerin, with an e.

This was the American way and clearly my parents' mantra was to assimilate, fit in, merge, leave your background behind, get ahead, and be successful. My father did precisely that. He went on to become a highly sought-after plastic and reconstructive surgeon straightening the noses of many wealthy Jewish women and face-lifting many entertainers and movie stars.

It should be noted that in addition to operating on these celebrities, he also fixed the noses of my mother, her two sisters, his brother, my sister, and myself. I was never clear as to whether this was merely to make us presumably "more attractive" or to assist us in appearing less Jewish or both (perhaps the motive was one and the same), but this was almost taken for granted as part of "getting ahead." It should be stated that I bought into this perspective hook, line, and sinker and never felt that I was losing anything in virtually abandoning my Jewish identity or part of my nose.

In retrospect, neither my parents nor I had any awareness of the sacrifice I was making since I placed no value at that time in being a Jew. I neither lied nor pretended to be another religion, but I never felt any pride in that aspect of my identity.

It was easy and relatively comfortable to be an upper-middle-class Jew in New York, but though safe, I never derived any satisfaction, meaning, purpose, or pleasure from being Jewish or from appearing to be Jewish.

To provide some broader historical perspective: in 1937, the year I was born, German authorities stepped up legislative persecution of Jews. The government set out to impoverish Jews and forbade Jewish doctors to treat non-Jews and revoked the licenses of Jewish lawyers to practice law.

Following the Kristallnacht pogrom (commonly known as "Night of Broken Glass") of November 9–10, 1938, Nazi leaders stepped up Aryanization efforts and enforced measures that succeeded increasingly in physically isolating and segregating Jews from their fellow Germans. Jews were barred from all public schools and universities, as well as from cinemas, theaters, and sports facilities.

In stark contrast, here in New York, after being briefly enrolled in the local public school, I transferred to the Hunter College Elementary School, a school for "gifted" students who were accepted on the basis of their IQ tests. I attended Hunter from grades 1 through 6. Of interest was the fact that in those days, the overwhelming majority of my class was Jewish. It was said that it was harder to get into this elementary school than into an Ivy League college. Indeed, most of my classmates went on to Ivy League colleges and then many became physicians and lawyers. Supreme Court Justice Elena Kagan attended Hunter Elementary along with many other distinguished graduates who became prominent scientists, inventors, and politicians.

All of this might have been possible in Germany between 1918 and 1933 during the Weimar Republic as Jews were achieving unimaginable heights, but, of course, it all changed as the undercurrent of anti-Semitism grew into the "Jew hatred" that fueled the flames of the Nazi movement eventuating in the Holocaust.

Meanwhile, except for occasional air raid drills, I was living a very safe and comfortable life on the Upper West Side of Manhattan attending Hunter College Elementary School. One of the amusing memories of those years was the image of one of my few non-Jewish classmates complaining that it seemed unfair to the Christian children in our class that the Jews had more holidays off.

The only memory of anti-Semitism I remember from my childhood occurred when I was around 8 years old.

Though it was nothing compared with what an 8-year-old Jewish child experienced in Europe, I still remember it with considerable pain and chagrin. My parents had a summer home on a lake in the area of Peekskill, New York, and there was still farmland up the road. My mother encouraged me to play with the neighborhood kids who lived on that farm. I still remember their name (De Maria) though I have probably forgotten everything I learned in elementary school. Perhaps this is because pain unresolved does not disappear but remains somewhere hanging heavily in the depths of the psyche and lasts a lifetime. The episode in simple terms was as follows. Four of these kids, who were older and larger than I was, picked me up and held me over a pile of horse manure on the farm and asked if I was Jewish. They said that if I was, they would push my face into the horse manure. I still remember my answer with some degree of shame. I said, "I don't know." As a consequence, they let me go. I had at least the integrity not to lie but lacked the courage to be fully honest.

Of course, I knew that I was a Jew but certainly not an observant Jew nor a proud Jew, simply a Jew by accident of birth. It is now 73 years later and if four men offered me the same choice today, I would not be able to plead ignorance. I have gradually reached the point where I can proudly say, "Yes, I am Jewish" and I hope with the heartfelt dignity of a Daniel Pearl who said before being beheaded, "My father's Jewish, my mother's Jewish, I'm Jewish."

At 81, I know I am a Jew and that it is a core aspect of who I am. I have gradually over many years and many experiences gained the deep sense of certainty, the courage, and the total acceptance to comfortably and non-defensively declare this aspect of my identity regardless of consequences. I remember the words of the distinguished Professor Simon Herman of Hebrew University who said 30 years ago at a seminar I attended at Yad Vashem on the subject of anti-Semitism, "The question historically in the mind of every Jew when he encounters a non-Jew is "Do they know I am Jewish?" And if they know, do they care?" What I feel should also be added when the issue is one of social acceptance, not life or death, is will their opinion affect my view of myself or my inner sense of security in the situation?

Sadly, my internal experience was even worse. I felt ashamed of being a Jew and wished that I had been born an upper-class WASP. This was an issue for many years. It is no longer a problem. I should add that this is a challenge for anyone who may be different than the presumably desired "norm." The challenge for anyone who is different or "other" is am I comfortable in my own skin? Clearly for many years I was not! I think the answer to this question depends on whether one's identity is solid and internally based or whether and to what extent it depends on how each of us believes we are perceived by others in any situation. For many years I projected my negative view of myself as a Jew onto others assuming that this would lead them to reject me or at the very least think less of me.

In years past, that was always my Achilles heel – being overly concerned with how I was perceived by "others." Given my parents' social ambition and concern with social acceptance, perhaps my concern was both neurotic and predictable.

Yet, as I grew older I often longed for the certainty, the commitment, and the courage of the great Rabbi Akiva who was executed by the Romans on the eve of Yom Kippur in the city of Caesarea where even today one can see the ruins of the Hippodrome where the Romans executed people publicly.

Even as they tortured him to death, he recited the final words and proclamation of faith, "Hear, O Israel, The Lord is our God; The Lord is one." "All my life," Akiva is reported to have said to his students, "I waited for the opportunity to show how much I love God, and now that I have the opportunity, should I waste it?"

Perhaps it would have been far easier for me to have proudly accepted my Judaism, despite my parents' march in the opposite direction, had I ever really believed in God!

When I finished sixth grade it was time to go to secondary school. I just took it for granted that I would be going to private school along with many of my friends from Hunter. The school of choice for bright Jewish boys whose parents could afford the tuition was Horace Mann. There was still a distinction at that time between the Jewish and non-Jewish private schools in New York.

The non-Jewish, church-affiliated schools such as Collegiate and Trinity were off limits for most Jews except those very wealthy or very well connected. But for those few Jews who attended these schools, the experience was not necessarily friendly. I recall an incident involving the son of friends of my parents who attended Trinity as one of the only Jews in his class. He made a presentation to the class after which the teacher told him to give it again "and this time don't use your hands like a Jew!"

Stories like that were repeated many times by my mother. This further diminished my comfort with being openly Jewish in non-Jewish settings. It further reinforced my discomfort with being a Jew and being seen as a Jew.

Those memories were painful because although I was comfortable at Horace Mann, I realized that Jews were not necessarily welcome in the larger, more elite community even in New York. Some of my friends who went on to boarding schools similarly encountered experiences of anti-Semitism. Of course, none of this compared with what had been going on in Europe during Hitler's regime. My problem was less about what anti-Semitism did to me externally but the harm that it created internally in terms of my perception of myself.

In understanding the impact of cultural anti-Semitism and my parents' striving for assimilation, I must say a word about my Bar Mitzvah.

Although my parents were moving further and further away from Judaism with the exception of the almost mandatory synagogue attendance on the High Holidays of Rosh Hashanah and Yom Kippur, my father wanted me to have a Bar Mitzvah at the time of my 13th birthday. By then we had left the Orthodox Spanish and Portuguese Synagogue and joined the reform Mount Neboh Synagogue. My Hebrew was limited but sufficient to the minimal requirements of Mount Neboh. For some reason I remember that I was proud that at least I read my portion from Hebrew and not from the English phonetics as had most of my friends.

What was very revealing about the direction of my parents' evolving values was that my mother wanted my Bar Mitzvah to be the first ever to be held at the *Maisonette* room of the very fashionable and prestigious St. Regis Hotel. Furthermore, when I requested that the band be Mark Towers, a band I had heard at a friend's Bar Mitzvah, I have never forgotten my mother's comment although it was made almost 70 years ago, "I don't want Mark Towers. He is too Jewish. I want Bill Harrington," a society band that played at many WASP debutante parties. Bill Harrington it was, and I never objected. In retrospect, I wish I had. That would have been a step toward self-acceptance.

As I moved into my teenage years, my parents moved to Park Avenue which was evidence that they had "arrived." I was attending dancing classes and encouraged to move in the "right" social circles and date "the right girls" which meant easing into what has become known as "Our Crowd" as described in the book of that title by Stephen Birmingham. The book told the stories of New York's upper-class Jewish families and their rise to prominence, wealth, and power.

Then it was time for college and my two favorite choices were Harvard and Princeton. Princeton was more attractive but I had a rude awakening when I visited and was told by a recent Horace Mann graduate, now at Princeton, that I would not be happy there as a Jew and suggested that I go to Harvard which is what I did in 1955.

Of course, at that time no Jew could possibly be a president of an Ivy League college. It is rather amazing in the many years since I graduated that not only has the president of Harvard been a Jew but even the president of Princeton from 1988 to 2000, Harold T. Shapiro, is a Jew.

Perhaps closer to home, in 1994 I had the honor of having dinner at the home of a friend and colleague who was a professor of psychiatry at Yale and guess who came to dinner? None other than Rick Levin, the new president of Yale who remained Yale's president for 20 years from 1993 until 2013. Perhaps it is revealing of a deeper yearning to ultimately embrace my own Judaism that I remember feeling profoundly moved and even thrilled to be able to welcome in Shabbat with President Levin and for us all at the dinner table to say a *Shehecheyanu* blessing acknowledging how far we and all Jews had come in America. That was long after I had graduated from Harvard in 1959.

I think that it is important to share that I avoided being identified as a Jew at Harvard and never attended religious services nor ever went to Hillel. Quite the opposite. Although I knew at that time that I would never be admitted to any exclusive WASP final club, there was still a wish to be a part of that world of upper-class preppiness. Things have changed greatly since I graduated in 1959 and these clubs now have a fair number of Jews as members which was not the case in the late 1950s when it was rare for any Jew regardless of his social status and credentials to be admitted to one of these "restricted" clubs.

I remember dating a girl from Wellesley who was not Jewish and being very uncomfortable about ever discussing religion, particularly mine. In fact, I was so insecure about being Jewish that I ended the relationship before that might have become a subject of conversation. I am now quite confident that had I been more comfortable in my own skin, it would never have become an issue. She liked me a lot and in retrospect I am certain that the problem was mine, not hers.

I entered medical school in 1959 at New York University/Bellevue almost by default. I remember being rather envious of my wealthy friends who went to work on Wall Street, but I think I lacked the courage to risk moving in a new direction and my father was a physician so this felt familiar and comfortable – hardly an admirable motivation to become a doctor of medicine.

When it came to Judaism, I had little or no interest. I was interested in dating girls "from the right social background" and married one my senior year in medical school. We were married at a very elite country club where I have remained a member for over 50 years.

The club was primarily made up of Jews of German origin who ruled Wall Street and are the core of the book *Our Crowd*. I remember one of my wife's uncles in recommending me for membership saying, "I hope you are not Russian."

I did not lie but I also did not confront him and say something that reflected any pride in my own historic origins. Indeed, most of the Jews in this club married their social equivalents and appeared to have little or no interest in being Jews.

Throughout that marriage which ended after 15 years, I had little or no interest in Judaism. I named my daughter Elizabeth and my son John, Jr. (contrary to Jewish tradition), and while I did not reject Judaism, I hardly embraced it.

My second wife who I married in 1982 was a Jewish physician who took Judaism seriously. Prior to that marriage I had travelled to Greece, Africa, and Egypt but never to Israel. I think that, in itself, speaks volumes.

Largely as a result of her influence, we went on a trip to Israel. While there I was so impressed by the experience that I enrolled my daughter in a summer program, *High School in Israel*, that dramatically changed her life. She became increasingly committed to Judaism, ultimately going to Brandeis and from there to live and study at a Jewish Yeshiva for women in Jerusalem.

My wife and I also began to celebrate all Jewish holidays. My trip to Israel and my increasing immersion in Judaism led to my pursuing and then enrolling in a summer 1-month program at Yad Vashem on the Holocaust and anti-Semitism. Though not an educator in the area of Holocaust studies like the other students, I was accepted into the program and returned two subsequent years. In the third year, a professor from Cambridge was not able to attend and give the lectures on the Psychology of Prejudice and the Psychodynamics of Anti-Semitism. I volunteered to give those lectures and as a result I immersed myself in learning and thinking about those issues in depth perhaps for the first time in my life. That experience had a profound effect on me.

Following this, in 1992 I qualified and then competed in the Maccabiah Games in the tennis over-55 Masters Division. This became a further turning point in my Jewish experience since both of my children were in Israel. My daughter had left Brandeis to enter EYAHT, the Aish HaTorah College of Jewish Studies for Women, having chosen totally on her own to move toward becoming an observant Jew. My son came to Israel to join me and see me compete in these sports events and decided to stay on and study at Aish HaTorah, a Yeshiva for young men who had grown up outside of the Orthodox tradition. The organization's stated mission is "providing opportunities for Jews of all backgrounds to discover their heritage." He stayed on for a number of months and subsequently has also pursued an Orthodox Torah-observant life.

There is an interesting irony to all of this unfolding family history. My parents sought to embrace a life of secular success in America. I followed the game plan by going to Harvard, then into medicine and on to psychiatry over my mother's objection and repeated comments, "Why don't you become a real doctor like your father." My children choose a totally different direction and today are both fully committed to a Torah-observant Orthodox way of life and both are very happy.

Both of my children in their 20s (over 20 years ago) experienced mood disorders serious enough to require hospitalization. The treatments were minimally successful, but I believe that what ultimately saved them – both are currently doing very well in their lives – has been a steadfast commitment to Judaism and its daily practices and observances.

While my daughter remained in Israel, I returned there to investigate this "cult" that she had chosen. In a word, I became *cultivated*. I was entranced by the study of

Torah, by its wisdom and its profound understanding of human nature. I loved the learning and so many of the people I met in the Torah-observant world. Though I never moved to a Torah-observant life, I joined the Conservative synagogue in Greenwich. I became involved in working with the leaders of the Jewish Federation to bring more varied Jewish education to Greenwich and did a fair amount of teaching myself.

In subsequent years I have made many trips to Jerusalem which have had a profound effect on me and which have increased my respect and love for Judaism. In so doing, my association with Judaism has become more and more positive and increasingly comfortable and emotionally centering.

Perhaps a parallel experience is more than relevant.

Although it has to do with my son's mental illness and my response to it, I believe it relates to deeper issues of shame and preoccupation with image and appearance versus true self-acceptance and authenticity. These were the deeper dynamics that colored my response to being a Jew.

The facts of my son's illness are these. His illness began over 25 years ago. I had been a board-certified psychiatrist for over 20 years and had treated hundreds of patients. Presumably I, of all people, should have been prepared for this challenge. The truth is I wasn't.

My son was diagnosed correctly with bipolar disorder which, at that time, was still called manic depression. His life was chaotic and several times he threatened privately and publicly to harm me.

He received the best available professional help – medication and psychotherapy– from a number of highly competent psychiatrists and was hospitalized three times at excellent facilities, all in the New York area. Sadly, and tragically for him and for me, none of this was effective.

At first, I was not prepared or honest enough to recognize and admit that it was not just my child who needed healing. I needed help as well. For quite a while, I chose not to discuss the issue of his illness rather than honestly facing my personal anguish, my fear that he might be killed or kill someone else, my helplessness, my anger, and, sadly but honestly, my shame about my son's illness and its seeming insolubility.

Sadly, 25 years ago I saw my Judaism as a liability, certainly not as a positive aspect of my identity that might bring meaning, purpose, or joy into my life. As I initially avoided facing my ambivalence about being a Jew, I also avoided facing my deeper feelings about my son's illness.

When I couldn't find any solution for my son's illness despite over a half dozen attempts at treatment and several hospitalizations which extended over a 10-year period, I thought that perhaps I might be able to do something more that might help others with this disease including suffering parents like myself.

As result, 20 years ago a few of us with the help of the Chicago national office of the Depression and Bipolar Support Alliance (DBSA) started a chapter and a support group in Greenwich, Connecticut, in my home office.

Since our first meeting in the fall of 1999, our group has held almost one thousand meetings which occur every Friday afternoon for 2 hours. Groups are regularly attended by 20–25 members who may be either suffering with depression or bipolar illness or may be a loved one of someone with these conditions.

My son is well aware that this group in Greenwich exists only because of his illness and that hundreds of patients and their loved ones have been helped. Neither of us now has any shame but rather we both have considerable pride in his recovery and in my commitment to facilitate a pro bono support group that has literally saved dozens of lives.

My primary goal at this stage in my life is to reduce stigma so that more people, whether they be colleagues or laymen, can accept this diagnosis in themselves or a loved one and commit to a regimen of recovery rather than hiding in the shadow of shame.

Perhaps this parallels my increasing commitment to Judaism, my travels to Jerusalem, my increasing desire to understand my Jewish heritage and discover its richness, and my evolving pride in being a Jew which grew exponentially as I began to increasingly immerse myself in the study of Torah and Kabbalah. I also became increasingly involved in Jewish education and in teaching others about many aspects of Judaism including becoming a speaker in the Greenwich community on Holocaust Remembrance Day.

All of this speaks to my personal journey as a Jew and my yearning for self-acceptance and authenticity, frequent themes in our support group which I have increasingly come to recognize as a displacement for my own deep desire for and journey toward self-acceptance and authenticity as a Jew, to accept my reality with pride and dignity rather than shame and avoidance. I might add that my and the group's mantra, often repeated, is "Shame is slavery, honesty is freedom."

Perhaps my commitment to fighting stigma and speaking out for people with mood disorders may have been an unconscious displacement of a yearning to own my humanity as a Jew and speak up and speak out.

One manifestation of this was when I designed a T-shirt for our support group. On the front of the shirt was a picture of Abraham Lincoln. Above the picture was the word DEPRESSED? and beneath the picture, PRESIDENT LINCOLN WAS. On the back of the shirt were the words SHAME IS SLAVERY, HONESTY IS FREEDOM.

I think this was all an unconscious way of getting closer to being honest about saying something like JEWISH with a picture of any number of distinguished Jews – from Maimonides to Einstein – and the same statement on the front of the T-shirt, HE WAS. And on the back, SHAME IS SLAVERY, HONESTY IS FREEDOM.

A very important event happened to me in 2003. I married for the third time – this time to an Episcopalian born in the United Kingdom. The irony is that this experience has served both to deepen my Jewish identification and my self-esteem. I never asked my wife to convert but she recognized that at a deep level this was important to me. She had previously been married three times, all to Jews who preferred that she remain "other" including a former pilot in the Israeli Air Force. She chose to have an Orthodox conversion and we were married by an Orthodox rabbi.

She has the most profound respect for Judaism and its teachings and has always had deep respect and compassion for the internal and wounded John Tamerin, that internal self who I spent years hiding but have gradually come to appreciate, embrace, and even love. Simply stated, her respect and love for my internal self has greatly assisted me on my journey toward self-acceptance.

Recently, someone made a remark that probably would have pleased me in the past. He said, "I didn't know you were Jewish." My answer was one I would never have given in the past. I said, "I am not Jewish, I am a Jew. Jewish means *sort of*, and I am not sort of Jewish. I consider myself a Jew, and a very proud one!" It seemed clear to me that the person felt a deeper respect for me, as I have developed a deeper respect for myself.

For many years I attempted to hide my Judaism fearing that it would in no way benefit me and could easily result in rejection. Now, both my attitude and position are precisely the opposite and I feel fortunate to have lived to be 81 and to have experienced this dramatic transformation in my behavior, in my attitude, and indeed in my self-concept about being a Jew.

Though not a Torah-observant Jew, I study the Talmud every Saturday at Chabad in Greenwich and find this experience to be central to my essence. For the past several years, I have co-facilitated a support group at Christ Episcopal Church with a minister as co-therapist, and I frequently talk about my experiences and feelings as a Jew within that group which enriches the conversation and is well-accepted and personally affirming for me.

I am currently in the process of developing a seminar entitled *The Kabbalah and Mental Health*, a unique integration which I will teach with a distinguished Orthodox rabbi in our community and which will be well publicized. This eight-session seminar will provide clinical and spiritual insights on how to deal effectively with emotional pain. Each session will focus on a specific, relevant insight from the Kabbalah followed by a professionally facilitated group dialogue.

This seminar represents the merging of my professional commitment to helping people reduce the emotional pain in their lives, specifically honoring and incorporating the wisdom of Judaism. My son is helping me assemble a reading list and is an enthusiastic supporter of this endeavor.

To return to the T-shirt that I designed for my support group (my brief excursion into the "shmatta" business) – SHAME IS SLAVERY, HONESTY IS FREEDOM. This statement epitomizes my personal journey and evolution as a man and a Jew.

I now wish to live my life with transparency, authenticity, and pride rather than secrecy, anxiety, and caution. Being a Jew is being bold but not brash. It is being strong, consistent, and resilient internally and far less concerned with my external image or the approval of others whether they be Jew or non-Jew.

Erik Erikson introduced the issue of identity in the 1950s as an antidote to feelings of alienation. After a long journey I have discovered the profound truth in that observation. It works for me!

My deepening identity as a Jew has not only increased my feelings of authenticity, self-acceptance, clarity, and personal empowerment but has also enriched every other aspect of my life as a husband, father, practicing psychiatrist, and human being. It has been a long journey from shame, repudiation, and denial to acceptance and joy. But the journey has made me who I am today and despite the valleys, it has permitted me to climb mountains and I am grateful to be where I am as I look forward to my 82nd birthday.

Finally, an issue that may be of particular interest to therapists or analysts who read this narrative is; was the issue of my Jewish identity addressed as a significant factor in personal psychoanalysis when I was a young psychiatrist in training?

The answer is NO. Perhaps other issues seemed more important to me or to my several analysts. Alternatively, perhaps many events needed to occur in my life to bring this issue to the center of my attention and the center of my internal life.

Also, readers may wonder how this change in my internal life has affected the way I practice psychotherapy. That could be a chapter in itself but is best epitomized by my increasingly encouraging patients gradually to remove their defensive masks of secrecy and shame and live their lives openly and honestly. This, of course, is paralleled by huge social changes which have occurred during the last 50 years. A number of psychiatrists with whom I trained and who married subsequently found the courage to own their authentic selves, divorce their wives, and marry men. By comparison, my owning and accepting myself as a proud Jew may seem relatively insignificant; however, it has had a profound effect on my view of myself and on the way in which I practice my profession.

A Psychiatrist's Life Journey Through Anti-Semitism

9

Saul Levine

Anti-Semitism and the Scourge of Prejudice

"I'm acutely aware that I'm hated by many people around the world."

I'd better explain that paranoid-sounding statement, especially because I'm a psychiatrist!

I actually think I'm personally well-liked by many, loved by a few, criticized by some, admired by others, and perhaps personally disliked by a handful, but I am *not personally hated*, at least to my knowledge.

I of course have frailties and faults but think I'm considered caring, sociable, and even (at times) wise. I've had fulfilling family and professional experiences, endured setbacks, and enjoyed achievements.

In short, I'm just like you and most everyone else, an amalgam of good, sometimes less so, and without a doubt, complex characteristics which often conflict.

A psychotherapist hearing those provocative words, "I'm hated by many people," might ask, "How long have you felt this way?," and my response would be, sadly but truthfully, "All my life."

You are not reading about my paranoid "delusions of persecution," but you are learning of my discomfort that I belong to a group of people who are intensely disliked. I am not *personally* disliked, mind you, since "my" haters don't even know who I am!

This form of hatred is entirely *impersonal*, and while it can take different forms, they all stem from deep hate-fueled-and-filled historical lore. These venal prejudices are based solely on a person's birthright and background, with "pre-judged" entrenched beliefs in the inferiority and evil of "lesser" human beings. Sadly, this hatred is directed against people of many religions, races, and ethnicities.

S. Levine (✉)
University of California at San Diego (UCSD), Del Mar, CA, USA
e-mail: slevine@ucsd.edu

© Springer Nature Switzerland AG 2020
H. S. Moffic et al. (eds.), *Anti-Semitism and Psychiatry*,
https://doi.org/10.1007/978-3-030-37745-8_9

In my own case, I had the "audacity," according to my haters, of being born into a family originating in Jewish genetics, religion, and culture. I learned early on that I was hated "merely" for being Jewish, the very definition of "anti-Semitism."

Jewish Life in a Shtetl and in an Immigrant Community

Prior to the Second World War, hundreds of thousands of Jewish people fled the rampant anti-Semitism prevalent in Eastern European countries for safer havens across the ocean. My father and some of his siblings emigrated from Lithuania and my mother's parents from Latvia to Canada (the United States had temporarily closed its doors). Both their families originated from impoverished backgrounds in "shtetls" (*shtetlach*, in Yiddish) like the mythical "Anatevka" in "Fiddler on the Roof," small towns with ghettoized Jewish enclaves in countries throughout Eastern Europe.

Their childhood experiences in the shtetls were rife with anti-Semitism, and vicious bullying and aggressive acts were commonplace. In addition, there were large-scale ritualized destructive attacks directed against Jews ("pogroms"), both organized and random, which could include vandalism, beatings, and arson. They often coincided with the Passover/Easter season when Jews were for centuries accused of drinking Christian children's blood (the so-called blood libel). These attacks were perpetrated by hostile ultra-nationalists and were often abetted by militias or police. But whoever the perpetrators, they were covertly encouraged and unpunished.

As hateful as these acts were, they were soon followed by much worse: The Nazis pursued their murderous onslaughts throughout Europe to fulfill Hitler's goal of "The Final Solution" (extermination!) to "The Jewish Problem" (their existence!). Millions of Jews, including members of my own extended family and other "inferiors," perished in the ovens and slaughterhouses of the Holocaust.

But many other Jews were more fortunate and were able to flee to countries as diverse as Russia, Ukraine, Poland, Hungary, Romania, France, the Balkans, and other regions. Their means of escape were often in overcrowded, disease-ridden steerage levels of old steam ships, but they were full of hope, as they were bound for safe havens across the seas and beyond.

As a young child, I lived with my immigrant father and mother in Montreal during the Second World War. I grew up in a household with a strong Jewish cultural identity, but my staunchly Jewish parents were decidedly non-religious. They had abandoned their beliefs in the God they were taught about in childhood who (they felt) betrayed them by "allowing" the atrocities perpetrated by the Nazis (my father was a loving and grateful man, but the one hate even he could not overcome was for the Nazis and their ilk).

Most of our social contacts took place within the insular world of that immigrant Jewish community. Given their background, it was understandable that establishing a safe homeland for Jews, or Zionism, was foremost in their minds.

Although not religious, our family was immersed in Jewish life. Yiddish was my first language (*mammehloshn*, which I speak, read, and write to this day), familiarly used by my parents, extended family, and the many neighbors who were also recent immigrants. We participated in the cultural aspects of Jewish lifelike religious holidays and rituals, like Brises (circumcisions), Bar Mitzvahs, and Shivas (mourning), and I attended a Jewish elementary school (courtesy of the Hebrew Immigrant Aid Society).

I was proud of my identity even as a young Jewish boy and of my heritage and culture.

Anti-Semitism in a Safe Haven

These immigrants had escaped the brutalities in Europe (*Dee Alteh Medineh*, "The Old Country"), and they generally felt much safer in Canada and the United States (*Dee Neiyeh Velt*, "The New World"). Other countries also offered refuge, like Mexico, Argentina, and South Africa. Wherever they landed, they soon learned in both subtle and overtly aggressive ways that some of their nativist "hosts" were less than welcoming and resented their presence or even their very existence. I'd been warned by my elders about this, but my personal experiences confirmed these very same lessons.

Even in our close-knit Jewish immigrant community, our neighborhoods were occasionally "visited" by angry groups yelling anti-Jewish slogans and epithets. There were Fascist rants on the radio, demonstrations, anti-Semitic posters and signs defaced with swastikas, and insulting stereotypic tropes (our noses, usury, evil, original sin). These were designed to sow the seeds of hatred and incite and rally others to their cause, and they were often successful.

I vividly recall being upset as a child when I saw signs on private properties with the words, "No Jews Allowed," or "No Jews or Dogs." The hatred was not limited to the general public; anti-Semitism infiltrated even "reputable" individuals who held public office. The mayor of Montreal at the time, for example, was incarcerated because of his expressed sympathies for Fascists and his urging of young Quebecers not to serve with the Canadian Army in the war raging overseas.

Our elementary school stood cheek-by-jowl to another (non-Jewish) school, and there were frequent schoolyard yells of "Dirty Jew!," threats, and a few skirmishes. I recall taking circuitous walking routes home to avoid gangs of louts.

As adolescents during the 1950s, my friends and I attended a local public high school with high academic standards. The student body population there was 95% Jewish, and we belonged to a Zionist youth group. Our ethnic identity was thus hardly a secret, and this clearly upset some people. We were occasionally harassed on skating rinks, the streets, parks, and other public areas, which sometimes ending in foot or car chases or in fights. On a few occasions when set upon by anti-Jewish gangs, we required the intervention of adults or the police to protect us.

When we applied for summer jobs, we sometimes experienced abrupt rejection when our Jewish names were spoken or written (not dissimilar from what adult Jews faced when trying to rent apartments at that time). In that vein, when I expressed an interest in a career in journalism, my mother, a socialist news junkie, strongly asserted "With your name, you'll never get hired by newspapers!"

During my first week in college, a mild-mannered seatmate in a crowded introductory lecture hall told me that he was Roman Catholic. When he asked about my background and I said, "I'm Jewish," he looked genuinely startled and remarked that he had never met a "real Jew" before. I remember that he studied me with wonderment. He told me he was surprised that I was friendly, as he'd been taught that "Jews killed Jesus Christ and are evil." This was a benign incident, but not unusual, which demonstrated some ignorance and incipient prejudice.

I am not saying that my childhood and youth years were unhappy. I was in a stable family, had good friends, and lived in a mostly safe community "cocoon." But we were aware of being different when we stepped outside that cocoon and were somewhat wary, "just in case."

I add that while these stories of anti-Semitism and turmoil are factual, they were not typical of the majority of the Montreal population who were respectful, tolerant, and even hospitable. But when these incidents occurred, our attention was riveted and we were vigilant.

There was also evidence of anti-Semitism elsewhere: There were newscasts and newspaper reports of pro-Fascist incidents in many American and Canadian cities (Los Angeles, Baltimore, Philadelphia, Milwaukee, New York, Chicago, Toronto, and elsewhere). These varied from hostile name-calling or threats to angry marches or demonstrations which occasionally escalated to physical altercations and even riots.

The common themes of these events were ostensibly hatred toward Jews, but they also encompassed unions, civil rights, racial inequalities, immigration, and other progressive causes, as Jewish people were strongly identified with these "dangerous" leanings.

Many Jews suffered worse indignities and experiences than we did, but whenever they occurred, we took each incident personally, as if our own families were under siege.

These memories are seared in my mind, imprinted in my consciousness. While extremely unsettling to me at the time, I would in later years occasionally recount these stories with some mordant humor. Readers can surmise whether this was a counter-phobic defense mechanism.

"Hiatus from Hate?"

In my college years well after the war, there seemed to be a period of reduction in overt anti-Semitism. It felt to me that there was more tolerance and acceptance in society, which I perceived as a respite, a "hiatus from hate." When I mentioned this in my parents' circle, they were aghast at my naïvete and said I'd been lulled into complacency with a false and dangerous narrative. Was I merely expressing my personal need for wish-fulfillment?

My experience at McGill University turned out to be eye-opening and rewarding, both academically and socially. There were Jewish students and faculty, but I had new opportunities to meet and enjoy relationships with people of different races, religions, cultures, and countries. There were occasional innuendos but no real anti-Semitic insults or attacks. That same equanimity persisted throughout my medical school and internship experiences.

There was a common sardonic saying back then that "Jewish boys go to medical school!" which was indeed borne out by many of my friends: A disproportionate number of us from similar poor Jewish immigrant backgrounds chose medicine as a career. This made some sense as it was an honorable profession, one could be assured of a comfortable living, and importantly, our mothers could be proud (tongue in cheek, yet valid)! It also fulfilled an ancient rabbinical and Jewish scholarly precept calling on Jews to pursue lives of generosity and noble calling by engaging in service to others.

When we were applying to Canadian and American medical schools, we were advised that it had only been a few years since the rescinding of the implicit (sometimes explicit) "quota systems," which had limited spaces for Jewish students in many public and private institutions of "higher learning" (you are no doubt aware that these themes regarding other immigrant or racial communities are being repeated in US university admissions policies today).

I came of age during those years. I learned more about human complexities and propensities to aggression. I recognized that by no means were we Jews the only victims of hateful prejudices, and we weren't immune to having our own prejudices. We were often overly ethnocentric, we too could be callous and cruel, and we certainly harbored our own biases and bêtes noires. We also had our own zealous reactionaries and intolerant fundamentalists. As horrific as the Holocaust was, other genocides had preceded (and have certainly followed) that infamous stain on humanity.

Like my activist mother, I was a "news junkie" and avidly followed the news in newspapers and television newscasts. I was keenly aware that despite the relative calm in my personal life and in society, there were hate-filled rampages being perpetrated against victims throughout the world. Even worse, these attacks were often righteously proclaimed in the names of the haters' avowedly peace-loving Gods.

In the roiling seas of conflict and conflagration, the ugly head of anti-Semitism seemed to have dipped beneath the surface. It was of course never completely submerged, and what I interpreted as a "hiatus" turned out to be a harbinger.

Choice of Psychiatry as a "Jewish" Profession

After my internship, my choice of specialization was fairly simple: My undergraduate major had been psychology, and it seemed a natural transition to the study of psychiatry, which I had once heard being likened to "the medical Talmud" (Jewish laws). There were also a disproportionate number of Jewish trainees, faculty, and practitioners in psychiatry throughout North America and Europe. Although unaware of this at the time, it was no accident that I felt comfortable in that professional community, not unlike my early experiences in my Jewish immigrant neighborhood cocoon.

Aside from this ethnocentric reason, my choice of psychiatry made sense for other reasons: I was interested in studying "what makes us tick" and enjoyed learning about and working with the "whole person," both the psyche and soma.

I don't have the "chutzpa" (unmitigated gall) to deny that my choice was in part an attempt to wrestle with my personal "tzoriss" (problems) and "dybbuks" (devils)!

The stimulating intellectual discussions in psychiatry and the cross-disciplinary nature of the studies were somehow familiar to me. They seemed in the traditions of ancient Jewish philosophers' and rabbinical discourses and debates about interpretations of the Talmud and precepts of human behavior.

I wanted to learn more about human concerns and conundrums, our commonalities and differences, and our weaknesses and strengths. Psychiatry helped me appreciate the remarkable complexity of our species: our inspiring creativity and benevolence vis-a-vis our primal moral failings and brutalities (often within the same individual).

The patients I encountered taught me about empathy as well as humility, as in "There but for the grace of God go I." I was captivated by the breadth and depth of human feelings, attitudes and behaviors, relationships and psychodynamics, and the interplay of socio-cultural and genetic factors (the nature-nurture diathesis).

Another personal impetus for my going into psychiatry was the diagnosis of my much younger brother with severe "early infantile autism" (as it was then called), which led to my further specialization in child and adolescent psychiatry, as well as my mother's lifelong struggles with recurrent depressions.

Finally, psychiatry offered me the privilege of making a positive difference in the lives of suffering people, which is what our Jewish heritage extols.

My career choice was thus a combination of rationality and serendipity, a fortuitous combination of interests and experiences, desires, and talent. Although I am not a traditional believer in God, I don't discount the role of synchronicity. That is, I am spiritually oriented and consider the possible influences of mysticism, "karma," and "other-worldly" or cosmic forces beyond our comprehension.

A Career in Psychiatry

The relatively peaceful existence I experienced in college and medical school continued during residency and fellowship years at Stanford. Anti-Semitic acts here and abroad were certainly being reported on the news (and especially by the Anti-Defamation League (ADL), the American Civil Liberties Union (ACLU), and the Southern Poverty Law Center (SPLC)); the current tensions were centered on prevalent racial conflicts at home and the controversial war in Vietnam.

Israel was as usual being both lauded and severely criticized, but it moved me when many Jewish colleagues in medicine and psychiatry volunteered to go to help Israel during the Six-Day War in 1967.

Toward the end of my training in 1968, I was fortunate to be awarded a Foundation Fund Travel and Research Fellowship, which included a stay of a couple of months in Israel. Aside from the psychiatric centers I visited, I met long-lost first cousins and their families. While Israel was a different cultural experience, it resonated in me as a natural "home."

Upon my return from abroad, I began my academic and clinical career in earnest in Toronto, where I eventually became a Full Professor and headed the Department of Psychiatry at one of the University of Toronto's Teaching Hospitals. The University Chair happened to be Jewish, as were four of the five other hospital heads of psychiatry.

It was in an anteroom just outside my office when I was presumed to be away that I overheard three of my non-Jewish colleagues – whom I liked and respected – discussing their strong resentment at the preponderance of Jewish senior faculty and residents, all the while using derogatory language and raucous laughter. So much for the equality and equanimity I thought I had engendered in the department I led!

For better or for worse, I never uttered a word of this to anyone and carried on working with these colleagues for a few more years. But it was never the same…

In addition to my teaching and research over the years, I was fortunate to have interesting clinical experiences with patients from very diverse racial, religious, and socio-cultural backgrounds. I met all kinds of personalities and professions, politicians, tradesmen, peacemakers, teachers, and yes, even haters. I learned about their lives and about "life."

I became schooled in the yin and yang of "the human condition": how we are by nature both social and tribal and generous and selfish, how we harbor loves and biases, how benevolences enhance us and prejudices harm us, how we are blessed and burdened, and mostly, how similar we all are, despite our visible differences.

I was also given the opportunity to spend a sabbatical year in 1980–1981 in Jerusalem with my young family, where I continued my research on young people involved in intense belief systems and taught in the Department of Psychiatry at Hebrew University Medical School.

It was a remarkable experience, enchanting and inspiring, though at times frustrating and challenging. Israel was familiar to me, yet foreign. It was serene and captivating, yet difficult and roiling. Thriving collective farms adjoining affluent and poor neighborhoods, large modern cities and small biblical towns, advanced educational and scientific institutions, creative arts vividly displayed, and always, the ubiquitous military, uniformed, armed young men and women, vigilantly on guard.

On an outing to an ice cream shop in Old Jerusalem with my son, we noticed the usual Saturday ("Shabbat") crowds of citizens, tourists, and soldiers and a rusty bicycle leaning up against a nearby wall close to where we were sitting. Not 15 minutes after we left, that very bicycle exploded, the tires having been filled with explosives detonated by remote control. There were pandemonium, deaths, and injuries, and we were in a state of shock, as we had come so close to…

The small land of Israel is made up of Jewish people from all over the globe as well as Arabs and Christians, unified in patriotism but torn by internal conflict, a bulwark of democracy in a sea of hostile dictatorships and kingdoms. A society under perpetual threat, yet creative and productive, alive and exciting, one felt at the center of humanity, a microcosm of the world's achievements and downfalls.

Adherents of four major religions (Judaism, Christianity, Islam, Greek Orthodox), all with their "homes" in Jerusalem, are living in a state of "flux," usually co-existing in tolerance and harmony, sometimes transforming into intervals of conflict and turmoil. Because of my research, I was afforded proximity and access to them. I met wonderful people there, but I also saw intolerance, prejudice, and extremism within each religious group, each believing and acting as if only they had the answers to life's eternal questions.

Israel enabled me to continue the studies I'd begun in the United States and Canada on young people who had become zealously attached to messianic religious movements and to their charismatic leaders. I interviewed devotees in *yeshivot* (Jewish theological seminaries) and similar religious schools and seminaries, as well as their religious and ideological leaders. My first book, *Radical Departures: Desperate Detours to Growing Up*, was "conceived" in Israel, though its "birth" was later in the United States.

After that year I returned to Toronto to raise my family and pursue my career.

My 25 years in Toronto were productive and enjoyable: academic, clinical, and media careers, articles and books published, three sons in professions and married, and grandchildren (*ayniklach*). A few years later I moved to San Diego where I remarried, and we adopted an infant girl in China (who is now a college freshman).

Moving from Toronto meant another cultural and professional transition: I became Professor of Psychiatry at the University of California at San Diego (UCSD) and Director of Child and Adolescent Psychiatry at Rady Children's Hospital, positions I held until I retired in 2012. I now have a private psychotherapy and consulting practice, write columns for *Psychology Today* and *San Diego Jewish Journal* magazines, and engage in other pursuits.

These columns attract readers' comments which are often laudatory and others which respectfully disagree. In this era (see below), however, it is no surprise that I also occasionally receive hateful "trolling" comments which are ad hominem and/or blatantly anti-Semitic.

Full Circle: Anti-Semitism Today

Over the centuries Jews have been persecuted by anti-Semites for our imagined iniquities. And wonder of wonders, here we are again, with anti-Semitic actions burgeoning in numerous countries.

Our "new" detractors still use the old vile and invalid tropes to portray us as greedy, deviant, evil sinners and usurers and invoke the blood libel and Christ-killer depictions. Militant Islamic texts still refer to Jews as "ancestors of dogs, monkeys and pigs."

When haters are confronted with evidence (real facts!) that Jews have been remarkably creative and beneficial to humankind and have made extraordinary contributions in the sciences, arts, music, literature, medicine, jurisprudence, philosophy, and business, the haters will scoff and invoke their hateful animus.

Jews today are confronted with a painful conundrum: Now that Israel ("Jewish homeland") exists as a major Middle East power, both loyal and hostile feelings toward its policies have complicated "purist" anti-Semitism. Provocative new questions have arisen: Can one be pro-Jewish and yet anti-Israel? Is criticism of Israel tantamount to anti-Semitism? Does support of Israel preclude its criticism? Is an authoritarian president's strong support good or bad for Israel? For Jews in general? Can one be a Jewish-American and avoid conflicted patriotism? Can descendants of Holocaust victims and survivors actually be cruel occupiers of innocent Palestinians? Is the Two-State Solution a desirable and attainable goal? Should Christian evangelists who strongly support Israel (Jewish, Old Testament) as the fulfillment of a biblical (Christian, New Testament) prophecy be praised or suspected?

These questions have inspired impassioned debates and even bitter conflicts dividing Jewry in Israel, the United States, and elsewhere. Major American Jewish lobby groups, like AIPAC (American Israel Public Affairs Committee) and J Street, hold deeply antagonistic political positions regarding Israel, as do other such groups. American Jewish religious movements (Orthodox, Conservative, Reform, and Reconstructionist) often have strongly differing opinions regarding their relationships with Israel. Authoritarian and nationalistic sentiments growing in the United States and many other countries are vividly mirrored in the polarized political battles between progressives and conservatives in Israel.

The Free Speech and BDS (Boycott, Divestment, and Sanctions) Movements in the United States and elsewhere are flashpoints on many university campuses, with vehement conflicts about using university endowment funds to participate in research in Israel or invest in Israeli businesses; which representative political perspectives should be allowed or refused permission to speak; which causes are to be tolerated, extolled, or criticized; and which comments or commentators are deemed as stimulating or provocative as opposed to inflammatory or dangerous.

As I write this, I am looking back at my past, examining my current existence, and thinking about my future. My family is healthy and engaged in their lives, my careers have flourished, my Jewish identity is strong, and I am grateful to the three countries which nurtured and facilitated my life's journey.

Yet, as a Jew, I feel uneasy.

Two thoughts reverberate in my mind:

The first may sound familiar because I started the chapter with this provocative statement: "I am aware that many people around the world hate me." I have thus come full circle in my own lifetime, living with the realization that overt anti-Semitism is again thriving in its uniquely wretched ways in many countries and that I am again personally affected (déjà vu?).

The second thought echoing in my ears is the sad expression my father would ruefully say, "Meh shlogt shoin veiter Yidn," meaning, "They're beating up on Jews, yet again."

Anti-Semitism is no longer surreptitious. Its virulent hate is professed loudly and proclaimed proudly in speeches, marches, and publications and on social media. Valid reports of anti-Semitic acts of harassment, vandalism, personal aggression, and deadly violence have increased dramatically in many countries, including the United States, France, Brazil, Germany, Denmark, England, Sweden, Poland, Russia, Hungary, South Africa, many Arab countries, and others.

Authoritarian and demagogic regimes stir up nativist and populist anti-Semitic, racist, and xenophobic sentiments. They thrive by spreading "fear and loathing" in the hearts and minds of worried and impressionable citizens, many of whom feel vulnerable and resentful at being "left behind" in this era of rapid technological change, globalism, and financial challenges, especially in the context of extreme wealth for the few. In looking for people to blame, Jews have always been one of humankind's "favorite" scapegoats. They are also, however, the "canary in the coalmine," meaning that when Jews are targeted for hateful attacks, this is an inevitable harbinger of vitriol and hate directed at different "others."

My studies of zealous religious and political cults have familiarized me with the phenomenon of susceptible people who become fervent "True Believers." They are mesmerized ("swept away") by charismatic and demagogic leaders and movements which promise simplistic answers to complex social and psychological issues.

There are a wide variety of intense ideological groups of True Believers who portray themselves as peaceful apostles of love, including most main-line religions as well as some so-called cults (Hare Krishna, 3HO, Unification Church). Others, however, are avatars of hate (fundamentalists, Ku Klux Klan, Fascists, anti-Semites) whose words and demeanors express rage and hatred through their words and behaviors for those deemed to be "dangerous," "lesser," or "foreign/alien."

Anti-Semites are in that cluster of groups whose members bond in hate, all the while keeping their eyes on their targets of revulsion. They are spurred on by their demagogic leaders and the energies of their fellow zealots. They are full of rancor, rage, and retribution, and they're often violence-prone ("spoiling for a fight!"). Nonetheless, we are aware that many avowedly peaceful religions have been subverted into brutal violence perpetrated in the names of their peaceful gods.

Paradoxically, the members of fervent hate groups feel better personally because they finally have *the* "causal enemies" whom they can blame for their previous frustrations and unhappiness. They have a cause celebre: By besmirching or harming those people who are clearly responsible for their problems, they now have "answers" (solutions!) to life's challenges.

"And everybody hates the Jews!" is a famous line from the satirical song ("National Brotherhood Week") by Tom Lehrer, the brilliant academic-turned-political and social troubadour in the 1950s and 1960s. His perceptive and sardonic lyrics skewered the haters of that day and, I dare say, today…

To borrow a phrase (from blood transfusions), we are a "universal recipient" of "malice-aforethought" from members of groups as diverse as Fascists, communists, white supremacists, populists, xenophobes, ultra-nationalists, Islamists, neo-Nazis, alt-rightists, extremist leftists, and others. All these people share an abiding hatred of Jews, which creates a bizarre and morbid paradox: anti-Semitism serving as a horrific "unifying" theme for humans! (forgive the counter-phobic humor).

Many people are startled by this information and disbelieve or ignore its implications. Many are surprised by the return of this ugliness, but my late father is not at all surprised. He is surely thinking, "I told you so," not with smugness, but with sad tears streaming down his face.

As a Jewish psychiatrist, I am deeply troubled by the current exacerbation of anti-Semitism. Although not religious, I am familiar with Jewish theology and liturgy and steeped in Jewish history and culture. I also have a reverence for cosmic forces beyond our understanding.

I am not single-minded. That is, while I do think about "big" issues like the "meaning of life," as do you, I also wish to enjoy my life with family and friends. In the current situation, however, I often find myself wrestling with how I can constructively deal with or counteract the growing anti-Semitism in my personal and professional life. I wonder what I can do in keeping with my sense of self, my expertise, and my Jewish heritage.

First of all, I shall continue to treat everyone I encounter – family, friends, patients, students, trainees, and strangers – with respect, tolerance, empathy, honesty, and compassion. And I shall expect the same from them. This is true to our Judaic teaching of honorable social behaviors.

Just as we are taught to welcome strangers to our Pesach Seder (Passover Dinner) table, I will in that same vein urge our country, as best as I can, to uphold this same tradition in welcoming deserving immigrants to our shores. The impassioned words of Emma Lazarus ("Give me your tired, your poor, your huddled masses yearning to be free…") ring out from our symbolic beacon of America, the Statue of Liberty. Perhaps they are particularly meaningful to me as I was welcomed here as an immigrant.

I shall embrace the lessons of countless generations of our Jewish forefathers (and mothers) in concentrating on personal growth through the loves of reading, learning, and teaching ("the power of the book"). This is as much for myself as it is for my children and my students.

I shall continue to "proselytize" about the importance that we humans act ethically to leave a "positive emotional footprint" as "our mark," both while we are here on this planet and long after we have passed on to dust and ashes or to a cosmic form of existence. Our spiritual energy and altruistic actions toward others enrich us and our self-worth.

I will try my best to live by, manifest the tenets of, and teach "the four Bs," as the cornerstone for living a life of quality, meaning, and worthiness: "being" (a sense of personal grounding and honesty), "belonging" (a sense of social engagement and communality), "believing" (a sense of overriding values to live by and pass on), and "benevolence" (a sense of meaningful altruism to others).

I will bear in mind that although we can aspire to leading inspiring and creative and generous and resilient lives, we are also fallible beings. We embody within our souls both strengths and frailties, magnanimity and selfishness, creativity and destructiveness, and love and hate. I will continue to strive for my own betterment and to teach these values to others.

I will try to convince national legislators that a mandated year of community service – like a domestic Peace Corps – for older adolescents to contribute to the needs of the country (the poor, the homeless, preschools, retirement homes, forests, waterways) might well captivate their energy and idealism, instead of being directed to sociopathic leaders and their hatreds.

I will support and promote dialogue and rapprochement as opposed to aggression and violence in my personal life, in the lives of my patients, and in my political expressions.

I will engage myself in the political process to achieve a better society. When I witness examples of cruel "isms," prejudices, or injustices, I shall speak out and write publicly about these malfeasances. I will be more outspoken about what is known about the destructive potential of authoritarian and demagogic groups.

Our hallowed species, *Homo sapiens*, long considered the most "evolved" of all Earth's creatures, has demonstrated remarkable heights of benevolence and creativity, while descending into depths of unimaginable hatred and brutality.

We ignore the recent rise in anti-Semitism at our peril. This dangerous and ugly side of humanity and other similar venal hatreds are truly scourges which bedevil our species and threaten our very survival.

In the present circumstances, with nativist authoritarianism and extremism on right and left being loudly promulgated, I am deeply concerned about the future of planet Earth. We need to be as vigilant and committed to "our emotional footprint" as we are to our "carbon footprint."

Failing this crucially important effort on the part of humanity, I fear for my children and grandchildren, for my patients and their kin, and for you and yours as well.

I do, however, have hope because there is indeed reason for some optimism: Research has shown that we have the capability to overcome our propensities to aggression and hate. It would take a major commitment on the part of humankind, but we can end violent conflict and achieve tolerance and peace. This is in fact what most of humanity fervently wants, and there is in fact no viable alternative.

My father's words again: "Mirken'n, un mir takeh muz'n, leb'n mit leebshaft un in sholom." ("We *can*, and indeed we *must*, live with love and in peace.")

I am optimistic that "we shall overcome."

Anti-Semitism: Social, Religious, and Clinical Considerations of a Jewish Psychiatrist

10

H. Steven Moffic

Serious thinkers… have to reinvent their messages; they have to put more of themselves in the story [1]. – Elaine Margolin

As a Jewish psychiatrist, how could I not be concerned with anti-Semitism during my career? Was being a physician, more specifically a psychiatrist, a haven from anti-Semitism? After all, psychoanalysis was thought to be a "Jewish science," even if that was sometimes a derisive term [2]. Freud was Jewish, as were most of his early followers. That early Jewish presence in psychoanalysis spread to the early years of psychiatry in the last century during the time when psychiatry was more psychoanalytically oriented than it has been in recent decades. This connection even led to Jewish psychiatrists being called psychiatry's "chosen people," mirroring the historical impression that Jews were God's chosen people when they accepted the covenant for an ethical monotheism [3]. Psychodynamics even helped to explain the evolution of anti-Semitism, such as when disliked aspects of oneself are projected onto – and identified in – Jewish people.

I grew up in Chicago in the 1950s in a small, entirely Jewish community. My family was Conservative Jews, situated between the more liberal Reform Judaism and the more traditional Orthodox Jewish religious traditions. However, I never seemed to embrace these religious aspects and only became a bar mitzvah at age 13 as a matter of parental expectation. In those days of second- or third-generation Jewish immigrants, the desire of many Jewish mothers was for their children, especially boys, to become lawyers or doctors. Jewish mothers of the time were noted for being able to influence their children by instilling guilt for not doing what the mothers expected. My mother had a chronic, life-threatening illness.

This time period was close enough to the Holocaust of World War II to emphasize careers that would be as safe and secure as possible. Moreover, being a doctor

H. S. Moffic (✉)
Private Community Psychiatrist, Milwaukee, WI, USA
e-mail: rustevie@mac.com

© Springer Nature Switzerland AG 2020
H. S. Moffic et al. (eds.), *Anti-Semitism and Psychiatry*,
https://doi.org/10.1007/978-3-030-37745-8_10

or lawyer would also fit the Jewish cultural value of tikkun olam, to try to make the world be a better place. Given that my mother's beloved brother died from Hodgkin's disease after he finished medical school, it later made sense to me that becoming a physician came first. I didn't particularly like biological science and so was drawn to psychiatry. This career quest solidified when I read Freud's *The Interpretation of Dreams* [4] during high school, an inspiration to understanding myself and others during the turbulent times of adolescent identity development. I wavered at times toward becoming a psychologist, but that would not be a medical doctor.

Freud was not religious in any sense. In fact, he felt that religion was an opiate for the masses. Nevertheless, he still embraced being part of the Jewish people and valued the Jewish organization B'nai B'rith [5]. This more secular orientation fits my own Jewish identity during high school. Most psychiatrists of that time, Jewish or not, were not particularly religious.

I certainly wasn't concerned with anti-Semitism then. I'm not even sure I knew what that was. And why should I have been concerned in the protective bubble of innocence where I grew up? It was the postwar boom of conquering America. Jews were assimilating, and didn't perennial anti-Semitism seem to have disappeared under a wave of collective guilt and responsibility for the Holocaust? Even the psychiatric profession, with an overrepresentation of Jewish psychiatrists, seemed to accept this promising new status quo and didn't look below the surface as psychiatrists were wont to do otherwise in the era of psychoanalysis.

As for me, even though I was reading Freud's *The Interpretation of Dreams*, learning how to analyze hidden meanings, I never thought of hidden meanings in the context of anti-Semitism.

Besides Freud, I came to be inspired by many other Jewish psychiatrists. Actually, technically speaking, Freud was not a psychiatrist, but a neurologist. Almost like the number of Jewish people winning Nobel prizes, Jewish psychiatrists and psychologists have been overrepresented in their contribution to psychiatry. According to one listing [6], these have included:

- Abraham Low (1891–1954), for self-help peer groups
- Victor Frankl (1905–1997), for coping with severe trauma (in concentration camps for him) and the establishment of logotherapy, a therapy focusing on the meaning of one's life
- Alfred Adler (1870–1937), for his work on the inferiority complex and self-esteem
- Albert Ellis (1913–2007), for developing rational emotive psychotherapy
- Erich Fromm (1900–1980) for his theories of personality and political insight
- Laurence Kohlberg (1927–1987) for his theories of moral development
- Abraham Maslow (1908–1970) for his pyramid of psychological needs
- David Wechsler (1896–1981) for intelligence testing
- Joseph Wolpe (1915–1997) for systematic behavioral desensitization

As apparent, none of these well-known Jewish psychiatrists and psychologists focused on Judaism and/or anti-Semitism. But one other did. To this list, I would at least add Robert Jay Lifton, MD, for his work on understanding brainwashing, the motivation of Nazi doctors, his political activism, and leadership in addressing the major threats to mankind of nuclear war and climate change [7]. As such, and because he was on the faculty while I went to medical school at Yale, he has been an ongoing role model [8]. Most fortunately, I was asked to introduce him when he received the first Humanitarian Award from the American Association for Social Psychiatry at an annual meeting of the American Psychiatric Association.

When I was accepted into Yale University School of Medicine in 1967 as sort of an experiment in admitting someone after three undergraduate years and no degree, many of my classmates were also Jewish. I had little inkling at the time that this was a dramatic change from the past, when Yale and other medical schools had a severe quota for admitting Jewish students. The dean of the medical school in 1967 was also Jewish and a psychiatrist, so perhaps it was not surprising that I had no sense of anti-Semitism there. Such psychological blindness must have been comforting.

However, I think that one of my classmates and a friend surely did recognize the underlying dangers and that helped to break through my ignorance and denial. As his required theses, he was among the first ever to make videotaped interviews with Holocaust survivors. He was indeed in touch with his Judaism and the associated anti-Semitic risks. I, instead, did a more mainstream research project on depression. In my defense, looking back, depression seemed to connect with the Holocaust, though that insight was lost to me at the time.

Similarly, the University of Chicago, Department of Psychiatry, where I trained to become a psychiatrist, also had a Jewish chair, a Jewish residency director, and a Jewish leader of the community psychiatry programs. Once again, though, Judaism and/or anti-Semitism was not discussed. This kind of organizational culture did not change for me until I served in the US Army for 2 years in 1975–1977. I was stationed in Fort McClellan, Alabama, and the first question most new acquaintances asked us was: "What church do you go to?" This question did not seem to reflect any overt or covert hatred of Jews; it was just an expectation of this cultural environment, with the assumption that Jews would be "saved" if they converted to Christianity. There was a small Jewish population which was served by a visiting young rabbi. Even so, my emotional involvement with Judaism still seemed superficial, and anti-Semitism was not a concern. Then, it was time to make my own choice for beginning my career as a psychiatrist.

Life lesson #1: Judaism and anti-Semitism inevitably affect anyone with a Jewish background, whether consciously aware of that or not.

Life lesson #2: With a strong congruence of values, Judaism and psychiatry have been a good fit.

Social Considerations

On the surface, it didn't seem to have little to do with being Jewish and/or anti-Semitism. Having been inspired by the community psychiatry programs during my residency training, I accepted a position in a new community and social psychiatry program at Baylor College of Medicine in Houston. As it turned out, this did have a lot to do with being a Jewish psychiatrist. Perhaps that even started with choosing a career in academics, as Jewish males traditionally focused on learning the Torah and Talmud, the traditional "academic" books of Judaism. Was this a modern secular manifestation of the traditional "Yeshiva Bookers"?

Baylor College of Medicine, of course, traced its origins to Baylor University, a Baptist school. However, my immediate boss was Jewish, who came from Castro's Cuba when he was a child, and the medical school seemed diverse culturally and religiously.

My wife and I joined a Reform Jewish congregation where my wife was active in the choir. However, for many years, I didn't attend often, mainly only for the High Holy Days of Rosh Hashanah and Yom Kippur.

Serendipitously, there was an anthropologist faculty member who was part of our program. Having already developed an interest in jazz music, which was an original music developed by Black Americans, with an assist from Jewish Americans like Benny Goodman, I was interested to learn more about the influence of Black culture in psychiatry. Moreover, I, as medical director of a community mental health center, had a Black woman social worker as the complementary administrative director. I was primarily responsible for the clinical services and she for the administration of the clinic. The anthropologist also helped to orient me to Mexican American culture, so prominent in Houston, including the common use of curanderos, or folk healers. Unless the kabbalists are included, there are not any such folk healers in modern-day Judaism nor exorcists such as those existing in some Catholic Churches, though Jewish clergy do some supportive counseling.

My interest in cultural aspects of psychiatry, or in how the values of any given culture influenced psychiatry, led to my being asked to develop an educational seminar series on cultural psychiatry. I made exploring the cultural identities of all the residents the initial process of the seminar series. In retrospect, that emphasis probably came from my own ambivalent cultural identity. How should I identify myself culturally? Was I just American? Jewish American? An American Jew? I ended up at that time embracing the concept of being both an American and Jewish male. The success of this seminar series led to ours being the first model curriculum on the subject in the United States [9]. My co-leader turned out to be one of the first residents to participate, a Black American male psychiatrist, as he labeled himself. Interestingly, in this time period well before September 11, 2001, and Islamic-related terrorism, we had many Muslim residents in training, and there was no sense of Islamophobia or discrimination toward them or toward Muslims in general.

Once again, organizational anti-Semitism did not seem to be a real concern at Baylor, possibly until there was an offer by Saudi Arabia for American physicians to spend time there educating their physicians. Given the conflict in the Middle East between Israel and the Muslim Arab nations, perhaps it should have been anticipated that Jewish faculty would not be allowed to be part of these stints. That, of course, by itself, didn't necessarily imply anti-Semitism on the part of the medical school. It did, though, have practical implications, because this was a lucrative sojourn and we Jewish physicians were not given any way to make up the lost financial opportunity. Because I was uncertain how I as a Jew would be viewed at Baylor, I didn't usually volunteer that I was Jewish, and no one suspected since I lacked a Jewish sounding name or appearance.

After a dozen years and a criminal conviction, my boss caused our community contract to be terminated, and we moved to the Medical College of Wisconsin in Milwaukee to be closer to our ill parents in Chicago and Milwaukee. There, too, a Jewish psychiatrist was the chair of the department, which had many other Jewish psychiatrists. The prominence of Jewish psychiatrists seemed to be continuing, at least in my professional social spheres.

It was not until the Jewish chair of the department retired that I started to wonder about anti-Semitism as a new, non-Jewish chair came in, and at the same time, the Jewish medical school dean was replaced by a non-Jewish one. Was this a realistic concern of mine or a newfound oversensitivity? At the very least, it helped to solidify my Jewish identity and concern for anti-Semitism.

Freud also went through a reassessment of his identity. In 1926, the Austrian native told an interviewer:

> My language is German. My culture, my attainments are German. I considered myself German intellectually, until I noticed the growth of antisemitic prejudice in Germany and German Austria. Since that time, I prefer to call myself a Jew [10].

Even so, Freud did not try to leave greater Nazi Germany until it was almost too late and his own daughter's life was in grave danger, despite his own theory of Thanatos, the self-destructiveness of humans [11].

Whether this was an influential variable in my ensuing departmental unhappiness never became entirely clear to me, but after some more years and another non-Jewish chair, I decided to retire in 2012. By then, as though Jews were no longer so highly represented in psychiatry, psychiatry had turned more toward a biological emphasis than psychological and social one.

It was around that time that anti-Semitism in Europe, and then the United States, started to escalate. Disapproval of Israeli policies toward Palestinians, anti-Zionism, became another form of anti-Semitism when it was not based on reality and practicality. Constructive criticism of Israel would otherwise not be anti-Semitism.

For me, this rising anti-Semitism became connected to the Holocaust and America's long history of anti-Semitism when I was asked to discuss a movie at the Milwaukee Jewish Community Center about the children of prominent Nazis. As I was considering my formal remarks, there suddenly was the unsettling epiphany that I would not have been born had it not been for escaping the Holocaust. Even though there seems to be an almost infinite number of variables leading to anyone's birth, my father was stationed in Dayton, Ohio, at the end of World War II. He was already a lawyer then. There, he met my mother and I was conceived right after the war ended and born on May 5, 1946. As far as I know, all the other members of the family of my grandparents stayed in Europe and were killed in the Holocaust.

It then became more important to me as a Jewish psychiatrist to focus on the Holocaust and anti-Semitism. What a small payback for being born that might be. That focus eventually led to the opportunity to edit this book, an opportunity that occurred not long after what was arguably the worst recent episode of anti-Semitism in the United States, the killings at a synagogue in Pittsburgh by a so-called white nationalist. Whether and when Jews are considered to be "white" in America is a never-ending moving target, especially with the increase of Jews who immigrate now coming from a variety of cultural backgrounds, including those "of color." In Israel, this became colorfully clear with the influx of dark-skinned Ethiopian Jews.

As an outcome of that epiphany, I became more involved with Jewish community organizations. One of them was the Jewish Community Relations Council of Milwaukee. This is an organization with widespread representation from various Jewish organizations, whose explicit goal is to improve intra-cultural and cross-cultural relationships in Milwaukee. One of its activities is to do an annual audit of anti-Semitic incidents in Wisconsin. The 2018 results were released to the public on March 5, 2019. There was an alarming rise in anti-Semitic incidents, with worsening tone and tenor, including the following trends:

- A 21% increase in such incidents
- A 166% increase in vandalism
- 45% of the incidents were online
- An increase in references to Nazism, the Holocaust, and white supremacy

Some examples (not including those of unprintable language) were:

- A message to a Jewish agency including the line: "These Zionists are without a doubt the most despicable religious (or cult) community in the world"
- A phone message left at a synagogue that included: "Hey king Jews, you know what 6 million times per is? Zero!"
- Spray-painted graffiti at a park that included a large swastika composed of penises as its four "arms"

Though I have not (yet) personally experienced any major traumas in relationship to anti-Semitism, these incidents feel like the microaggressions of perpetrators that cause microtraumas in the recipients, many of them previously reported by discriminated against groups [12]. They add up. They can disrupt sleep. And they can provide concern for the future. Repeated exposure to them over and over can cause subclinical post-traumatic stress disorder (PTSD) symptoms and, if the intensity increases to life-threatening trauma, contribute to full-blown PTSD.

My wife has always stated: "keep your bags packed," meaning be ready to go to Israel. Looks like time to repack those bags, no?

Life lesson #3: Appreciating and respecting the cultural identities of the patient and clinician are essential to providing competent care.

Life lesson #4: Whether philo-Semitism or anti-Semitism becomes institutionalized in psychiatry and society often depends on the leadership.

Religious Considerations

My own religious Jewish identity started to evolve at the end of our time in Houston, in the late 1980s. As part of being involved to some extent in our Reform congregation, I decided with the senior rabbi to offer a seminar on psychotherapy and Judaism. My role was to present on how psychotherapy reflected such Jewish values as tikkun olam, as well as how Freud seemed to adapt Jewish mysticism, the hidden meanings of self-understanding of the Kabbalah. The renowned Jewish educator, the late Eugene Borowitz, approached the topic from the standpoint of Reform Judaism.

Also near the end of my time in Houston, I volunteered some time at the local Jewish Family Service, which had been established nationwide to provide mental health services to poorer Jews and non-Jews. When I came to Milwaukee, I dedicated a half day a week to pro bono service at Milwaukee's Jewish Family Service.

Our family joined another Reform synagogue in Milwaukee. I became more active there over time, which led to being asked to do a special lecture sermon on Maimonides, the prominent Jewish physician and rabbi of the Middle Ages, also renowned for his Jewish medical ethics and psychological insights [13]. By then, one of my special areas of interest was medical and psychiatric ethics. Traditionally, Judaism is looked upon as the first religion to be based on ethical monotheism. Saving a life was a dominant value, which obviously was reflected in medical ethics.

More important for the Jewish religious perspective, our son decided to become a rabbi. For a psychiatrist of any religion to have a clergy child is a rarity, but this spurred me to learn more about the religious aspects in Judaism in order not to embarrass him. That came mainly in the weekly study of Torah, otherwise known as the "Old Testament," the essential text said to be given to the people when they became a Jewish people [14]. Every year, Jews over the world study the same passages, though of course how one responds to a particular passage may vary year by year as one's life changes. Just recently, I attended a Torah inscription ceremony on the top of Masada in Israel; Masada was where the Jews held out much longer than expected against the mighty Roman army centuries ago. Though questions about whether there were suicides at the end and suicides are generally prohibited in Judaism religious beliefs, Masada is usually viewed as a symbol of Jewish heroism [15].

What I found in this Torah study was descriptions of leaders and families which seemed to have similar conflicts and narcissistic challenges as I encountered in my psychiatric practice. Among the examples I found:

- Sibling rivalry in the murder of Abel by his brother Cain
- The alcohol abuse of Noah after his journey on the Ark during the flood and his return to land
- The Oedipal conflict reflected in the father of Judaism, Abraham, when God apparently asked him to sacrifice his beloved son, Isaac, only to be stopped by an angel of God

- The apparent traumatization of Isaac from the almost sacrifice, possibly to the level of post-traumatic stress disorder
- Jacob's son Joseph becoming his favorite, exhibiting narcissistic characteristics as a teenager but also an ability to interpret prophetic dreams, thereby possibly qualifying for being a predecessor of Freud and the first psychiatrist
- Moses struggling with his self-esteem and anger
- The Jewish people's struggle to lose their slave mentality in their escape and journey from Egypt to the promised land of Israel, immortalized in the annual Passover service;
- Hearing the voice of God by several historical leaders, which nowadays might at first bring up the question of psychosis
- The golden rule of loving thy neighbor as thyself and its relevance to cultural competence in psychiatry, especially if you revise the rule a bit to not doing unto others as you would wish to be done to you, but doing to others as they would wish.

In these family vignettes, we see the need for a future of the interpretation of conflicts in dreams, family therapy, cultural competence, and the role of the Jewish religion in the well-being of the Jewish people. Moreover, the recommended way of studying the Torah is to look at the layers of meaning from the surface to the deeper, just as in psychodynamic psychotherapy.

Life lesson #5: Psychiatry and religion can overlap in a father and son.

Life lesson #6: The levels of interpretation in studying the Torah can correspond to the levels of psychodynamic interpretation in psychiatry.

Clinical Considerations

For a field with an initial overrepresentation of Jewish psychiatrists, as well as a long history of psychological mindedness on the part of Jewish people, one would expect to find literature on modern Jewish mental health. However, there is actually a paucity of relevant research. Moreover, though Jews as a whole have embraced psychotherapy as a helpful service, shame and stigma seemed to surround more severe mental illness, substance abuse, domestic violence, and incest.

With this relative lack of research about Judaism and psychiatry, most of what is known was put together by an expert on religion and psychiatry, Harold Koenig, MD. Here is a synopsis of what he found and concluded [6]:

- Jews, particularly those in Israel and those from the Orthodox branches, frequently use religion to positively cope with life stressors.
- Jews in the United States and Canada, particularly the less Orthodox, experience more depressive symptoms and clinical depression than non-Jews, perhaps since they tend to not cover it up with alcohol.
- There seems to be lower suicide rates and attempts in Jewish people.

- The more traditionally religious Jews, most apparently in Israel, seem to have greater anxiety, especially of the obsessive-compulsive nature.
- With the terrorism more common in Israel than elsewhere, post-traumatic growth was significantly higher in the more religious Jews.
- Substance abuse seems to be generally lower in Jews.
- Jews in the United States tend to see mental health clinicians more often and still tend to be more likely to be mental health professionals themselves.
- A careful spiritual history should be taken as part of an evaluation of all Jewish patients and if religion is important in their lives, to try to integrate that into treatment, including involvement and consultation with their rabbis.

However, it should be noted that what is not addressed in this review of Judaism and mental health is any mention of the psychological effects of anti-Semitism. One might assume that the more a Jewish person is confronted with anti-Semitism, the higher the anxiety and, at extreme, the development of post-traumatic stress disorders.

Also not covered are the most seriously ill mental disorders, such as bipolar disorder and schizophrenia. Those may be the most stigmatized illnesses and hence less available for research study.

On the more humorous diagnostic side is a Jewishly oriented diagnostic classification, called *The Diagnostic Manual of Mishegas*, DSOM [16]. This is a culturally congruent parody of the American Psychiatric Association's DSM and bases the manual on Mishegas, a Yiddish word for troubles or craziness. Some of these "Jewish" disorders are nervous conditions of everyday life and tsuris addiction. Tsuris refers to worries. Humor can often be a positive coping mechanism for low levels of stress and uncertainty, as in the saying "laugh to keep from crying." Jewish comedy and comedians were numerous in the United States after the Holocaust [17].

There is also a more colloquial diagnostic term applied to Jews, called the "self-hating Jew." In other words, this term could refer to a Jewish anti-Semite. The term can be traced back to the modern Zionist desire to return to Israel, led by Theodore Herzl [18]. He called his opponents "disguised anti-Semites of Jewish origin." "Self-hating Jews" came to be applied to academics opposing Zionism, that is, the return to Israel. Currently, the term is most often applied to liberal Jews who support the BDS (boycott/divest/sanction) movement against Israel. A prominent anti-Semitism scholar recommends that the term be abandoned [19].

Another internal Jewish perspective on anti-Semitism comes from occasional Orthodox clergy who view increasing anti-Semitism as a "wake-up call." This wake-up call is not to awareness of external danger but a message from God that Jews should be doing better regarding their covenant with God. That same sentiment was conveyed at times after the Holocaust.

In actual clinical practice, what matters most for any patient is the relationship with the therapist. Though each patient is an individual, cultural background is an influence [9]. Neglecting that can result in cultural incompetence and worse outcomes. Of course, the clinician has to know the cultural background of the patient to understand its influence in treatment. Ask the patients for their connection to any culture and the associated values. If choices of clinician are available, ask if the patient has any cultural preference.

Problems are more likely at the cultural extremes, when the clinician is too different from the patient or too similar. The former makes understanding of the patient harder, whereas the latter can tend to lead to cultural assumptions which might not hold true. Depending on the clinician's own cultural background and history, countertransference needs ongoing monitoring [20].

There may even be some particular Jewish influence on the most common type of psychotherapy nowadays, cognitive behavioral therapy. This technique seems to have similarities to ancient Jewish teachings [21].

Life lesson #7: Jewish people differ in their mental health risks and care-seeking.

Life lesson #8: Jewish people can contribute to their own anti-Semitism.

Conclusions

There is a complex web of social, religious, and clinical signposts of anti-Semitism that any Jewish person and psychiatrist encounter in their lifetime. Understanding them can not only lead to better understanding of how to address anti-Semitism but perhaps how to reduce stigma in psychiatry. Such signposts should also remind us that anti-Semitism should always be kept in mind collectively, as I as an individual neglected to do for much of my life. Given that anti-Semitism of varying degrees of intensity can be uniquely traced back thousands of years, the resilience and ethical values that sustain the Jewish people are admirable and the coping mechanisms perhaps of use for other discriminated groups of people. Such recognition and use may thereby increase philo-Semitism.

Life lesson #9: Anti-Semitism is ultimately hatred of aspects of people that are disowned and then projected onto Jewish people as a universal scapegoat.

Life lesson #10: Psychiatry may have an important role in healing society of its group conflicts.

As I finish writing my second draft of this chapter, the media reports that two rockets were launched from the Gaza Strip toward Tel Aviv. I landed and took off from Tel Aviv only 2 weeks ago. Although I have never been close to a gun duel that cost Alexander Hamilton his life, there are other dangers for Jews today. And, as well, there are other opportunities for safety, peace, and achieving our ethical ideals. I will try to continue to do my part and avoid anything like a gun duel!

Each of us, psychiatrists or not, Jewish or not, has to find our own ways to reduce anti-Semitism and its harm not only to the Jewish people but all who may be scapegoated. We can do some of this work ourselves, but often our endeavors are enhanced by others. I had the particular benefit of having my wife be my Jewish muse for 50 years, lacing the pathway with gold. In times of challenge, she often conveys this Jewish saying:

Be strong, be strong, and let us strengthen one another.

References

1. Margolin E. A moderate approach to antisemitism. The Jerusalem Post. 2019 Jan 31. https://www.jpost.com/Magazine/A-moderate-approach-to-antisemitism-579313.
2. Frosh S. Hate and the 'Jewish science': Anti-Semitism, Nazism and psychoanalysis. London: Springer; 2015.
3. Kay B. Psychiatry's chosen people. The Walrus. 2017 Jan 19. https://thewalrus.ca/author/barbaa-kay.
4. Freud A, Strachey J (translater). The interpretation of dreams: the complete and definitive text. New York: Basic Books; 2010.
5. Philips A. Becoming Freud: the making of a psychoanalyst. New Haven: Yale University Press; 2016.
6. Koenig H. Judaism and mental health: Harold G. Norwalk, Connecticut: Koenig; 2017.
7. Lifton RJ. Witness to an extreme century: a memoir. New York: Free Press; 2011.
8. Moffic HS. Book review: witness to an extreme century: a memoir. Psychiatr Times. 2011;28(11):46–72.
9. Moffic HS, et al. Cultural psychiatry education during psychiatric residency. J Psychiatr Educ. 1988;12(2):90–101.
10. Gay P. Freud: a life for our time. New York: Norton; 1998. p. 448.
11. May U. Freud's beyond the pleasure principle: the end of psychoanalysis or its new beginning? Int Forum Psychoanal. 2013;22(4):208–16.
12. Clay R. Did you really just say that? Here's advice on how to confront microaggressions, whether you're a target, bystander or perpetrator. Monit Psychol. 2017;48(1):46.
13. Nuland S. Maimonides. New York: Schocken; 2008.
14. Plaut WG, editor. The Torah: a modern commentary. New York: Union of American Hebrew Congregations; 1981.
15. Schwartz B, et al. The recovery of Masada: a study in collective memory. Sociol Q. 1986;27(2):147–64.
16. Neugeboren J, Friedman M, Sederer L. The diagnostic manual of Mishegas DMOM. North Charleston: CreateSpace Independent Publishing Platform; 2013.
17. Dauber J. Jewish comedy: a serious history. New York: W.W. Norton & Co.; 2017.
18. Troy G. The Zionist ideas: visions for the Jewish homeland – then, now, tomorrow. Philadelphia: The Jewish Publication Society; 2018.
19. Lipstadt D. Antisemitism: here and now. New York: Schocken; 2019.
20. Traub-Werner D. A note on counter-transference and anti-Semitism. Can J Psychiatr. 1979;24(6):547–8.
21. Rosmarin D. Spirituality, religion, and cognitive-behavioral therapy: a guide for clinicians. New York: Guilford Press; 2018.

Anti-Semitism: A Christian Psychiatrist's Perspective

11

John R. Peteet

The past two millennia have seen untold injustice and cruelty perpetrated on Jews in the name of Jesus. What accounts for this, since Jesus was a Jew? In this chapter we consider the history of the fraught relationship between Christians and Jews, its theological dimensions, the psychological aspects of "Christian" anti-Semitism, and their clinical implications, before exploring constructive approaches to the worsening challenge of anti-Semitism today.

History

The chapter in this volume by Mary Boys describes the transformation of anti-Judaism into anti-Semitic attitudes toward Jews who rejected Jesus' claims to be the Messiah and subsequently killed him – a major justification for anti-Semitism over the centuries. In the Middle Ages, local rulers and church leaders restricted the access of Jews to most occupations; those who went into finance, one of the few fields open to them, were then depicted as insolent and greedy (this negative stereotype has been caricaturized in popular culture and perpetuates anti-Semitic attitudes in the mainstream). Christians conducted pogroms during the first crusade. Martin Luther called for burning synagogues, and his publication *On Jews and Their Lies* was cited by Nazi propagandists. Shakespeare contributed the character of Shylock, Wagner considered Jews corrupt, and Grimm featured them as villains in his fairy tales thus planting the seeds of anti-Semitism into the fertile minds of children. Discrimination against Jews in employment and membership in clubs, professions, and organizations was a prominent part of American life well into the twentieth century, and Jews continue to be vilified by "Christian" identity hate groups, whose

J. R. Peteet (✉)
Department of Psychiatry, Brigham and Women's Hospital, Boston, MA, USA
e-mail: jpeteet@partners.org

© Springer Nature Switzerland AG 2020　　　　　　　　　　　　　　　　　137
H. S. Moffic et al. (eds.), *Anti-Semitism and Psychiatry*,
https://doi.org/10.1007/978-3-030-37745-8_11

activities have recently been increasing [1], notably in the October 2018 attack on the Tree of Life synagogue in Pittsburgh.

Theology

While the Gospel of John is often singled out as referring to "the Jews" in a negative light, many passages in Luke and Acts also present Jewish rulers as primarily responsible for the death of Jesus [2]. 1 Thessalonians 1:14–16 continues the theme. While these verses played a significant role in forming Christian attitudes toward the Jews, scholars such as Krister Stendahl [3] have shed new light on their meaning in the context of their time – suggesting that Jesus was one of thousands of Jews and others the Roman Empire crucified as a deterrent against dissent, rather his being then a lone victim of Jewish hostility to the Son of God.

Other scriptures call into question the interpretation that the New Testament is anti-Jewish. For example, Jesus maintained he came to fulfill, and not to contravene the law, and grieved over Jerusalem "as a hen over her chicks." The Apostle Paul expressed a willingness to be damned if it somehow meant his fellow Jews could find salvation in Jesus.

A related theological question dividing Jews and Christians is whether the "new covenant" with God ushered in by Jesus supersedes and replaces the old covenant established with Abraham. David Novak has contrasted "hard" and "soft" supersessionalism [4], arguing that while the former prevents dialogue, the latter does not. A soft Christian supersessionist could see Jews as tenants in the first floor of a house, free to occupy the second or not, still having a place created by its maker. Conversely, a soft Jewish supersessionalism, unlike a hard one, does not need to identify Christianity with an idolatrous, pagan past superseded by the Torah. He further points out that both contemporary Christians and Jews descended from a "Hebraic monotheism" and as such share many commonalities, including a conviction that we should all be superseded by God in his final judgment.

Similar questions surround efforts to convert Jews to Christianity. Does being a Christian entail evangelizing Jews and is doing so anti-Semitic? While Judaism is not a proselytizing religion, Christians have generally felt a scriptural mandate to share (though not necessarily to impose) the "good news." Conservative and evangelical Christian denominations such as the Southern Baptists, Assemblies of God, and Lutheran Church-Missouri Synod have organized programs for reaching out to Jews, and Jews for Jesus, the largest single ministry of this type, founded in 1973 by Moishe Rosen, spent $15 million in 2008 to convert Jews to Christianity [5]. Several organizations such as Jews for Judaism and Outreach Judaism have arisen to counter these efforts. However, Messianic Judaism, which combines elements of Jewish and Christian traditions, exists in over 100 congregations in Israel, and data from the Pew Research Center show that, in 2013, 1.6 million American Jews also identified as Christians [6]. Most progressive and mainline Christian denominations, on the other hand, have pointed out that New Testament writers give Jews a special status as God's chosen people whom he has not forgotten and have proscribed proselytizing Jews as anti-Semitic. In 2015, 50 years after its *Nostra Aetate* statement officially condemned anti-Semitism, the Vatican's Commission for Religious Relations with the Jews released a statement saying that Catholics should not evangelize Jews. The same year, a group of Orthodox rabbis released a signed statement acknowledging that "Christianity is neither an accident nor an error, but the willed divine outcome and gift to the nations" [7].

Other contentious theological questions concern the Holy Land. Do Jews have a divine right to the land, and what does this mean for the rights of Palestinians living there? While many evangelical Christians have linked arms with Jews to support Israel through organizations such as the International Fellowship of Christians and Jews, others (both Christians and Jews) who have advocated for Palestinian rights have sometimes been accused of being anti-Semitic [8]. An adequate discussion of this issue is beyond the scope of this chapter.

Psychology

Several theories have been advanced to explain the intensity and the persistence of anti-Semitism. Freud, who experienced systematic discrimination by the Catholic establishment in Vienna and was eventually forced to leave by the Nazis, argued in *Totem and Taboo* for the importance of envy. "I venture to assert that jealousy of the people which declared itself the first-born, favourite child of God the Father, has not yet been surmounted among other peoples even today: it is as though they had thought there was truth in the claim" [9]. As further evidence he cites "the fact that the Gospels tell a story which is set among Jews, and in fact deals only with Jews." Conversely, both Freud and many contemporary Jews see Christians as forsaking monotheism for paganism.

Consistent with Freud's insight, one can see in Jewish-Christian relations a rivalry of siblings for a close relationship with the Father and a valued shared tradition, complicated by feelings of betrayal and the dynamic of projective identification, in which each side is tempted to react to what they perceive in the other. Historically, for example, Jews were confined to arenas such as finance and administration and then resented as "shrewd." Jews, for their part, can experience as hostile the efforts of well-meaning Christians to convert them to what they believe to be the one true faith.

Other chapter authors highlight the power of tribalism in Christianized Europe to otherize and scapegoat Jews. Some evidence also supports the theory of secondary anti-Semitism, according to which, for example, reminders of the German atrocities and the victims' suffering still evoke aversive feelings of guilt and thus increases a defensive anti-Semitism [10], as reflected in the quip "Germans will never forgive the Jews for Auschwitz." Finally, fundamentalist, authoritarian ways of coping have been shown by Pargament et al. [11] to be associated with greater religious prejudice such as anti-Semitism ("they killed our Lord").

In 2018, the Southern Poverty Law Center listed a record number of 1020 hate groups in the USA which malign or attack an entire class of people, typically on the basis of an immutable characteristic. Many, including the Ku Klux Klan, neo-Nazi, white nationalist/supremacist, racist skinhead, Christian Identity, and neo-Confederate groups, are virulently anti-Semitic. The Christian Identity movement (not affiliated with any Christian denomination), for example, developed in the early 1900s a white supremacist theology, notably among prison gangs, that only Aryan races were descended from Abraham, that Jews are a lower race descended from Satan, and that all non-whites will be exterminated or enslaved to serve the white race in the heavenly kingdom to come. A plausible explanation for the pervasiveness of anti-Semitism among hate groups is the appeal of a conspiracy to account for the failure of white nationalists who perceive themselves as disenfranchised to achieve domination in this life [12].

As Cooper-White [13] points out, Freud saw it as no accident that his new, persecuted religion of psychoanalysis was made up primarily of Jews, who brought to its early development "a long history of valuing intellectual work, a capacity to work from a position of marginalization (so that it was easier as social outcasts to also be intellectual outcasts), a rejection of mysticism in favor of abstraction (as in the refusal to depict G-d in images), and an emphasis on the ethical life" (p. 77). Freud's break with Jung, whom he had hoped would bring more widespread acceptance of psychoanalysis, has continued to influence the way that some Christians view the field. An example is the recent warning of a prominent evangelical regarding secular therapy, with its debt to Freud that "much of those disciplines are built on a faulty worldview and must be (at least partly) rejected" [14].

Clinical Implications

As Knafo [15] illustrates in her description of three psychodynamically treated patients, anti-Semitism may serve a range of complex defensive purposes, including compromise formations and restitutive functions. Consistent with Freud's theory, experience suggests that envy is prominent in the anti-Semitism of paranoid patients – for example, the illusion that successful Jewish colleagues somehow enjoy unfair advantages (a paranoid, conservative Catholic patient revealed to me his conviction that Jews were dating all of the attractive women he met.)

Historical contributions have particular relevance to the treatment of a patient by a clinician coming from another tradition. Many non-Jewish German successors to the Holocaust experience inter-generational shame and guilt [16]. The fact that the Holocaust took place in Christianized Europe left many deeply suspicious that Christianity had an anti-Semitic core and/or was motivated by an agenda of conversion. For example, Sloan has recently criticized Christian psychiatrists such as Koenig for inappropriately advocating the integration of (Christian) spirituality into treatment [17].

Conversely, although the anti-religious, naturalistic bias of early psychoanalysis has waned, Freud's well-known characterization of religion as pathological made many Christians suspicious of psychiatry as hostile to their religious faith. This is despite the claims of some such as David Bakun that Freud's technique of free association can be traced to roots in Jewish mysticism [18].

These dynamics influence the kinds of clinicians whom both conservative Christians and Orthodox Jews [19] trust to treat them and are reflected in the growing prevalence of the option for "Christian therapy" on health insurance menus in the USA.

Suspected or actual anti-Semitism can play an important role in transference and countertransference. Daniele Knafo [15] observes that most analysts are reluctant to engage anti-Semitism for countertransference reasons and cites her own early refusal to work with a blatantly anti-Semitic patient and her belated recognition of how the treatment of a self-hating Jewish patient elicited profound conflicts about her own Jewish identity. These considerations can also influence decisions about self-disclosure, as Ringel [20] discusses in her treatment as an Israeli American therapist of a Palestinian. In my own clinical practice, I have felt, at times, reluctant to identify as a Christian psychiatrist when first seeing a Jewish patient, both out of guilt for the historical contribution of Christians to anti-Semitism and out of fear of being suspected or blamed for this legacy.

Finally, the preferred virtues of therapists of different faiths can differ, influencing the direction of treatment in ways that are not explicitly acknowledged [21]. For example, Jews and Christians typically share commitments to altruism and love but differ in whether they believe forgiveness should be unconditional or framed within a context of reconciliation [22–24]. This has potential clinical relevance because some Christians in secular therapy have been shown to be sensitive to therapeutic goals of their therapists differing from their own, despite rating their personal characteristics quite favorably [25].

Ways Forward

What can be done to mitigate and overcome the historical and contemporary reality of Christian anti-Semitism? First, Christians can examine, confess, and try to redress their own contributions. In the wake of the Holocaust, several such initiatives have taken place, which have been intent on promoting interfaith dialogue. In 1947, the Seelisberg Conference explored the relationship of Christianity to anti-Semitism. Its ten points later became the basis for the International Council of Christians and Jews (ICCJ), an umbrella organization of 38 national Jewish-Christian organizations founded in 1987. In 1993 the ICCJ published *Jews and Christians in Search of a Common Religious Basis for Contributing Towards a Better World.*

In the 1960s, the Second Vatican Council issued the declaration *Nostra Aetate* ("In Our Time"), which officially rejects the charge of deicide; "decries hatred, persecution, displays of anti-Semitism directed against Jews at any time and by any one"; and calls for "mutual respect and knowledge" between Catholics and Jews. Pope Paul II, elected in 1978, went further, apologizing for past church sins and emphasizing that without Judaism, Christianity would not exist.

In 1991, the European Lutheran Commission on the Church and the Jewish People issued the Driebergen Declaration, which rejected the traditional Christian "teaching of contempt" toward Jews and Judaism, including the anti-Jewish writings of Martin Luther, and called for changes in church practice in the light of these insights. There is some evidence that such initiatives may be having an effect. A 2008 survey of American Christians by the Pew Forum on Religion and Public Life found that over 60% of most denominations believe that Jews will receive eternal life after death alongside Christians [26].

Members of Jewish communities have responded with their own initiatives. In 2000, rabbinical and academic leaders from different denominations issued a statement called Dabru Emet, "Speak the Truth," which acknowledged Christian attempts to improve interfaith relations and called on Jews to learn about and likewise affirm the positive changes. Its eight points on which Jews and Christians could base dialogue included "Jews and Christians worship the same God," "a new relationship between Jews and Christians will not weaken Jewish practice," and "Nazism was not a Christian phenomenon."

And in 2015, over 25 (and, since, over 60) prominent Orthodox rabbis from around the world signed the Orthodox Rabbinic Statement on Christianity, *To Do the Will of Our Father in Heaven: Toward a Partnership Between Jews and Christians*, initiated by the Center for Jewish-Christian Understanding and Cooperation (CJCUC) to encourage more partnership between Jews and Christians.

Second, having clarified where they agree and continue to differ, Christians and Jews can collaborate in areas that they share, such as human rights and social justice. The civil rights marches of Martin Luther King and Rabbi Abraham Heschel and the activities of the Greater Boston Interfaith Organization provide examples.

Third, where their differences are more about faith than about ethnicity, clinicians can come together around a concern for truth and the needs of patients. A good early example is Oskar Pfister, the Swiss pastor, analyst, and lifelong friend of Freud whose ability to see in Freud's passion for truth a religious, even godly basis for common ground and to demonstrate a generous acceptance of Freud as a person even when they disagreed openly. This was probably responsible for their rare and unbroken friendship.

Within the American Psychiatric Association (APA), the tradition of dialogue between religion and psychiatry has continued, with an annual lectureship named in his honor, and also in the faith and mental health partnership established in 2014 by Paul Summergrad, the Jewish then president of the APA, and a Baptist pastor to promote better mental health care within faith communities – diminishing the perception of many Christians that these fields as begun and dominated by secular if not atheist Jews are hostile to their faith. *Mental Health: A Guide for Faith Leaders* continues to find wide readership among clergy of various faiths.

APA workshops have also brought attention to the mental health needs of marginalized conservative Christian and Orthodox Jewish communities and in the process have brought together Christian and Jewish clinicians, whose understanding of one another and of their traditions grows in the process. Similar initiatives have also been launched by the Royal College of Psychiatrists (RCPsych) in the UK (i.e., through events organized by the RCPsych Specialist Interest Group in Religion and Spirituality).

Conclusion

The relationship between Christians and Jews is complicated both by diversity within each tradition [13, p. 78] and by tribalism which has contributed to centuries of injustice perpetrated on Jews. All clinicians can help to explore the roots of anti-Semitism in individual patients and work toward a greater understanding of diverse traditions, with the goal of mutual respect for their common relationship to a loving God and shared mission of improving the world.

References

1. https://yr.media/news/tracking-the-rise-of-anti-semitism/.
2. Levine A-J, Brettler MZ, editors. The annotated Jewish new testament. New York: Oxford University Press; 2011.
3. Boys MC. Turn it and turn it again: the vital contribution of Krister Stendahl to Jewish Christian relations. J Ecumenical Stud. 2016;51:281–94.
4. Novak D. Supersessionalism hard and soft. First Things. 2019;290:27–32.
5. https://web.archive.org/web/20090910201443/; http://jewsforjudaism.org/faq-quick-links-157.
6. http://www.pewresearch.org/fact-tank/2013/10/02/how-many-jews-are-there-in-the-united-states/.
7. https://www.christianitytoday.com/ct/2015/december-web-only/orthodox-rabbis-and-vatican-exchange-olive-branches.html.
8. https://www.counterpunch.org/2019/02/06/the-empathy-of-the-irish-for-palestinians-is-in-no-way-anti-semitic/.
9. Freud S. Moses and Monotheism. In: Strachey J, editor. Standard edition of the complete works of Sigmund Freud, vol. 23. London: The Hogarth Press; 1939/1964. p. 91.
10. Ongoing victim suffering increases prejudice: a case of secondary anti-Semitism. Psychol Sci. 2009;20:1443–47.
11. Pargament KI, Trevino K, Mahoney A. They killed our lord: the perception of Jews as desecrators of Christianity as a predictor of Anti-Semitism. J Sci Study Relig. 2007;46:143–58.
12. https://www.politicalresearch.org/2017/06/29/skin-in-the-game-how-antisemitism-animates-white-nationalism/.
13. Cooper-White P. Old and dirty gods: religion, Antisemitism and the origins of psychoanalysis. New York: Routledge; 2018.
14. Stetzer E. Mental illness and the Christian: scripture and science. Christianity Today. 2014 June 3. https://www.christianitytoday.com/edstetzer/2014/june/mental-illness-and-christian.html. Accessed 1 Jan 2019.
15. Knafo D. Anti-Semitism in the clinical setting: transference and countertransference dimensions. J Am Psychoanal Assoc. 1999;47:35–62.
16. Rothe K. Anti-semitism in Germany today and the intergenerational transmission of guilt and shame. Psychoanal Cult Soc. 2012;17:16–34.

17. Sloan RP, Bagiella E, VandeCreek L, Hover M, Casalone C, Jinpu Hirsch T, Hasan Y, Kreger R, Poulos P. Should physicians prescribe religious activities? N Engl J Med. 2000;342:1913–6.
18. Bakun D. Sigmund Freud and the Jewish mystical tradition. London: Free Association Press; 1990.
19. Schnall E. Multicultural counseling and the orthodox Jew. J Couns Dev. 2006;84:276–82.
20. Ringel S. To disclose or not to disclose: political conflicts in the countertransference. Smith Coll Stud Soc Work. 2002;72:347–8.
21. Peteet JR. What is the place of clinicians' religious or spiritual commitments in psychotherapy? A virtues based perspective. J Relig Health. 2014;53:1190–8.
22. Balkin RS, Freeman SJ, Lyman SR. Forgiveness, reconciliation, and *Mechila*: integrating the Jewish concept of forgiveness into clinical practice. Couns Values. 2009;53:153–60.
23. Fortune MM, Marshall JL. Forgiveness and abuse: Jewish and Christian reflections. New York/London: Routledge; 2002.
24. Drach M. Forgiving the unforgivable? Jewish insights into repentance and forgiveness. J Relig Abuse. 2003;4:74.
25. Cragun CL, Friedlander ML. Experiences of Christian clients in secular psychotherapy: a mixed-methods investigation. J Couns Psychol. 2012;59:379–91.
26. Many Americans say other faiths can lead to eternal life. Pew Forum on Religion and Public Life. Published 2008 Dec 18. https://www.pewforum.org/2008/12/18/many-americans-say-other-faiths-can-lead-toeternal-life/. Accessed January 2, 2020.

Anti-Semitism from a Hindu Psychiatric Perspective

12

Shridhar Sharma, Rama Rao Goginene, and H. Steven Moffic

Relatively little attention has been given to the interaction of Jews and Hindus over history, certainly when compared to the consideration given to relationships among Jews, Christians, and Muslims. Hinduism isn't even mentioned in the religious section of a recent long catalogue of policies to combat anti-Semitism [1]. As a result, there is a relative paucity of information about how Jews and Hindus have lived together over the years [2]. On the other hand, this may simply reflect the fact that Jews and Hindus have lived together harmoniously, with relatively little friction. There is no word for anti-Semitism in the Hindu language. Yet, Jews have lived among Hindus, and, as is known, anti-Semitism is even seen in countries like Japan where no or few Jews have ever lived [3]. It may be that the world can learn from any general Hindu philo-Semitism.

A Brief History of Jews in India

The major Jewish populations in India over at least 2000 years have settled primarily on the coasts [4]. They are not well known by the Jewish or Hindu public, let alone mental health professionals, and are therefore described in the following paragraphs. Notable is a lack of any anti-Semitism described in the interactions with their Hindu neighbors.

S. Sharma
Department of Psychiatry, National Academy of Medical Services & Sciences Institute of Human Behavior and Allied Sciences, Delhi, India
e-mail: sharma.shridhar@gmail.com

R. R. Goginene (✉)
Department of Psychiatry, Cooper University Hospital and Health System, Camden, NJ, USA
e-mail: rgoginenimd@yahoo.com

H. S. Moffic
Private Community Psychiatrist, Milwaukee, WI, USA
e-mail: rustevie@mac.com

© Springer Nature Switzerland AG 2020
H. S. Moffic et al. (eds.), *Anti-Semitism and Psychiatry*,
https://doi.org/10.1007/978-3-030-37745-8_12

The oldest of the Indian Jewish communities was in the erstwhile Cochin kingdom, situated at the southern tip of India. It started around 562 BCE. After the destruction of the Second Temple in Israel in the year 70 CE, there was an influx of exiled Jews. The earlier settlers recounted stories of settling in India during the time of King Solomon. It was after the death of King Solomon and the breakup of his kingdom that the dispersal of the lost tribes of Israel apparently began.

The Jewish community in the Cochin area was called Anjuvannam. Jews lived there peacefully for over a thousand years. In Mala, Thrissur district, and in neighboring areas, the Malabar Jews built a synagogue as well as a cemetery. There are at least seven existing synagogues in Kerala, although they no longer serve their original purpose. In recent years, there has been an increase in Jewish tours to India, particularly to this area.

The Nagercoil Jews arrived soon after the Common Era began. They came from the region of Syria. Most were merchants and tended to settle around the town of Thiruvithamcode. Their language skills were useful to the Travancore kings for trading. From the Jewish perspective, selecting Nagercoil as their place of settlement had to do with the town's salubrious climate and its significant Christian population. By the twentieth century, most of these Indian Jewish families had made their way to Cochin from where they eventually emigrated to Israel.

The Chennai Jews arrived in Madras during the sixteenth century. They were diamond traders and of Sephardic heritage, coming from Spain and Portugal. Although they spoke Ladino, a form of Judeo-Spanish, in India, they learned Tamil and spoke Judea-Malayalam.

The Jews of the Goa area were Portuguese Jews who fled after the commencement of the Inquisition in Portugal. This community consisted mainly of "New Christians" who were Jews historically and had converted under the duress of the Inquisition. This group was the target of heavy persecution with the start of the Gao Christian Inquisition, a Portuguese Catholic inquisition that took place between the sixteenth and nineteenth centuries to punish heresy against Christianity in Asia. It persecuted Hindus, Muslims, Bene Israels, New Christians, and the Judaizing Nasranis. Among others, a famed Sephardi Jewish physician, herbalist, and naturalist working in Goa was put on trial. While taking place in India, this Inquisition was not against Jews by Hindus, but by Christians against Jews and Hindus.

The Bene Israel date at least from 1768 when Yechezkel Rahabi wrote to a Dutch trading partner that there were many Jews in Maharatta province. He described two Jewish observances: recital of the Shema and the Shabbat day of rest. This group of Jews claimed that they were descended from 14 Jewish men and women who survived a shipwreck just south of Mumbai some 17–19 centuries previously. They built the largest synagogue in Asia outside of Israel in Pune, called the Ohel David Synagogue. Mumbai had a thriving Bene Israel community until the late 1950s when many emigrated to the fledging state of Israel. In Israel, they came to be known as the Hodi'im (Indians). The Bene Israel community has since risen to many positions of prominence in Israel.

Small groups of Jews in India trace their roots to the sons of Joseph in the Old Testament Torah. The Bnei Menashe means "sons of Manassah." They are an ethnolinguistic group living in India's northeastern border states of Manipur and Mizoram. This group claims ancestry to one of the ten lost tribes of Israel and adopted the practice of Judaism. Most of those who now identify as Bnei Menashe had converted to Christianity. Similarly, the small Telugu-speaking group, the Bene Ephraim, meaning "sons of Ephraim," claims ancestry from Joseph's other son, Ephraim. They observe about 450 ancient halakhic customs such as burying the dead, eating kosher animal meat, entering marriage under a chuppah, going through bar/bat mitzvahs, and using Hebrew words and sayings. They hope to find ancient Torah scrolls when the government conducts digs in the new capital for Andhra Pradesh state. Since 1981, they have practiced a modern form of Judaism.

Although India, like the United States, refused to accept many Jews who were trying to flee the Holocaust, that also seemed due more to the political reasons of Muslim opposition rather than any substantial Hindu anti-Semitism [5]. Since the creation of the modern state of Israel in 1948, the majority of former Indian Jews have made Aliyah to Israel, not to escape anti-Semitism, but to join their people in their ancestral homeland. Over 70,000 Jews now live in Israel, over 1% of Israel's total population. Of the remaining 5000 in India, the largest community is concentrated in the large city of Mumbai, formerly known as Bombay, where 3500 have remained from the over 30,000 Jews living there in the 1940s. The majority of Jews from the old British-Indian capital of Calcutta (Kolkata) have also migrated to Israel.

Though kept under wraps, the political relationship between the new states of Israel and India has been quite positive and now seems better than ever before. It is a measure of success that in spite of domestic political considerations, India has managed to strengthen its ties with Israel, while continuing to support the Palestinian cause, just as it has managed to strengthen its relations with the United States without weakening its relations with the Russian Federation.

Anti-Semitism in Modern Independent India

Sometimes it is thought that a terrorist attack that took place in Mumbai in 2009 was anti-Semitic. However, this attack on a Chabad House was not carried out by Hindus. The Chabad House was run by Chabad-Lubavitch emissaries Rabbi Gavriel Noach and Rivkah (Rivky) Holtzberg, who had moved to Mumbai in 2003 to serve the small local Jewish community. One or two terrorists took hostages and made demands of the Indian government. Indian commandos began a full-fledged assault on the Chabad House. Gunshots and grenade explosions were heard throughout the day. The terrorists were killed. So were the rabbi and his wife, as well as several other visiting Jews. The Holtzbergs' 2-year-old son, Moshe, was saved by his Indian nanny, Sandra Samuel. An Israeli air force plane transported the bodies of those killed to Israel. Also on the plane were Rivky's parents and their now-orphaned grandson, as well as Sandra Samuel, the Indian nanny who was deemed a heroine.

Despite what seems like historical philo-Semitism, there may be danger ahead in India. Newer polls indicate some increase in anti-Semitic feelings, up to 20% on the anti-Semitic global index, which is higher than many other countries [6]. Militant national Hinduism now promotes some bigotry and prejudice against Muslims, Christians, Dalits, and anybody, including Jews, who eats beef.

Why has there, thus far, or at least until recently, been relatively little anti-Semitism among Hindus in India? Gary Weiss, one of the major writers about this phenomenon, after spending 25 years visiting India, poses a possible explanation [7]. He attributes it to a long history of religious tolerance in India. Even so, he found that anti-Semitism as a concept has mystified Hindu Indians, as it did him to some degree. However, that explanation is open to criticism because of the long, intermittent conflict and bloodshed between Hindu Indians with Muslim Indians. Other reasons must be responsible. Interreligious conflicts and wars may be caused more by a quest for power than prejudice. The small number of Jews in India prevented any likelihood of their obtaining any significant political power.

Gandhi and Anti-Semitism

What about Gandhi? Gandhi was one of the world's greatest humanitarians, as his writings and actions so clearly reveal [8]. He could not be anti-Semitic, could he? Yet, often when the possibility that Hindu India was not anti-Semitic is brought up in informal conversation, his comments are brought up as a refutation. We conclude that no, he was not anti-Semitic, but a selection of his comments about – and to – Hitler and the Nazi regime could mistakenly lead one to conclude otherwise [9]. Instead, in continuing to advocate for passive resistance, he may have been naive about the extent of the German genocidal goals, as indeed Freud seemed as well as many other national leaders seemed to be.

Gandhi's viewpoint has importance because he led the modern emergence of an independent India from its colonization by Great Britain. He is still quite revered by many around the world. Moreover, given the coincidence in timing of the establishment of modern India, modern Israel, and the immediate aftermath of World War II, his comments on Nazi Germany and the Holocaust are pertinent, though not entirely clear. His emphasis on nonviolent resistance suggests what he thought Jews should or should not do:

> I would claim Germany as my home even as the tallest gentile German may, and challenge him to shoot me or cast me in the dungeon; I would refuse to be expelled or to submit to discriminating treatment.

Gandhi argued for passivity in civil resistance as he had done in other countries:

> Herr Hitler will bow before the courage which he has never yet experienced in any large measure in his dealings with men.

Gandhi went even further in his belief in nonviolence by saying:

> I can conceive the necessity of the immolation of hundreds, if not thousands, to appease the hunger of dictators…

On the other hand, he supported the German Jews' right to be treated as equal citizens in any country in which they lived. For this reason, he could see no reason for Jews having their own homeland. He argued, as indeed Theodore Herzl had made decades previously, that a Jewish demand for a national home would provide justification for subsequent banishment. It is interesting to speculate in which direction his views would have evolved; he might have been against Israel, but he expressed great sympathy and concern for the historical persecution of the Jews and called anti-Semitism "a remnant of barbarism."

Moreover, there are also many more comments that support of love and admiration of Gandhi for the Jews [10]:

> My attitude towards Jews is one of great sympathy. I am very much attracted to the Jew firstly, because of selfish motives since I have very many Jewish friends; secondly, for a far deeper one - they have got a wonderful spirit of cohesion… Moreover, they are a people with vision.

He went on in this exclusive interview, available in the JTS's historical archive, and posited a solution for anti-Semitism:

> The remedy? My ready is twofold. One is that those who profess to be Christians should learnt the virtue of toleration and charity, and the second, is for Jews to rid themselves of the causes for such reproach as may be justly laid at their door.

Perspectives of Hindu Immigrants to the United States

To try to supplement the limited information on Hinduism and anti-Semitism, the authors surveyed Indian immigrants, mainly Hindus but also Muslims, in the United States for their views on anti-Semitism. Here are their anonymous responses, along with our recommendation for formal future surveys of more Hindus in the United States, as well as adding on Hindus in Great Britain, Israel, and India, supplemented by Jews in India.

> Here are some of my thoughts – I believe so too that there is no Anti-Semitism in India or anti any-religion views that are deeply rooted in India. Hindus strongly believes in one God, the God that belongs to all humans. India has always respected all other human beings regardless of any differences. The positive feelings I have towards Jews usually are related

to sympathizing with sufferings that the Jewish community had in various parts of the world, including the Holocaust. I feel Hinduism has been a victim in a very similar way and there are historical facts supporting this… the number of Hindus who died due to aggressive views of others purely based on religious belief differences is very high and may exceed any other killings according to many estimates. This is where I feel that Jews and Hindus share a common bond that religious aggressiveness shouldn't, can't, and won't survive – united against Anti-Semitism! – a 35-year-old male immigrant.

I was trying to think, 'did I ever have any positive or negative feelings while I was in India?" but since I was too young to think critically about anything at the time, I wasn't aware what the general sense is but talking to my parents as well as my extended family in the recent times there is a sense of familiarity in terms of the repression since the British rule. The general sense that I get is that it's mostly positive and most people tend to side with the oppressed or suppressed group with sense of familiar feelings felt under British rule. Again I think I have very poor knowledge in this topic. – a 34-year-old 1.5 generation female immigrant.

I personally don't have many feelings towards the Jewish people (that aren't criticisms of Israel's policy itself). I've sometimes felt a kinship with Jews as an immigrant group with similar values as Indian immigrants, aka valuing family, career, and education. I've felt culturally closer to them than some of my other Caucasian friends or peers due to these similarities. Beyond this, I don't really have other thoughts. – a 30-year-old second-generation female Indian immigrant.

We are not Anti-Semitic. We have lots of Jewish friends. But we don't like the plight of Palestinians under Israel rule. – two Muslim Indian Americans in their 50s.

I am a psychiatrists and psychoanalyst, trained by many Jewish teachers and psychoanalysts. Many of my colleagues are of Jewish faith. They all took good care of me. So, my feelings may be contaminated with positive feelings. I have a lot of respect, and positive feelings about Jewish people and their faith. I can identify with them wanting a homeland. I do have to admit at times I feel bad about the Palestinian plight and get upset at Israeli leadership for Palestinian suffering. I can definitely say I have no Anti-Semitism. – a 61-year-old male Indian immigrant.

Despite the small number of responders, and only from America, they point to various factors involved in the evolving view of Hindus toward Jews. Among them:

- The plight of Palestinians in Israel may be beginning to produce some anti-Zionism concern, with the ensuing challenge of separating legitimate criticism of the Israeli government from masked anti-Semitism.
- There seems to be common familial and work values that may inhibit the development of anti-Semitism due to mutual identification.
- Both Hindus and Jews have suffered immensely from religious persecution and thereby should have mutual empathy and compassion.
- Any claims of not having any anti-Semitism likely need confirmation by an anti-bias test as it is known that such bias can be unconscious.
- Knowledge about any Hindu anti-Semitism is limited, just as the journalist Gary Weiss found [7].

Conclusions

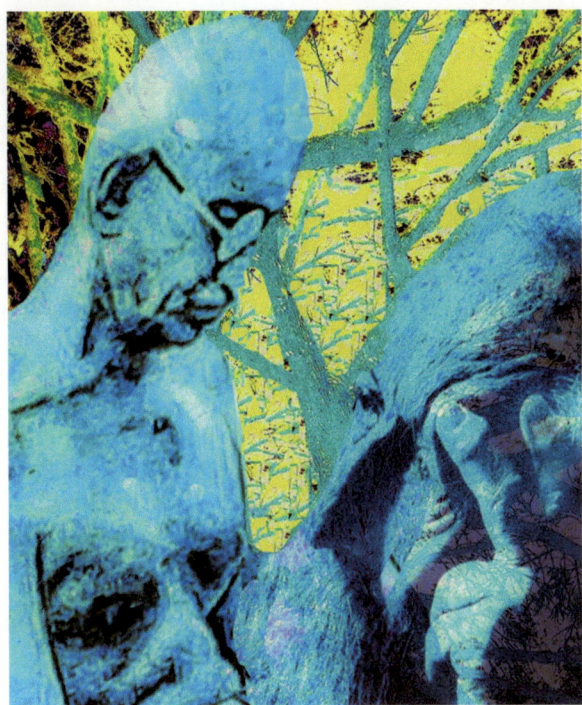

Judaism and Hinduism are rooted in respect for education and in cherishing the light that emerges from the darkness. Martin Buber and Mahatma Gandhi, depicted in this digital collage, see "eye to eye" as seekers and scholars reflecting upon the source of the tree of life. Image by Barry Marcus (barmar46@icloud.com).

For better or worse, information about the relationship between Hinduism and anti-Semitism is sparse. More historical study, updated research, and personal narratives are needed to flesh out what we already have. Nevertheless, the remarkable absence of any clear-cut anti-Semitism seems impressive and perhaps unique.

An analysis of the overlapping principles of the Jewish philosopher Martin Buber and Gandhi may explain some of this success [11]. Buber, who moved to Palestine in 1938, found his inspiration in Judaism, whereas Gandhi found his in Hinduism. Buber sought a fundamental transformation of practical I-It relationships to holier I-Thou relationships. Satyagraha offers a "soul force" for truth as an alternative to "brute force." Their philosophies thereby share a unity of spirit and a remarkable affinity.

This distinction does not necessarily suggest that Hinduism is a better religion, but that some aspects of its essence have led to more positive relationships with the Jewish people. Perhaps that essence also has something to do with the general Hindu belief in Brahman as an uncreated, eternal, transcendent, and all-embracing principle [12], which thereby does not favor or separate one people from another. Perhaps this is what Gandhi meant when he told Louis Fisher in 1942 [13]:

I am a Christian, and a Hindu, and a Muslim and a Jew.

However, there is concern about the recent rise of Hindu nationalism in India and its implications for the development of anti-Semitism [14], let alone its impact on Islamophobia and the well-being of Muslims in India. Perhaps this Hindu nationalism is not true to the essence of Hinduism, but it is nevertheless rising, as is India as a global power. Given that Nazi Germany was an extremely nationalistic state and that "white nationalism" is on the rise in the United States and Europe, whatever we can learn to reduce anti-Semitism is crucial.

We can speculate further why anti-Semitism has seemed to be virtually nonexistent in Hindu India over the centuries, but that question also needs more psychiatric analysis. There was apparently no historical Oedipal-like rivalry or competition between Hinduism and Judaism, the first major religions to emerge in what is often called the East and West, respectively. Both religions emphasized doing good deeds. More study might find other overlapping components in the two religions.

Given this philo-Semitic heritage of Hindus, it may be useful to develop more formal and informal interfaith interactions among Jews and Hindus wherever they co-exist. That can be a model for other Jewish interfaith relationships. One place to start is a potential coalition between Jewish and Hindu psychiatrists, perhaps called the Jew-Hindu psychiatric group to undo anti-Semitism.

This chapter and its authors may be a start in that direction.

References

1. Lange A, et al. An end to antisemitism!: a catalogue of policies to combat antisemitism. European Jewish Congress, 2018.
2. Katz N. Who are the Jews of India? Berkeley: California University Press; 2000.
3. Goodman D. Miyazawam: Jews in the Japanese mind. New York: Free Press; 2004.
4. Israel B. The Jews of India. New Delhi: Mosaic Books; 1998.
5. Aafreedi NJ. The impact of domestic politics on India's attitudes towards Israel and Jews. In: Singh P, Bhattacharya S, editors. Perspectives of West Africa: the evolving geopolitical discourses. Delhi: Shipra Publications; 2012.
6. Tausch A. The new global antisemitism: implications from the recent ADL-100 data. Middle East Rev Int Affairs. 2014;18(3):46–72.
7. Weiss G. India's Jews. Forbes. August 5th, 2007.
8. Gandhi MK. The selected works of Mahatma Gandhi, volumes one to five, translated from the original in Gujarati by M Desai. India: Navajivan Publishing House; 1968.
9. Tripath S. Gandhi and the Jews: should the Jews, as Gandhi counselled, have submitted willingly to their Nazi oppressors? Prospect Posted February 29, 2008.
10. JTA Historical Archive. Gandhi and the Jews. October 2, 1931.
11. Murti W. Buber's dialogue and Gandhi's Satyagraha. J Hist Ideas. 1968;29(4):605–13.
12. Doniger W, et al. Hinduism. Encyclopedia Britannica. Last updated June 26, 2019.
13. Fisher L. The life of Mahatma Gandhi. London; 1951. p. 360.
14. Truschke A. Anti-Semitism of Hindu nationalists made me a target of their attacks. India Abroad November 5, 2018.

Anti-Semitism: The Jungian Dilemma

13

Aryeh Maidenbaum

Introduction

If we have learned anything from the past, it is that even perfectly brilliant and cultured leaders and artists – individuals from whom we would expect more given their overall values and publicly pronounced thoughts on the need for a more ethical world – had extreme biases toward Jews. Over the centuries, just a few such examples have included Popes, Queen Isabella of Spain, and Martin Luther from the world of theology; noted poets and composers such as Ezra Pound, T.S. Eliot, and Richard Wagner; and business and political leaders like Henry Ford and Ernest Bevin among many others.

In the field of psychiatry and mental health, one of the luminaries accused of being anti-Semitic has been Carl Gustav Jung – at one point the designated heir of Sigmund Freud. The shadow of anti-Semitism cast over Jung's reputation has prevented many from delving deeper into the immense contributions his psychology and ideas have made – from the field of psychology, and psychoanalysis, to literature, theology, art, and history. Accusations against Jung is a topic I spent considerable time investigating, writing about, and presenting at international conferences on, which ultimately resulted in several articles and two books: *Lingering Shadows: Jungians, Freudians and Anti-Semitism* and *Jung and the Shadow of Anti-Semitism*, and a letter in the *New York Times* (5/21/88).

This is a topic that I had not wanted to investigate, about a man whose psychology and ideas have played a pivotal part in my own personal and professional development. I was raised in an Orthodox Jewish environment, spent many years in Israel, and earned my PhD at the Hebrew University of Jerusalem. To this day, Jewish history, culture, and tradition are a paramount aspect of the world in which I live. Moreover, professionally, I am a Jungian analyst, a trained diplomate in analytical psychology from the C.G. Jung Institute in Zurich, and founder and director

A. Maidenbaum (✉)
New York Center for Jungian Studies, New York, NY, USA
e-mail: amaidenbaum@gmail.com

© Springer Nature Switzerland AG 2020
H. S. Moffic et al. (eds.), *Anti-Semitism and Psychiatry*,
https://doi.org/10.1007/978-3-030-37745-8_13

of the New York Center for Jungian Studies. Furthermore, on a personal level, given my still active involvement in both the Jewish and Jungian worlds, writing about Jung and anti-Semitism is neither an easy nor a dispassionate task.

Was Jung an Anti-Semite?

My first indication that Jung's attitude and reputation toward Jews was an issue arose when the Hebrew University of Jerusalem awarded me a postdoctoral grant. When I announced that I intended to use it to study at the Jung Institute in Zurich, I was put on notice that this was not acceptable. One of the committee members insisted that Jung had not only been anti-Semitic but also been a Nazi. I soon learned this was a widely held view. Nevertheless, I was able to convince the committee – with the testimony of Dr. Rivkah Scharf Kluger and Zwi Werblowsky – that Jung was not personally anti-Semitic. Since both were highly respected academics and acknowledged experts in the field of Judaica, who had participated in programs at Eranos – an annual, inter-disciplinary conference in Switzerland where Jung played an active role – their firsthand support played a pivotal role in my application being approved. Ultimately, I was able to obtain the postdoctoral grant, spent several years in Zurich training at the C.G. Jung Institute, and was fortunately able to meet and study with the first generation of Jungian analysts who were connected with the institute.

The question of Jung being anti-Semitic lingered and kept resurfacing in public. It motivated me to delve deeper into Jung's personal relationship with Jews and Judaism and come to some understanding as to whether there was truth to this accusation. One of my mentors at the Jung Institute, knowing my involvement and commitment to the Jewish world, handed me a photocopy of a secret document limiting Jewish membership in the Analytical Psychology Club which was founded by Jung and composed of first- and second-generation Jungian analysts in Zurich who were disciples of Jung. This document was given to me in confidence, with the understanding that I was free to make it public but not reveal who gave it to me. These, and other factors, compelled me to continue exploring the disturbing allegation that Jung was an anti-Semite.

A Brief Biography of Jung

Carl Gustav Jung, MD (1875–1961), began his professional career at the Burgholzli Mental Hospital in Zurich – one of the leading psychiatric mental hospitals in Europe. Through the encouragement of his mentor, Dr. Eugen Bleuler (best remembered for defining and introducing the term, schizophrenia), Jung read Freud's groundbreaking book, *The Interpretation of Dreams*. Shortly afterward, he began a correspondence with Freud, which lasted until their break in 1912. The correspondence, punctuated by several powerful meetings between the two, which included a joint trip to the USA in 1909, led to a strong bond between Jung and Freud for the next decade.

Jung's exposure to the field of depth psychology came through his initial work in the realm of psychiatry – treating psychoses and working with institutionalized patients. During the course of his long and fruitful career, some of the many concepts for which he is best remembered include archetypes, the collective unconscious, the process of individuation, psychological types, synchronicity, shadow, animus and anima, and the role that complexes, symbols, and myths play in dream interpretation.

Though many in the field of "mainstream" psychology portray Jung as a mystic and philosopher rather than credit his work in the field of psychiatry and psychology, until their break, Jung was considered by Freud to be his "crown prince," his "heir apparent." In effect, at the time (the first decade of the twentieth century), Jung was considered among the leading Freudians in the world. Indeed, one of the basic tenets of psychoanalytic training originated with Jung's suggestion to Freud that analysts should themselves undergo a "training analysis." In short, Freud looked to Jung not only as his successor but also as one who would lead the psychoanalytic movement into the future and ultimately validate Freud's own work. In a letter dated January 19, 1909, Freud writes to Jung:

> We are certainly getting ahead; if I am Moses, then you are Joshua and we will take possession of the promised land of psychiatry, which I shall only be able to glimpse from afar. [1]

The fact that Jung was not Jewish was important to Freud, who was understandably concerned that his work would be dismissed as a Jewish psychology. Jung, in addition to being well placed in the field of mainstream psychiatry and the son of a Protestant pastor, represented credibility and acceptance – a position Freud himself clearly acknowledged to his early followers. In a letter to Karl Abraham as early as 1908, Freud stated:

> ...you are closer to my intellectual constitution because of racial kinship, while he [Jung] as a Christian and a pastor's son finds his way to me against great inner resistances. His association with us is the more valuable for that. [2]

As Sanford Drob has noted:

> Jung had been placed by Freud in the unenviable position of playing guarantor that psychoanalysis would not be looked on as a "Jewish national affair." [3]

Jung and Freud Part Ways

The break between Jung and Freud has been well recorded. To truly appreciate this more fully, it is important to understand the nature of their personal relationship – one that, psychologically, was clearly that of father-son. Additionally, perhaps another issue that lurked beneath the surface was the fact that many of Freud's (primarily Jewish) disciples resented Freud catapulting Jung into the leadership of this new and exciting movement. Here was this gentile, a stranger (someone to whom Freud referred to as, "not like us") from another country, Switzerland, being brought in and instantly promoted to "crown prince" of the movement. Freud's inner circle resented Jung and did not find it easy to relate to him personally. In turn, Jung felt alienated and snubbed, adding fuel to the fire of his need to break free of Freud, the father.

Following his break with Freud, Jung spent several years in withdrawal from professional activities and in deep contemplation. He referred to this period as the "dark night of his soul" with much of his inner turmoil revealed in his recently published *The Red Book*. During this incubation period, many of his ideas germinated; ultimately, he resurfaced and began to take his place in the wider world of psychoanalysis, though clearly disconnected from the mainstream Freudian-dominated world.

By 1933, well after Jung and Freud had ended their personal and professional relationship, Jung accepted the presidency of the General Medical Society for Psychotherapy. By then, Jung had, in effect, reversed roles with Freud and become the "outsider." Along with Adler (in 1911) and Stekel (in 1912), Jung was depicted as a traitor to the movement and marginalized by those close to Freud. Some of these men included Ernest Jones, Sandor Ferenczi, Otto Rank, Karl Abraham, and Max Eitingon, unofficial members of a "secret society" that had been proposed by Jones to protect Freud.

In effect, the decision by Jung to accept the presidency of the society at this time gave credibility to the rumors and accusations that Jung was anti-Semitic – even a Nazi sympathizer. Throughout his life, however, Jung steadfastly insisted that, by taking this honorary post, he could be of help to many of his German Jewish colleagues. In fact, Jung was responsible for having the society renamed (it became known as the International General Medical Society for Psychotherapy) and for permitting Jews, who were barred from the German national section, to join as individual members. This seemingly small change was quite an important distinction since, up until that time, one could only become a member through a local society – clearly eliminating all Jewish members.

Here the plot thickens, so to speak, as, in the December 1933 issue of the society's journal, the "Zentralblatt," an editorial was published praising Nazi ideology and using Jung's theories of archetypal, cultural patterns to justify the superiority of the Aryan race. These theories, some of which Jung admitted as his own to Dr. Sigmund Hurwitz (a Jewish colleague trained by Jung), were broad generalizations and not Jung's final words on the subject of collective psychologies [4]. They were taken out of context by the Nazis and over the years have come back to haunt Jungians. They were stereotypical in nature – ideas that Jung thought and theorized about and that pertained not only to Jews but also to American Indians, women, and other ethnic and racial collectives.

Both Jung and C.A. Meier, Jung's assistant and chief editor of the journal, insisted that this editorial had been inserted without Jung's or Meier's permission by

Dr. Matthias Göring (leader of institutional psychotherapy in Nazi Germany and cousin of the infamous Hermann Göring). During the course of my research, I personally interviewed Dr. Meier (an interview I have on tape and intend to donate to an appropriate archive) and was informed that Jung was not involved in any of the details of the journal's publications. Indeed, Meier took personal responsibility and told me that Jung had delegated the task of compiling and editing the journal to him since Jung did not want to be bothered by such tasks. According to both Jung and Meier, the editorial in question was written by Dr. Göring, and Jung's name had been inserted as author without the permission of either Meier or Jung.

In hindsight, it is clear that Meier and Jung should have written a second editorial in a subsequent issue renouncing the first and disassociating the society from its views – or resigned their posts. However, in my interview, Meier made it clear that Jung did not work on the journal at all and that Jung felt it was better simply to ignore the incident in order to avoid risking the breakup of the society. According to Meier, Jung felt that, under his leadership, the society was better able to protect some Jewish psychotherapists from Nazi persecution by including them in the reorganized international society. Meier, who was the first president of the Jung Institute in Zurich and closer to Jung than any other Jungian at the time, ascribes Jung's inaction to naivete and insists that one has to understand Jung in this light.

> Jung was naïve… particularly when it came to political things… He was always looking for the healing aspect of any disturbing neurosis or psychosis or whatever it be, and he always tried to help the patient or cure the patient… and so, he accepted this German movement as a disease, as the collective disease which maybe even had a chance to do something good to the German Nation… But of course, he was rather naïve…. [5]

Nevertheless, naivete alone cannot explain Jung's take on what was transpiring in Germany at the time. To do so is at best a rationalization and at worst willful ignorance. In this context, one cannot help but attribute Jung's motivation at the time to his own personal ambition. If seen in this context, it is not a far stretch to understand that Jung, caught in his own issue of feeling unappreciated by the psychoanalytical world, saw the presidency of the society as an opportunity to put his psychology and ideas foremost and center in the world of psychoanalysis. To my mind, based on interviews with many who knew and worked with him personally, he was not anti-Semitic, but rather a victim of his own grandiosity in believing he could easily handle Göring and the Nazi machine and promulgate his theories and ideas to a wider public. Jung's various political activities in the 1930s were no doubt some combination of good will, the need for ego gratification, and political naivete on a large plane. For, as Meier acknowledges, in that particular time in his life, he [Jung]:

> …suffered from the impression that he was not sufficiently accepted- his ideas were not sufficiently accepted in the world – so he had a sort of, a kind of minority complex in that respect and when the Germans started to condemn Freud he had a hope that maybe now, Jungian ideas may have a better chance…. [6]

But Jung's difficult relationship with Jews and Judaism went beyond that one editorial. In 1934, Jung himself wrote an article, "The State of Psychotherapy Today," which discussed the differences between what he called the Jewish psychology and the German psychology:

> The Jewish race as a whole [Jung wrote]… possesses an unconscious which can be compared with the 'Aryan' only with reserve. Creative individuals apart, the average Jew is far too conscious and differentiated to go about pregnant with the tensions of unborn futures. The "Aryan" unconscious has a higher potential than the Jewish; that is both the advantage and the disadvantage of a youthfulness not yet fully weaned from barbarism. [7]

Much in this article offended his Jewish followers, and other troubling writings followed during the 1930s. Nevertheless, while many Jewish Jungians were, and are, offended by Jung's insensitivity to the plight of Jews during that decade and disappointed by his failure to speak out against the Nazis, they generally do not consider Jung anti-Semitic on a personal level – especially given the many instances in which he helped Jewish people with money and other forms of support. Later in his life, Jung would tell Dr. Hurwitz (a good friend, observant Jew, and at one time Jung's dentist who ultimately became a Jungian analyst) that:

> I have written in my long life many books, and I have also written nonsense. Unfortunately, that [the 1934 article] was nonsense. [8]

Anti-Semitism and Psycho-analytical Society in the Era of Jung

During this same period, and for years afterward, Jewish quotas existed in leading universities of the USA, including Yale, Harvard, and Princeton. Somehow, this does not bother me as much as finding out that a quota existed in the Psychological Club fostered by Jung. The official policy of the club was to claim that this was solely the secret policy of the executive committee and that the club members were unaware of any quotas [9]. This was clearly not the case. Indeed, the reaction of several older club members with whom I spoke with was that an unwritten understanding among members limiting Jewish participation existed all along – a position that they justified as a means of protecting Jung should the Nazis invade Switzerland. The quota, however, was put in writing in 1944 and not rescinded until 1950, by which time the danger of Nazi invasion had well passed – a fact that casts doubt on this justification and paints a poor picture of some of the Jungian followers of Jung at that time.

One must, of course, place Jung and the Swiss Jungians within the culture of anti-Semitism that was pervasive in Europe at the time. European anti-Semitism depicted Jews as lacking spirituality and being by nature materialistic. Indeed, this stereotype not only made open hostility toward Jews acceptable but also gave it social respectability. This negative depiction of Jews was widespread and existed among varied layers of European society and the USA as well. It is not far-fetched to think that, at one time, Jung held similar views. Indeed, in Freud's *The History of the Psychoanalytic Movement*, Freud notes:

...He [Jung] seemed to give up certain racial prejudices which he had previously permitted himself. [10]

In any event, while Jung in all likelihood identified with a collective bias against Jews, from all the testimony of many Jewish colleagues, patients, and friends, he was not personally anti-Semitic. Indeed, the Jewish founders of the London, Los Angeles, and Tel Aviv Jungian societies were all disciples, analysands, and close colleagues of Jung. Aniela Jaffe, Jung's personal assistant and acknowledged co-author of Jung's autobiography, *Memories, Dreams, Reflections,* was a refugee from Germany and a committed Jew.

Nevertheless, and possibly due to Jung's personal issues with Freud and his Vienna followers (most of whom were Jewish), after his break with Freud, one could surmise that anti-Jewish sentiments resurfaced. "According to Freud, after the two parted ways, Freud accused him of anti-Semitism." Among the reasons listed by Jung as to why he broke with Freud was Freud's inability to tolerate dissent and his own inability to accept what he called Freud's "soulless materialism" [3]. Accusations of anti-Semitism against Jung still survive in the many and varied accounts of the reasons behind the Jung/Freud split.

Personal Reflections on the Accusation of Jung Being an Anti-Semite

What has troubled me personally has been the absence of a clear, distinct public statement by Jung dealing with his questionable pronouncements and actions during the 1930s. While he did disassociate himself from Nazism and by the late 1930s was writing scathing and incisive articles interpreting the mass hysteria that had taken hold in Germany, even in later years, he did not unequivocally express regrets regarding his own early naive attitudes. And, while Jung personally admitted to Rabbi Leo Baeck that he had "slipped up," he never said anything that would lead us to believe that he had come to terms with his own "Jewish shadow" issue of earlier years, for Jung's attitude toward Jews cannot be discerned either in his writings or in his public pronouncements. One could easily make the case that some of what Jung wrote about collective psychologies of different peoples – among them Jews – was not only ill timed but blatantly incorrect and biased. Jung himself referred to some of his earlier thoughts on a Jewish collective psychology as "nonsense." His closest collaborator for many years, C.A. Meier, in a personal conversation with me, attributed the failure to clarify this issue to Jung's "wooden-headed Swiss stubbornness" which always prevented him from admitting he was ever at fault.

To me, it is apparent that Jung underwent a personal change in his understanding of "the Jewish question." The Holocaust came as a harsh reminder to him of the dangers of his own as well as the collective's shadow. Nevertheless, he did himself, the Jungian community, and especially Jewish Jungians a huge disservice by not speaking or writing about the cloud surrounding his alleged anti-Semitism. Private statements, even to Jewish leaders, that he "slipped up" are not enough, and criticism of him in this context is deserved. As a result, Jung damaged his credibility and set back acceptance of his magnificent contributions to the field of depth psychology by picking an inappropriate moment in history to discuss the Jewish psyche or, as he put it, "cultural form." Nevertheless, notwithstanding his description of "Jewish collective psychology," one cannot accuse him of being personally anti-Semitic, an attitude that is defined as "a belief or behavior hostile toward Jews just because they are Jewish."

Conclusions

1. Jung was neither a Nazi sympathizer nor an anti-Semite as some have accused him of being.
2. Jung, as a consequence of accepting the presidency of the General Medical Society for Psychotherapy, was able to reorganize that predominantly Christian German group and enable German psychiatrists and psychotherapists to join a newly formed international organization, with Jung as president.
3. While Jung seems to have been initially genuinely taken by what he took to be a potentially positive resurgence in German nationalism during the early 1930s, he did, in fact, help many Jewish colleagues, both personally and professionally – throughout his life, including during the period when the Nazis were in power.
4. As part and parcel of his political activity in the international psychotherapy society, Jung had his own, opportunistic agenda: to promote his ideas and himself; this was ambition, not anti-Semitism. His interest was in seeing his own work and his own psychology and ideas, and in gaining widespread recognition.
5. Notwithstanding the shadow aspect of Jung's personal ambition, there are lingering shadows among Freudians and mainstream psychiatry in their accusations that Jung was an anti-Semite. In this context, there is an, perhaps unconscious, area where many Jungians and Freudians meet in resisting exploration of this topic. In Jungian terms, we might say that the collective shadow of Jung's followers lay in zealously protecting the man and his public image for fear of uncovering some faults. At the same time, it is just as clear that the Freudian shadow, so to speak, consists of keeping the emphasis on Jung the man, while just as strongly denying the importance of his psychology and ideas. There is no doubt that Jung was one of the giants and pioneers in the field of depth psychology. He would have been the first to point out that the message is more important than the messenger. In short, it has been easier to discredit the man than to deal with his psychology and ideas.
6. Jung himself said: "The greater the light, the greater the shadow." Jung, being indeed a "great light," had quite a large shadow, some of it revolving around his break with Freud as well as his attitude toward Jews – more on a larger, cultural level than on a personal one. As a result, Jung chose an inappropriate moment in history to discuss the Jewish psyche at a time when he still knew very little about

Jewish history, tradition, mysticism, or even – as he put it – "cultural form." This gap in his knowledge was something he corrected later as a result of his interest in Kabbalah, Hasidism, and the Jewish mystical tradition.

7. His complex and ambivalent attitude toward Jews was influenced by his personal experience with Freud's Vienna circle – many of whose members were Jewish.

I hope that this chapter will add to the information contained in my other writings on this complicated and nuanced subject [11].

References

1. Freud-Jung Letters. Princeton University Press, Bollingen Series; 1974, p. 197.
2. A Psychoanalytic Dialogue: The Letters of Sigmund Freud and Karl Abraham, referred to by Sherry J. The case of Jung's alleged anti-Semitism. In: Maidenbaum A and Martin SA, editors. Lingering shadows: Jungians, Freudians and anti-Semitism. Boston/London: Shambhala Publications; 1991, p. 120.
3. Drob SL. In: Maidenbaum A, editor. Jung and the shadow of anti-Semitism. Berwick: Nicolas Hays; 2002. p. 190.
4. Interview with Sigmund Hurwitz, Maidenbaum A. The shadows still linger. In: Maidenbaum A, editor. Jung and the shadow of anti-Semitism. Berwick: Nicolas Hays; 2002. p. 201.
5. Filmed Interview with C.A. Meier, Maidenbaum A. The shadows still linger. In: Maidenbaum A, editor. Jung and the shadow of anti-Semitism. Berwick: Nicolas Hays; 2002. p. 201.
6. Filmed interview with C.A. Meier, Maidenbaum A. The shadows still linger. In: Maidenbaum A, editor. Jung and the shadow of anti-Semitism. Berwick: Nicolas Hays; 2002. p. 202.
7. Appendix A. In: Maidenbaum A, editor. Jung and the shadow of anti-Semitism. Berwick: Nicolas Hays; 2002. p. 229.
8. Sigmund Hurwitz, filmed interview, quoted in Jung and the Shadow of anti-Semitism. Maidenbaum A, editor. Berwick: Nicolas Hays; 2002. p. 211.
9. Bernstein J. In: Maidenbaum A, Martin SA, editors. Lingering shadows: Jungians, Freudians and anti-Semitism. Boston/London: Shambhala Publications; 1991. p. 330.
10. Sherry J. The case of Jung's alleged anti-Semitism. In: Maidenbaum A, Martin SA, editors. Lingering shadows: Jungians, Freudians and anti-Semitism. Boston/London: Shambhala Publications; 1991. p. 120.
11. Maidenbaum A, editor. Jung and the shadow of anti-Semitism. Berwick: Nicolas-Hays; 2002; Maidenbaum A, Martin SA, editors. Lingering shadows: Jungians, Freudians and ani-Semitism; Boston/New York: Shambhala; 1991; Carl Jung and the question of anti-Semitism: struggling with the historical record. In: Jewish currents. Accord: Autumn; 2012.

Anti-Semitism: A Psychoanalytic Perspective

14

Andrew (Nachum) Klafter

The specific questions this chapter seeks to answer are the following:

- Do psychoanalytic theories offer any insight into the question of why Jews have so frequently become the object of fascination, hatred, and persecution throughout world history?
- When anti-Semitism erupts throughout an entire society or population, does psychoanalysis have anything to offer in explaining this phenomenon?
- Can anti-Semitism present itself in individual patients as a clinical symptom of psychopathology which can be treated with psychoanalytic therapy? If so, what is it a symptom of?

Case 1: Individual Patient

Mr. A was a 55-year-old man when he first came to see me for chronic unhappiness, anxiety, and feelings of resentment and anger. He was raised in a northeastern American city, had obtained an extensive education, and enjoyed a successful career. He was married, though not happily. He was superficially gregarious but reported having no real friends and no one whose company he genuinely enjoyed. After a year of productive psychotherapy treatment, he reported a dream to me: he said that I was flying an Israeli fighter plane while he was aboard the USS Liberty. (The USS Liberty was an American spy ship which conducted clandestine surveillance on Israel and its Arab enemies during the Six-Day War in June, 1967. Because the vessel bore no US flag or other markings, Israeli pilots mistook it for an enemy ship and attacked it, provoking a diplomatic crisis with their greatest ally and

A. (N.) Klafter (✉)
Cincinnati Psychoanalytic Institute and University of Cincinnati Residency Training Program, Cincinnati, OH, USA
e-mail: andrew@klafter.com

© Springer Nature Switzerland AG 2020
H. S. Moffic et al. (eds.), *Anti-Semitism and Psychiatry*,
https://doi.org/10.1007/978-3-030-37745-8_14

supporter.) "I am embarrassed to tell you that I have always been very uncomfortable around Jews." He shared that when he first met and saw my *yarmulke*, he nearly turned around to leave. "But I decided to stay. I have always been ashamed of being an anti-Semite, and I felt maybe this was a chance for me to get rid of this problem." He reported a long history during childhood and adolescence of brutal physical abuse and emotional intimidation by his volatile, alcoholic father. By contrast, "Jews indulge their children, and because of this, they become confident and assertive, like you." He pointed out the bar mitzvah ritual, where an entire synagogue congregation takes seriously the ideas and insights of a 13-year-old boy. He also cited the Passover Seder custom where young children are encouraged to ask questions about the reasons behind the festival's religious rituals. "You give your children so much power and attention." Jews, we discovered during in the course of his analytic psychotherapy treatment, had become a symbolic embodiment in his mind of the loving, supportive, and nurturing parent relationship which he had been deprived of, causing him to suffer from lifelong feelings of inadequacy and insecurity.

Case 2: Individual Patient

Mr. B has been in psychoanalytic treatment for the last 5 years. He was referred for a history of depression and suicidality since childhood, fear of humiliation and rejection by others, and fragile self-esteem. His fear of failure inhibited him from making any efforts toward professional or academic success and greatly interfered with his ability to form social or romantic relationships. There has been significant instability in his identity and belief systems. At different times, he has identified himself as a devout conservative Catholic, a Jehovah's Witness, a non-denominational born-again Christian, and a Muslim. He also shows shifts in his pattern of sexual preferences. During the first evaluation visit, he had for several months identified himself as a "neo-Nazi skinhead," and prior to this, he had affiliated with a chapter of the Ku Klux Klan. His parents are not racists and have long been horrified and puzzled by his attraction to hate groups. He stated he was not sure he would be willing to work with me, as a Jew. I recommended that we put this important question aside for the moment and simply proceed with an evaluation so I could offer him and his family recommendations for a treatment plan. Then, later, we would consider the question of whether I should be the person who works with him or whether he would prefer a therapist who is not Jewish. I made the diagnosis of borderline personality disorder and, at his request, spent a full appointment explaining to him and his parents what this meant and what the treatment would involve. Like many patients suffering from borderline personality, he had been previously misdiagnosed with many different disorders and started down several misguided treatment paths. Concluding that I am "a different kind of Jew," he stated his willingness to work with me. Over time, Mr. B and I have come to learn that his affiliation with extremist groups provides a sense of belonging. "They accept anyone as long as you accept their doctrines." We have also learned that he is attracted to groups which preach hatred toward others and who also incite hatred by others. Dehumanization of other ethnic groups gives him a sense of superiority, and being part of a group that is hated by others provides him with a rationalized group narrative which neutralizes his personal fear of humiliation and scrutiny: "If people hate me because we are preaching the truth, then I no longer feel like people are rejecting me because I'm a stupid loser." He now sees that his bigotry has served as a means to evade uncomfortable feelings of inadequacy and fears of rejection, and this awareness has led to both a relinquishing of racist beliefs and a recognition that many of the other members of the hate groups he has identified with are, themselves, suffering from psychological problems similar to his.

Case 3: Nations and Societies

Following World War I, Germany is ruled by the Weimar Republic, a democratic parliamentary government which passes the Weimar Constitution, granting equal rights to all Germans, including Jews. In fact, a Jewish industrialist and banker serves as Germany's foreign minister until 1922. In 1933, President Paul von Hindenburg needs the Nazi Party to join his weakened coalition and therefore appoints Adolf Hitler as chancellor as a concession. Through a series of ingenious and manipulative political maneuvers, Hitler obtains emergency powers and terminates the civil liberties guaranteed by the Weimar Constitution. German Jews are subject to a constant barrage of written racist propaganda, as well as hate speech at huge rallies and assemblies. Through anti-Semitic legislation passed between 1933 and 1938, Jews in Germany are shut out of all government positions, barred from the professions and academic posts, forbidden to marry Aryans, expelled from German schools, stripped of citizenship, dispossessed of property, and targeted by government policy for forced emigration. Next, they are subject to government-instigated violence, where marauding mobs of Germans burn synagogues, destroy Jewish businesses and property, and commit physical assaults and murders. Between 1938 and 1941, Germany annexes Austria and Czechoslovakia and then invades Poland, Denmark, the Netherlands, France, Belgium, Greece, Yugoslavia, the Baltic states, Belarus, Ukraine, and Russia. Jews under Nazi rule are ghettoized, stripped of all rights, dispossessed of property and citizenship, forced to wear identifying symbols, and subjected to random acts of brutality. Subsequent military occupations by Soviet and Nazi forces throughout Eastern Europe entirely destroy the legal and social institutions of those societies, creating lawless zones of chaos where no civilians are protected from violence or murder. In 1941, the systematic mass murder of Jews begins in Lithuania and quickly spreads to Latvia, Belarus, Ukraine, and Russia in carefully orchestrated mass shootings. Centers for industrialized killing are built, mostly in Poland, where the remaining ghettoized Jews under Nazi occupation are transported to be shot, gassed, or worked to death. Nearly 6,000,000 Jews are murdered, including 1,500,000 children. The degree of collaboration with or resistance against Nazi mass murder by non-Germans varies by region. Historians continue to debate the degree to which collaboration was willing or coerced, and

European society continues to reconcile itself two generations later with the legacy of mass murder of Jews and other civilians.

What Can Psychoanalysis Teach Us About History, Politics, and Religion?

Given the limited exposure among many general psychiatrists nowadays to psychoanalytic thought, a brief review may be helpful for most readers of this book before turning back to its specific relevance to anti-Semitism and a discussion of the case examples described above.

Psychoanalysis is a large and diverse set of psychological theories about (1) conscious and unconscious mental activity ("unconscious" means automatic and outside of the person's awareness), (2) personality, (3) human motivations, (4) interpersonal relationships, (5) normal and abnormal psychological development, (6) the etiology of certain mental disorders, and (7) the mechanisms by which psychotherapy treatments can re-catalyze healthy development in order to effect enduring and beneficial changes in the patient's subjective experience and objective social and occupational functioning. As a professional discipline, psychoanalysis is now about 120 years old. Like other disciplines, new observations challenge old theories, and familiar concepts are refined or discarded.

People whose main exposure to psychoanalysis has been as part of general courses in psychology have mostly learned about Sigmund Freud's early ideas about sexual conflicts and the Oedipus complex, his symbolic understanding of dreams, and his classification of mental functions as id, ego, and superego. As psychoanalytic thought evolved over time, analysts felt that sex and aggression, though powerful motivations in all people, just could not adequately explain the basis of all human behavior. They became divided into different schools of thought according to their views about human motivation and how psychotherapy works. "Ego psychologists" believed that most psychological problems are the result of inevitable conflicts between the person's instinctual wishes and his internalized values or moral beliefs. The goal of treatment, according to this approach, was to help people become less uncomfortable or anxious about their needs and desires and more effective in finding ways to gratify them within the framework of their responsibilities to others and the expectations of their social environments. Psychoanalysts who were influenced by "object relations theories" believed that our personalities and most of our emotional problems are shaped by how we have come to understand and feel about ourselves and others through our experiences in close relationships. According to the object relations school, the primary motivation in human beings is to be involved in intensive, loving relationships with others and to avoid their disruption or loss. "Self-psychologists" believed that the need to feel like a good, likeable, and significant person is the most powerful, central, and organizing concern for most people's motivations; conversely, they felt that most emotional problems are caused by the inability of people to regulate their self-esteem in response to narcissistic injuries (i.e., events which cause people to feel disliked, rejected, disrespected, incompetent, or insignificant). "Relational analysts" and "intersubjectivists," the most recent innovators in psychoanalytic theories, agreed with many of the ideas of object relations and self-psychology, but they felt it was important to emphasize that the processes by which change occurs during treatment are, at least in significant part, the result of the emotional impact of a new and unprecedented relationship between the therapist and the patient. They pointed out that the analyst is not an inert spectator, dispassionately examining the patient's individual mind; rather, the therapist and the patient are mutually influencing one another in profound ways, and that their relationship has more in common with other real-life relationships (parent-child, teacher-student, or close friends) than analysts had previously acknowledged.

A state of polarized disagreements between psychoanalysts who identified with these contrasting theories of the mind and approaches to treatment largely ended with the close of the twentieth century. Nowadays, most psychoanalysts would not identify with one particular psychoanalytic school or movement and would more likely say that they gain important insights and helpful treatment techniques from each approach. They draw from the ideas of each theoretical system, according to its relevance to each patient or for each clinical encounter. What all psychoanalytic approaches share in common is the following assertions:

1. Human motivations are more emotional than rational; people are driven by love, attachment, sexual pleasure, power, aggression, domination, wealth, fear, vanity, the pain of loneliness, the need to feel important, and the need to avoid shame and humiliation.
2. Knowledge that one's own motivations are tied to these very messy emotions is often distressing and uncomfortable, and therefore people may often be unaware that they are hurt, angry, attracted, falling in love, insulted, hateful, intimidated, ashamed, or embarrassed. They may even be unaware of what has triggered these powerful and sometimes unpleasant emotional experiences.
3. Early life experiences and relationships have long-lasting effects on a person's personality, interpersonal relationships, and general mental functioning, in both positive and problematic ways.
4. When psychological problems result from these emotional experiences, which are often at least to some degree outside of the person's awareness, psychoanalytic therapy offers special therapeutic techniques which can help relieve symptoms of mental distress and, more importantly, expand a person's emotional freedom to live his or her life the way he or she wishes to and believes in [1].

Although many psychoanalytic theories and treatment interventions have been validated by scientific research, psychoanalytic ideas are accepted by analysts largely due to their clinical usefulness as established by the consensus of the community of psychoanalytic practitioners. For example, a very important concept in psychoanalysis, referred to as "transference," is the observation that people experience themselves and others in stereotyped, repetitive ways that were originally established through their early relationships [2]. A child whose parents and older siblings are frequently annoyed at him may internalize this as a belief about of himself that he is inherently annoying, may frequently assume that others are annoyed with him, and may therefore feel rejected by others before he has even interacted with them. Even worse, this unpleasant "reality" (i.e., his internal sense that he is annoying and that others find him to be annoying) may cause him to be hypersensitive and defensive, which are traits that can truly be annoying. The patient may not have much insight into the fact that he feels and experiences people in this stereotyped and distorted way; it is simply what life has always been like for him and how he has always felt. If this patient begins psychotherapy treatment, an attuned psychotherapist would sense that he fears that the therapist will not find him interesting or that he feels like he is a burden and waste of the therapist's time and energy. The same theory of "transference" helps the therapist to develop a sense of how the patient's experience of others as being annoyed with him developed over time. The way this personality trait plays itself out in the therapy is understood by the therapist as an illustration of how this patient typically relates to people in his real-life relationships. Related psychoanalytic theories ("enactment," "countertransference," and "projective identification") predict that a patient who expects people to reject him may cope with these unpleasant feelings by acting aloof and uninterested in relationships or even by adopting critical and rejecting attitudes toward others. Even though this perpetuates his sense of isolation, it helps him feel safe from rejection. The therapist working with an aloof, hostile, rejecting patient will need to sort through a series of confusing, contentious interactions with the patient before understanding why the patient is acting like this.

All of the above has been scientifically validated through very sophisticated research studies conducted by a team of investigators at the University of Pennsylvania [3]. But, as mentioned above, psychoanalysts for the most part are not terribly interested in the scientific evidence confirming the theory of transference or the related theories of countertransference, enactment, and projective identification. They are convinced by the usefulness of these theories as a result of how it has been demonstrated in the course of their close work with patients during many thousands of psychotherapy sessions. Some psychologists and psychiatrists are uncomfortable with making use of clinical theories before they have been scientifically studied, and it is certainly easy to understand the sensibility of mental health providers who prefer to rely on "hard science." Nevertheless, the reality remains that psychoanalysts, by and large, accept theories based on whether they are practically helpful in their clinical work. In fact, most analysts do not even read the scientific psychological literature where controlled experiments examining the validity of psychoanalytic concepts and interventions are reported.

Taking psychoanalytic ideas out of the clinical setting and into the world of anthropology, religious studies, politics, literary interpretation, and history began with Sigmund Freud himself. "Applied psychoanalysis" is the term which now refers to the use of psychoanalytic concepts in nonclinical contexts. If we believe that all human beings are motivated by specific unconscious wishes, as well as the forces in the mind that aim to keep these unpleasant truths hidden from awareness, then we cannot help but speculate about the motives of characters in novels and films, as well as those of historical personalities. Freud authored a number of speculative essays on religion, morality, and history, some of the most famous being *Totem and Taboo, Moses and Monotheism, Civilization and Its Discontents*, and *The Future of an Illusion*. The plausibility of Freud's grand theories of religion and the history of civilization is seen by most contemporary scholars in those areas of the humanities as tenuous. But the application of psychoanalytic ideas to other disciplines has, over time, been extremely fruitful. Erik Erikson's *Young Man Luther* [4] was perhaps the first psychoanalytically oriented biography. Erich Fromm's *Escape from Freedom* is a psychoanalytically informed attempt to understand how the German people allowed their society to become overrun by a totalitarian regime [5]. Psychoanalysis has become an important perspective and resource for philosophers, literary critics, historians, and religious scholars.

The degree to which psychoanalysis can teach us about nonclinical topics is a fascinating and controversial question. Can we really reconstruct the unconscious motivations of historical figures based on information gleaned from their diaries, public speeches and writings, testimony of relatives and friends, and other artifacts that have caught the attention of historians? Psychiatrists and psychoanalysts have caused controversy in the past by offering their opinions about the emotional health or unconscious motivations of political candidates whom they've never examined [6]. It would be wise to proceed with caution when using psychoanalytic tools to assess the motivations of someone we do not know, have never assessed, cannot interview, and who has not come to our offices with an assurance of confidentiality and the motivation to be open and honest in order to receive relief from the suffering caused by psychological problems. In this spirit, I will attempt to present a contemporary and modest view of what I think psychoanalysis can and cannot offer in helping us understand the phenomenon of anti-Semitism.

Previous Attempts at a Psychoanalytic Understanding of Anti-Semitism

The psychoanalytic literature on anti-Semitism is vast. For example, a title search (conducted April 15, 2019) of the peer-reviewed psychoanalytic journals included in the Psychoanalytic Electronic Publishing (PEP) database for "anti-Semitism" or "antisemitism" yields 78 original psychoanalytic papers whose primary subject is a psychoanalytic understanding of hatred of Jews. An examination of the references in these papers reveals that there have been many hundreds of additional psychoanalytic contributions to this topic in books or journals which are not included in the PEP database. Nazism is overrepresented in this literature, probably due to the high numbers of European Jewish refugees among psychoanalytic authors, and the fact that the Holocaust was the most catastrophic chapter of persecution in Jewish history. Therefore, other historical contexts and more subtle expressions of anti-Semitism are not as well represented in this literature. Exploring anti-Semitism was not a theoretical or academic interest for many of these authors, but a burning (figuratively and literally) issue that needed to be addressed urgently. Some of these authors struggled to understand the Nazi madness as the towns they grew up in were being destroyed and as their loved ones were being murdered. For this reason, I have chosen to include publication dates as I review this literature in order to frame the historical context of each author's contributions, both in terms of their proximity to the Holocaust and their place in the evolution of psychoanalytic ideas. The following common themes emerge in this literature as important factors in understanding the causes of anti-Semitism: the primitive wish in all people during times of crisis for a scapegoat, projection of unwanted urges onto another ethnic group, the blood libel myth (i.e., the myth that Jews commit ritual murder of Christian children), the myth that Jews are "Christ killers," Jewish cultural and religious customs which project an air of superiority and may trigger resentment by gentiles, and the tendency to target a defenseless minority in order to gratify or displace aggressive impulses. I think it is worth mentioning that the quality of these contributions is very uneven; some propose ideas which are nuanced and plausible, but others, particularly earlier papers written from the perspective of sexual conflict theory, are unpersuasive and apply psychoanalytic concepts to entire societies or nations as though they were individual people. I observe a few psychoanalytic authors who, employing impressive literary sensitivity and interpretive skill, make use of Jewish historical events and biblical passages as metaphors for psychoanalytic ideas; although these papers are fascinating to read, a careful examination reveals that these contributions do not and cannot explain the origins or reasons for anti-Semitism as an actual phenomenon in any concrete, specific historical or cultural contexts [7, 8]. Finally, I am struck that very few psychoanalytic contributions identify anti-Semitism in individuals as a treatable phenomenon [9]; the current chapter is an attempt to help fill this gap.

A comprehensive review of all psychoanalytic ideas about anti-Semitism is beyond the scope of this chapter and would require its own book. I will instead highlight the contributions of several authors because of their merit, because they were landmark publications, or because they are representative of larger trends in the psychoanalytic literature on this subject.

Sigmund Freud's *Moses and Monotheism* is a lengthy, speculative monograph which makes provocative claims about the nature and ancient origins of Judaism. Anti-Semitism is not the main subject of this work, but Freud has a good deal to say about it. He sees in anti-Semitism evidence that the Jews are perceived by the world as the symbol of a punitive, rejecting father figure. The Jewish ritual of circumcision, in Freud's view, may cause "castration anxiety" (a classical psychoanalytic conception of guilt over sexual impulses) to become linked to Jews, thereby creating an association between Jews and feelings of dread and fear [10]. He attributes some animosity toward Jews to what he sees as real characteristics in many Jews which he believes were adapted for their survival, including stubbornness, resiliency, and their determined refusal to accept the religious tenets of Christianity [11]. He also attributes Christian anti-Semitism to a form of collective sibling rivalry and jealousy (i.e., Judaism being the "older brother" of Christianity and being God's "favorite child" as the "chosen people") [12]. Some of the assertions in *Moses and Monotheism* about the origins of Judaism have been appraised by modern scholars as trite, implausible, "uncomfortable," [13] and even "painfully absurd." [14] In a more balanced passage, Freud states: "A phenomenon of such intensity and permanence as the people's hatred of the Jews must of course have more than one ground." [15] Freud published this work in July, 1939, exiled in London after the Nazis had annexed Austria, just several weeks before the Germans invaded Poland on September 1, and only 2 months before his death on September 23. Freud makes explicit reference to the Nazi movement in this essay. His sisters were stranded in Europe under Nazi rule and would be murdered in 1941, as would countless of his friends, colleagues, students, former patients, and more distant relatives. Therefore, Freud's ideas on anti-Semitism and his provocative theories about the Jewish religion cannot be separated from the chaotic emotions he must have experienced in his anticipation of personal death and collective devastation.

Jean-Paul Sartre (1948), the French existentialist philosopher, though not a psychoanalyst by career or training, offered an influential psychoanalytic theory of anti-Semitism in his monograph, *Anti-Semite and Jew,* originally published in French as "Reflections on the Jewish Question." Sartre's understanding begins conceptually with the observation that anti-Semitism is not a logically derived ideology based on an empirical study of world events. Rather, it is a primitive passion, which throws the anti-Semite into a state of mind where he is willing to adopt values or beliefs that he knows, on some level, are untrue. In such a state, people convince themselves to accept falsehoods as truth because believing in them is emotionally appealing. The particular falsehood embraced by anti-Semites is to blame their economic and political problems on Jews, which leads them to propose expulsion or even extermination of the Jewish people as a solution to their misfortune. Sartre is obviously using the historical events leading to the Holocaust as his model. Sartre concludes with a postmodern critique of the idea of "Jewishness." One's identity as a Jew is determined by anti-Semites who will not allow him to assimilate and become a member of surrounding society. Anti-Semitism is not caused by any inherent, essential characteristics of Jews. Using contemporary terminology, we would say that Sartre argues that Jewishness is "socially constructed." What makes someone Jewish is simply that he is defined as "Jewish" by anti-Semites. Therefore, it is not Jewishness that provokes anti-Semitism, but anti-Semitism which creates Jews. If the Jews would no longer exist, anti-Semites would find a new group to hate and define them as "Jews." [16]

Fenichel (1940) was an original psychoanalytic thinker and influential writer. In the middle of World War II, though before mass killings had begun (and before most people imagined they would happen), he authored a nuanced and balanced assessment of anti-Semitism, in which he soberly notes the following:

Is the instinctual structure of the average man in Germany different in 1935 from what it was in 1925? Surely not. The psychological mass basis for antisemitism, whatever that may be, existed in 1925 too, but antisemitism was not a political force then. If one wishes to understand its rise during these ten years in Germany, one must ask what happened there during these ten years, not about the comparatively unaltered unconscious. [17]

In other words, the rise of a specific anti-Semitic historical movement cannot be accounted for by a change in the human psyche. To the contrary, according to Fenichel, what anti-Semitic movements teach us about the human psyche is the susceptibility to outrageous propaganda of ordinary people under conditions of poverty and crisis and the desirability of blaming a scapegoat for a nation's misfortune and vulnerability. Fenichel also points out that governments, in times of crisis, have an interest in providing the masses with a defenseless scapegoat which they can abuse in order to displace rage and blame more appropriately directed toward their own political leaders. Thus, persecution of Jews provided the German nation with a scapegoat and provided the Nazi government with an outlet for the people's frustration, which might have otherwise led to a violent revolution (as it had in Russia). He notes the vulnerability and defenselessness of the Jewish people to persecution and the long history of anti-Jewish sentiment in European culture, which have kept the Jews available for the "condensation [and displacement] of the most contradictory tendencies." [18] He identifies these contradictory tendencies as (1) the instinct for violent rebellion against authority and (2) the urge to cruelly punish the self for this forbidden desire to rebel. Fromm-Reichmann (1942), writing while Final Solution was being carried out, noted that, unlike other thinkers, Fenichel did not fall into the trap of trying to explain historical events and social change in large populations on the basis of individual psychodynamics [19].

Lennard (1947) [20] in the immediate aftermath of the Holocaust attempts to offer an expanded theory of how the Jew serves, for anti-Semites, as a symbolic embodiment of guilt and punishment, consistent with Freud's theory. He describes modern anti-Semitic myths (capitalism, socialism, control of the world's economies, etc.) as being updated versions of medieval myths about Jews as sorcerers with magical powers. Lennard does not address how or why the Jews became the objects of these myths. Similarly, Lennard suggests that the Jewish ritual of circumcision may have accounted for the myth of Jewish ritual murder of Christian children, though the evidence for this hypothesis is lacking. Despite its methodological flaws, Lennard's paper is noteworthy for his identification of an important feature of anti-Semitism which is difficult to explain and neglected by most other analytic authors, namely, that Jews have been dehumanized by portraying them as demonic and Satanic in anti-Semitic propaganda [21, 22].

A. Brenner (1948), in the same time period, cites numerous biblical passages and historical events in an attempt to support his overarching thesis that the Jews serve as a symbolic embodiment of unwanted unconscious conflicts, which he describes in theoretical, classical psychoanalytic terms [23]. What this lengthy paper lacks, in my opinion, is plausible evidence that his literary and historical insights can account for historical anti-Semitism. As mentioned above, this tendency to use biblical proof-texts and isolated historical events without the guidance of historians and experts in religious studies is a common shortcoming among some analytic authors.

Schoenfeld (1966) describes two trends in psychoanalytic attempts to understand anti-Semitism: (1) anti-Semitic beliefs as signs or symptoms of emotional disorders and (2) Jewish behavior as inviting or provoking anti-Semitism. He cites the ideas of dozens of analytic thinkers and notes that there is no consensus on the psychological origins of anti-Semitism. Schoenfeld, in my judgment, gives more credibility than most other authors to Jewish provocation [24]. He suggests that certain Jewish religious rituals, including the dietary laws and purity laws, may convey an air of exclusivity and superiority which triggers resentment among non-Jews. He cites Ernest Jones (1951) in identifying a Jewish "superiority complex in respect to brain power" (i.e., a Jewish sense of being more intelligent than others) [25]. Other analysts observe that hostile reactions to arrogance are so predictable that what passes as arrogance may be better understood as a masochistic, unconscious but purposeful triggering of anti-Semitism [26].

Székely (1988) describes the analytic treatment of several patients with anti-Semitic prejudices. He sees in all forms of anti-Semitism a belief in secret societies and a mystical belief that these secret societies of Jews wield magical powers that control the world. He attributes such beliefs to infantile fantasies about secret powers and magical abilities [27].

Rubin (1990) published a psychoanalytic book [28] on anti-Semitism which was reviewed by Remen [29]. In addition to many themes also explored by other psychoanalytic authors, Rubin offers another interpretation which I believe is unique: he claims that the anti-Semite's most guarded secret is that he secretly wishes to become a Jew. He also includes a chapter on Jewish self-hatred as a form of anti-Semitism [30].

Kestenberg and Brenner (1996), in their fascinating book, *The Last Witness: The Child Survivor of the Holocaust*, propose a novel theory for Nazi aggression toward the Jews. Citing psychoanalytic case-histories from the treatment of the children of Nazi officers and leaders, they report that these children frequently believed or fantasized that they were in fact Jews who had been kidnapped from Jewish families during the Holocaust and that their German parents hated them and wanted to kill them. Kestenberg and Brenner suggest that Nazism functioned as an extreme projection of unwanted weakness and vulnerability. Projection of vulnerability is often expressed in stoic cultures as a hatred for children, who are in fact weak and vulnerable. But in the case of the historical circumstances of the Nazi movement, it was displaced instead onto the vulnerable and defenseless population of European Jews [31]. Consistent with this theory, Rosenman (1998) claims that anti-Semitism seems to rear its head in social contexts where there is brutal, abusive parenting. For example, the blood libel myth of ritual murder occurs in the context of a *murdered child*. Rosenman sees child abuse and brutality to children as key factors in the cultivation of hatred of Jews [32].

Ostow (1996) summarizes the findings of a distinguished psychoanalytic study group composed on analysts and historians about the origins of anti-Semitism, which is noteworthy for collaboration with experts from other disciplines. The analysts in this group note that they have had very few anti-Semitic patients in treatment over the course of their careers. Studying the phenomenon of anti-Semitism historically, the group traced the development of Christian anti-Semitic propaganda from the first century through the medieval period and observed the following features: the deicide of Jesus; images of Jews as unclean, sexually perverse, and financially corrupt; and blood libels. Modern propaganda identified by this group includes the following: *The Protocols of the Elders of Zion*; Shylock in Shakespeare's *The Merchant of Venice*; Nazi racial ideology portraying the Jews as threats to the survival of humanity; Islamic literature in which the Jews as the source of "cosmic evil;" and highly biased criticism of Zionism and Israel that in their view can only be explained by hatred of Jews. He also notes that the blood libel myth is still alive in contemporary times. What all of these myths have in common is that Jews are to blame for most of suffering and evil in the world. Ostow notes the impact of these anti-Semitic myths on the psyche; he states that anti-Semitic myths have shaped apocalyptic, fundamentalist, millenarian movements (including Nazism), which justify persecution of the Jews as punishment for the evil they have wrought [33].

In a paper titled, "What if anything can be done about my anti-Semitism?," Young (2003) describes his lifelong attempt to rid himself of the racism and anti-Semitism he was raised with and shares his psychoanalytic and common sense interpretations of a wide range of relevant political, economic, religious, and historical issues. Young is certainly not what any of us would consider to be an anti-Semite. He is clearly very comfortable around Jews, has a cultivated rich personal and professional relationships with Jews, is married a Jewish woman, writes glowingly of the Jewish children raised as Jews, and articulates a strong set of moral arguments against anti-Semitism. (With anti-Semites like this, who needs friends?!) What remains is perhaps a latent discomfort and tension over an automatic tendency to think of Jews as inferior which he was indoctrinated with during his childhood and a persistent awareness of cultural and ethnic alienation. Young emphasizes that even people who demonstrate real virtue in many aspects of their lives nevertheless can harbor racist attitudes and beliefs [34].

Kressel (2007) investigates the recent intensification of anti-Semitism in Arab and Muslim societies. He attributes it to four factors: (1) anti-Semitic elements of Muslim religious history and theology; (2) political and economic frustration, leading to scapegoating; (3) socialization of hate ideologies in contemporary Muslim societies; and (4) the political context of the Israeli-Arab conflict [35]. This paper is a good illustration of how contemporary psychoanalysts recognize the limitations of psychoanalytic theories. To analyze historical and cultural trends, analysts must turn to the tools and expertise of religious studies, anthropology, sociology, and history.

Böhm (2010) traces how primitive mechanisms, present in all individuals, can grow into various forms of hostility, including racist and xenophobic ideologies. This process is shaped by a fundamentalist belief system in absolute truths which cannot be questioned and a preference for purity and simplicity over complexity and messiness. An "alienated self " results from deficient nurturing during early childhood. Primitive and infantile myths which were internalized in later childhood without subsequent reflection or refinement easily become prejudices about specific ethnic groups. Such beliefs further toxify the alienated self, resulting in a xenophobic preference for one's own race or ethnicity and envious resentment of others. He identifies specific historical factors that have encouraged the emergence of myths about Jews: the Jewish concept of being the "chosen people," collective blame for the murder of Jesus, the blood libel myth, religious indoctrination with perverse ideologies which justify racism and persecution, regression to more primitive states when individual identity is subservient to a group, and authoritarian political systems which undermine the individual rights and dignity of specific minority populations [36]. Thus, Böhm identifies anti-Semitism as a cause, more than a symptom, of psychopathology.

A Contemporary and Integrative Psychoanalytic Understanding of Anti-Semitism

1. Do psychoanalytic theories offer any insight into the question of why Jews have so frequently been the object of fascination, hatred, and persecution throughout world history?

One feature of Jewish history, which to my knowledge of world history is unique to the Jewish people, is that since the Roman conquest of the Second Jewish Commonwealth in the year 70 CE (or perhaps a better starting point is the Babylonian exile in 586 BCE), Jews have been scattered throughout the Western Hemisphere in tiny communities as a distinct, ethnic minority group. Not only have the Jews been vulnerable and defenseless in these communities, but they have often been conspicuous. The reasons for this are varied: they dressed in distinctive and identifying clothing (usually by choice, but occasionally by coercion); they rejected conversion and resisted assimilation into the surrounding, majority religious cultures; for their own cultural and religious reasons, they established insular neighborhoods or enclaves; they resisted intermarriage and often limited social contact with their gentile neighbors; and they spoke and wrote in their own primary languages (Yiddish, Ladino, and Aramaic), making meaningful social relationships difficult or impossible for most non-Jews. In some cultures and historical contexts, Jews achieved disproportionate professional, political, economic success and social prominence. This became particularly pronounced in liberal democracies after the Enlightenment. Whether this was due to a cultural predilection for education and professional training or an average IQ among Jews significantly higher than most other populations [37–39], what resulted is that in nearly every Western society since the High Middle Ages through contemporary times, Jews became conspicuously identifiable and remained vulnerable. (In my mother's words, "We may be only 2% of the population in America, but we seem to be the 2% that you notice.")

Achieving disproportionate influence and success was at least one impetus for the development of conspiracy theories that branded the Jews as scapegoats. Myths developed and circulated about Jews committing ritual murders of Christian children, controlling world finances, and spreading the black plague. Their refusal to accept Jesus as a Prophet, Messiah, Son of God led to the church doctrine of the "inveterate obduracy of the Jews" (the stubborn refusal to accept faith in Jesus), which both motivated and fomented persecution. This background of myths and conspiratorial preoccupation with Jews was fertile ground for anti-Semitism.

The refusal by the Jews under Islam to accept Mohammed as the Seal of the Prophets and their faithfulness to their religious norms led to a more nuanced form of anti-Semitism under Islam. A few depictions of Jews as apes and swine in the

Quran and other sacred Islamic texts are not representative of Islam's view of Judaism. Because the Jews were monotheists and preserved prophetic scriptures which Mohammed and his followers recognized as legitimate (albeit "corrupted") revelations, Islam granted Jews a protected, second-class citizenship. It is true that on rare occasions, fanatical Islamic movements subjected the Jews to religious persecution, forced conversion, expulsion, and genocide. However, for most of Judaism's 2600 years under Arab rule and 1400 years under Islam, the Jews were protected from discrimination and violence, owned property, operated businesses, established synagogues, operated religious Jewish schools and academies to train rabbis, and were granted autonomy to appoint their own communal leaders and judges. During many periods, Jews were appointed to powerful government positions under Arab and Islamic rule and flourished economically, intellectually, religiously, and politically. 1400 years of Jewish life under Islam came crashing to an end after the establishment of the State of Israel in 1947, at which time anti-Semitism erupted throughout the Islamic world. In the next three decades, about 900,000 Jews fled or were expelled from Muslim nations. I submit that it is unnecessary to invoke psychoanalytic theory to understand Islamic anti-Semitism. It is well explained on the basis of religious, cultural, political, and military history.

Certainly, there are other ethnic groups who have suffered genocide, slavery, discrimination, expulsion, economic exploitation, religious persecution, and other forms of racial injustice. There are certainly unique aspects to the Holocaust, including the of targeting an entire ethnic group for extermination and the construction of elaborate industrial complexes devoted to mass murder, which included murdering Jewish babies. But would anyone claim that the Cambodian genocide, the Soviet starvation policies of 1932–1933 in the Ukraine, or the African slave trade were "less" atrocious? What is different (not worse or more severe) about the persecution of the Jews is the duration of Jewish vulnerability as members of defenseless communities in a large diaspora for 2600 years over such a vast cultural and geographic expanse. Therefore, "why the Jews?" seems to be a question that can be best explained by historians, religious scholars, and political scientists. Anti-Semitism became a fact of Western culture, but not a fact of the human mind. Psychoanalysis helps us understand the dark, violent urges inside human beings that are expressed openly when social conditions allow it. These conditions include civil wars, violent revolutions, and apocalyptic religious movements, which have led to horrific episodes of anti-Semitism, among other forms of racial persecution. But how and why these conditions come about is a question of history, not psychoanalysis.

2. When anti-Semitism erupts throughout an entire society or population, does psychoanalysis have anything to offer in explaining this phenomenon?

A few psychoanalytic theorists posit aggression as a secondary, rather than primary, instinct [40, 41]. In other words, this subset of analysts sees anger, hostility, rage, violence, and other expressions of aggression as phenomena which occur only in response to an injury or stressor. But the majority of psychoanalytic thinkers view aggression as a primary and basic instinct in all human beings which seeks expression even under normal, peaceful circumstances [42, 43]. The urge to attack, dominate, harm, or kill is ubiquitous in every culture and requires containment in every society. No group has ever been able to create a community without violence. Normal childhood development includes fights and violence. Over the course of development, children are required by their caregivers to learn to contain their aggressive impulses. In healthy individuals, creative outlets allow for the channeling of aggression into socially acceptable activities, athletics being a good example. Even purely intellectual endeavors can serve as a battleground for competition, such as grades in school, chess competitions, political debates, or legal disputes. Most societies need militaries to protect the country. Even during war, under normal circumstances, there are rules and laws. Nations do not expect their enemies to torture and murder captured soldiers. But, of course, the scenarios I have described above, not uncommonly, can devolve into aggressive violence. Fights break out on the baseball field, fans riot during soccer matches, soldiers rape and murder civilians, and prisoners of war are in fact tortured and murdered.

What is it that causes civilization to break down? One factor identified by psychoanalysis is the regression of individuals when they are in groups [44]. Paradoxically, groups seem to confer "permission" to individuals to commit aggressive acts they never would have performed while alone. Although "peer pressure" may be one factor, more central to the hypothesis of group regression is the fact that people surrender their autonomy and sense of morality. It is easier for a group to commit a crime than it is for an individual, because, while part of a group, one's sense of responsibility has been dissipated among group members or given over to the group leader. Observers of the Nuremberg trials were shocked to hear the common refrain, "I was just following orders." At the time, many simply considered this to be a weak excuse for their culpability in crimes against humanity. But it is also true that "just following orders" is an actual psychological mechanism which can help explain how deviant acts are committed by normal people when their individual selves have dissolved into the identity of a group.

Milgram [45] conducted a series of famous experiments where subjects were repeatedly instructed to inflict pain on others. He showed that normal, civilized human beings under relatively benign circumstances can be persuaded with no actual coercion by an authority figure to perform acts of aggression which are contrary to their morality. In fact, he demonstrated that the individuals being instructed to "continue the experiment" were in fact in great distress over the pain they were being instructed to inflict. But most nevertheless complied with those instructions. Milgram also demonstrated how proximity to or distance from the victim had an effect on the percentage of subjects willing to continue shocking people who were pleading with them to stop, which brings us to another important factor: dehumanization. When perpetrators of racial persecution have been indoctrinated with myths and propaganda that undermine the very humanity of their victims, additional restraints on the aggressive instinct are lifted [45].

In studying the Holocaust, analysts can learn a great deal about the factors that allowed this horrible chapter of destructive violence to unfold. The historian, Timothy Snyder [46], has demonstrated that the geographic regions where the mass killings took place during the Holocaust were the nations situated between the Soviet Union and Germany [46]. As mentioned above in Case 3, those societies had been utterly devastated, with no rule of law, no protection for civilians, dismantled courts, no functional police – nothing. Paradoxically, the murder of 1.5 million Jewish children did not occur and could not have occurred, in Germany, where there was still an intact (albeit totalitarian) society with intact institutions. The German public would never have tolerated it. In Central and Western Europe, where societies were still intact, Jews were deported onto trains and transported to the stateless zones of death and destruction, where mass murder was possible. What psychoanalysis has learned from the history of the Holocaust is that civilizing the human being not only requires a humane upbringing and the cultivation of an intact personality structure but also requires the continuity of an intact civilization. When the structure of civilization breaks down, the moral structure of the individual breaks down as well.

3. Does anti-Semitism present as a symptom of psychopathology, which can be treated by psychoanalytic therapy? If so, what is it a symptom of?

The two patients presented at the opening of this chapter both, at the time of their original presentations, harbored many anti-Semitic beliefs and feelings. They both endorsed many negative and inaccurate stereotypes about Jews. They felt uncomfortable around Jews and would claim that, generally speaking, they did not like people who are Jewish. Upon careful investigation, both in fact had positive experiences and good relationships with numerous Jews. Mr. A had been involved romantically with Jewish women, for whom he still felt affection. He had many Jewish clients whom he appreciated and hired Jewish professionals whom he admired. Mr. B had Jewish teachers in school whom he respected and felt were kind to him. He also had known family friends who were Jewish, about whom he had positive feelings. Mr. B would later also become deeply attached to me, as his analyst. Both of these men explained away their positive experiences with Jews as "exceptions," rationalizing that each of the Jewish individuals for whom they felt positive regard were "atypical" or "not like most other Jews."

To hold onto an irrational belief despite evidence against it should be seen as a symptom of psychopathology. This is all the more so true for a belief that is not endorsed by the majority of people in one's culture. In particular, Mr. A wanted help getting rid of his anti-Semitic feelings. From a psychoanalytic perspective, we wish to know what emotional discomfort would be provoked if this belief were relinquished. Why is it so important to hold onto these stereotypes and prejudices? The answer to this question will always be unique for each individual person. As mentioned above, Mr. A felt envious of the assertiveness and confidence he believed Jews are endowed with through their religious culture and upbringing. Mr. B's anti-Semitism was a price he paid for the sense of belonging that was provided by his fellow, neo-Nazi skinheads.

Mr. A's hatred of Jews helped him avoid feeling his own sense of weakness, passivity, and insecurity. His father, a bigot, held racist beliefs about many different groups, including, but not limited to, Jews. Mr. A later revealed that he also harbored prejudices against blacks, Italians, Irish, Indians, Muslims, and Latinos. There was virtually no group for which his White Anglo-Saxon Protestant father did not harbor significant antipathy, and he realized that he had absorbed much of this. As the therapy unfolded, Mr. A revealed that he felt like he had been a great disappointed to his father. His father wanted an athletic, self-assured, macho son. Mr. A was bookish, sensitive, hated sports, and excelled in his studies. During the beatings he endured, which lasted into his late adolescence, he sensed that his father was testing to see if he had finally grown into a real man. "But I never did. It was always humiliating and painful, and it always made me cry." His jealousy and resentment of Jews and their confidence gave way during the therapy to rage at his father for abusing him. He ended therapy saying, "I will never feel normal around Jews, but at least I know now that I'm the crazy one and they simply love their children."

Mr. B's was not raised to be a racist. His family members were deeply disturbed by his affiliation with hate groups. His wandering from one group to another has continued. He abandoned his neo-Nazi affiliation and then joined another extremist Christian group. Most recently he has expressed interest in becoming an Orthodox Jew. Dream material and free association have allowed the two of us to realize that his interest in conversion to Judaism represents both a fantasy that he might join my family and also a fear that I am going to reject him by telling him he is not allowed to become a Jew. For people unfamiliar with psychoanalytic treatment, fantasies like this may sound psychotic, but Mr. B is fully aware that these are only fantasies and retains full insight into this as he shares this material. Over the course of the therapy, Mr. B has shared many anti-Semitic jokes with me. Recently, he said, "Hey Dr. Klafter, I just found out that my grandfather died in Auschwitz... [pause]. He fell out of a guard tower!" I actually found this to be funny and laughed. As I considered with him the deeper meaning of this joke, I offered to him my interpretation that it expresses both his wish to be part of my family (relative "died in Auschwitz") and also his disavowal of his wish to be part of my family (grandfather was a Nazi) because he fears he will be rejected.

I believe that both of these cases illustrate how in fact anti-Semitism and other forms of racism can be understood as symptoms of specific forms of psychopathology and that in some individuals these problems can be treated. Prejudice allows narcissistic patients with fragile self-esteem to blame their disappointments or failures on others and to cultivate a sense of superiority. In cases of trauma, victims of abuse sometimes absorb the beliefs and abusive patterns of their tormentors. Prejudice can also function in the mechanism of splitting seen in borderline personality pathology as it provides a basis for devaluation and dehumanization. Freud, Fenichel, Lennard, and A. Brenner all identify specific "projections" of unwanted parts of the self, which they believe anti-Semites see in Jews. What is problematic about their hypotheses is that they proposed for all anti-Semites very specific conflicts and emotional problems. While it is certainly true that racists project unwanted parts of themselves onto the objects of their prejudice, it is each person's individual and unique psychological conflicts which determine what will be projected.

On an individual basis, a psychoanalyst can discover how specific issues and emotional problems have led to the development of racist beliefs, including anti-Semitism. Jews, for the reasons mentioned above, are easy and frequent targets for racism and prejudice. The successful treatment of whatever underlying emotional conflicts have influenced the development of a racist or anti-Semitic schema should give the patient greater emotional freedom, allowing him to address his actual problems and vulnerabilities and no longer need to resort to prejudice or discrimination as a means of regulating a fragile sense of self.

References

1. Wallerstein RS. Psychoanalysis: the common ground. Int J Psychoanal. 1990;71:3–20.
2. Joseph B. Transference: the total situation. Int J Psychoanal. 1985;66:447–54.
3. Luborsky L, Crits-Christoph P. Understanding transference: the core conflictual relationship theme method. 2nd ed. Washington, DC: American Psychological Association; 1998.
4. Erikson EH. Young man Luther: a study in psychoanalysis and history. New York: Norton; 1993.
5. Fromm, Erich H. Escape from freedom. Holt Publishers, 1941. New York
6. Kohut H, Anderson AR, Moore BE. A statement on the use of psychiatric opinions in the political realm by the American Psychoanalytic Association. Bull Am Psychoanal Assoc. 1965;21:450–1.
7. Stein HF. The binding of the son: psychoanalytic reflections on the symbiosis of anti-Semitism and anti-Gentilism. Psychoanal Q. 1977;46:650–83.
8. Weill TL. Anti-Semitism: selected psychodynamic insights. Am J Psychoanal. 1981;41(2):139–48.
9. Ackerman NW, Jahoda M. Anti-Semitism and emotional disorder: a psychoanalytic interpretation. New York: Harper; 1950.
10. Freud S. Moses and Monotheism: three essays. The standard edition of the complete psychological works of Sigmund Freud, Volume XXIII (1937–1939): Moses and Monotheism, an outline of psycho-analysis and other works, 1–138; 1939. See p. 87–92.
11. Freud S. Moses and Monotheism. p. 105–106.
12. Freud S. Moses and Monotheism. p. 91.
13. Morpurco VE. Why does Moses and Monotheism still make us uneasy? Freud, psychoanalysis anti-Semitism. Italy Psychoanal Annu. 2007;1:203–20.
14. Williams R. Freudian psychology. In: Richardson A, Bowden J, editors. A new dictionary of Christian theology. London: SCM Press; 1983. p. 220.
15. Freud S. Moses and Monotheism. p. 90.
16. Sartre J-P. Anti-Semite and Jew. New York: Schocken Books; 1948.
17. Fenichel O. Psychoanalysis of Antisemitism. Am Imago. 1940;1B(2):25.
18. Fenichel O. p. 31.
19. Fromm-Reichmann F. Psychoanalysis of antisemitism: Otto Fenichel. Amer. Imago, I, 1940, pp. 25–39. Psychoanal Q. 1942;11:130.
20. Lennard HL. The Jew as symbol. Psychoanal Q. 1947;16:33–8.
21. Trachtenberg J. The devil and the Jews. New Haven: Yale University Press; 1943.
22. Smith DN. The social construction of enemies: Jews and the representation of evil. Sociol Theory. 1996;14(3):203–40.
23. Brenner AB. Some psychoanalytic speculations on anti-Semitism. Psychoanal Rev. 1948;35(1):20–32.
24. Schoenfeld CG. Psychoanalysis and anti-Semitism. Psychoanal Rev. 1966;53A(1):24–37.

25. Jones E. The psychology of the Jewish question. In: Essays in applied psychoanalysis, vol. 1. London: Hogarth; 1951.
26. Simmel E. Anti-Semitism: a social disease. New York: International University Press; 1946.
27. Székely L. Tradition and infantile fantasy in the shape of modern antisemitism. Scand Psychoanal Rev. 1988;11(2):160–77.
28. Rubin TI. Antisemitism: a disease of the mind. Lanham: Barricade Books; 2010 (Reprint, first release 1990).
29. Remen S. Anti-Semitism: a disease of the mind, by Theodore Isaac Rubin, MD. Am J Psychoanal. 1991;51(1):83–6.
30. Rubin TI. p. 91–94.
31. Kestenberg JS, Brenner I. The last witness: the child survivor of the Holocaust. Washington, DC: American Psychiatric Press; 1996.
32. Rosenman S. A critique of classical psychoanalytic theories of anti-Semitism: a commentary on M. Ostrows myth and madness: the psychodynamics of anti-Semitism. Am J Psychoanal. 1998;58(4):417–33.
33. Ostow M. Myth and madness: a report of a psychoanalytic study of antisemitism. Int J Psychoanal. 1996;77:15–31.
34. Young RM. What, if anything, can be done about my anti-Semitism? Free Assoc. 2003;10(3):360–81.
35. Kressel NJ. Mass hatred in the Muslim and Arab world: the neglected problem of anti-Semitism. Int J Appl Psychoanal Stud. 2007;4(3):197–215.
36. Böhm T. On the dynamics of xenophobic prejudices: with antisemitism as an illustration. Scand Psychoanal Rev. 2010;33(1):32–9.
37. Entine J. Abraham's children: race, identity, and the DNA of the chosen people. New York: Grand Central Publishing; 2007 (Published October 24, 2007).
38. Lynn R, Longley D. On the high intelligence and cognitive achievements of Jews in Britain. Intelligence. 2006;34(6):541–7.
39. Cochran G, Hardy J, Harpending H. Natural history of Ashkenazi intelligence. J Biosoc Sci. 2006;38:659–93.
40. Kohut H. Thoughts on narcissism and narcissistic rage. Psychoanal Study Child. 1972;27:360–400.
41. Posner BM, Glickman RW, Taylor EC, Canfield J, Cyr F. In search of Winnicott's aggression. Psychoanal Study Child. 2001;56:171–90.
42. Arlow JA. Perspectives on aggression in human adaptation. Psychoanal Q. 1973;42:178–84.
43. Meerloo JA. Human violence versus animal aggression. Psychoanal Rev. 1968;55(1):37–56.
44. Mitscherlich A. Group psychology and the analysis of the ego—a lifetime later. Psychoanal Q. 1978;47:1–23.
45. Milgram S. Obedience to authority: an experimental view. New York: Harper & Row; 1974.
46. Snyder T. Black earth: the Holocaust as history and warning. New York: Tim Duggan Books; 2015.

Part III

Specific Clinical Challenges

Jewish Stereotypes in Psychiatric Diagnosis and Treatment

15

Kate Miriam Loewenthal and Barry Marcus

Introduction

I was once told that a social worker, watching Jewish boys praying in school, remarked on the fact that they were swaying backwards and forwards. This is culturally normative behaviour for boys in a cheder or Jewish school: the swaying is believed to aid concentration in prayer. Unaware of its religious roots, the social worker saw it as a sign of a culturally specific psychological disturbance. This points to the problem of the culturally naive observer who sees normative behaviour and misjudges it as pathology. Mislabelling can increase the risk of psychiatric disturbance [1].

Attending a conference on mental health some years ago, and chatting to one of the other attenders, I said that I was doing research on mental health in the Jewish community. "Aha" they said, "That would be OCD!" My colleague was convinced that "all those religious rules and regulations" must predispose Jews, especially the religiously observant, to obsessionality.

This incident set me thinking. What is the evidence with respect to Jews and the prevalence of obsessive-compulsive disorder (OCD)? Does Jewish religious observance and OCD frequently co-occur? And supposing Jews, especially religious Jews, are stereotyped as more prone to OCD than others, could this influence the accuracy of any diagnoses they are given or the effectiveness of any treatments they receive? And are there other stereotypes regarding Jewish mental illnesses?

This chapter will look at hypotheses and evidence regarding Jews and psychological disorders and consider implications for diagnosis and treatment. I will look at mood disorders, psychosis, alcohol use and abuse, OCD and scrupulosity,

K. M. Loewenthal (✉)
Department of Psychology, Royal Holloway, University of London, Egham, UK
e-mail: c.loewenthal@rhul.ac.uk

B. Marcus
Bainbridge Island, WA, USA
e-mail: Barmar46@icloud.com

stereotypes of Jewish women, eating disorders and some other stereotypes. Some stereotypes may result from subtly or blatantly anti-Semitic motives.

Stereotypes of Psychological Disturbances Among Jews

The first stereotype that I would like to examine, that Jews are more prone to **mood disorders** than people from other social-cultural groups, has a basis in reasonable scientific findings [2, 3]. Careful examination of epidemiological data has shown that Jewish *men* are more likely than men from most other groups to suffer from major depressive disorder. There were no noteworthy differences in the prevalence of depression for Jewish women compared to other women. A close examination of the data suggests that this effect is largely – possibly solely – the result of a culturally carried norm among Jews against the recreational use of alcohol [4]. Where recreational alcohol use does take place, generally among the less religiously observant, Jewish men show a similar prevalence of depression to men in other groups [5]. Although Jews form a relatively inbred community, the low prevalence of alcoholism in Jews is not explained by genetic intolerance to alcohol (as in many Asians and indeed present in a minority of Jews) but rather in an association of alcohol with religious rites and a cultural tradition that opposes drunkenness [4, 6].

It has also been noted that Jewish men may be more willing than men from Protestant backgrounds to disclose/discuss symptoms of depression [7], perhaps because, from a historical perspective, they have always had much to be depressed about. This may also help to account for the relatively high prevalence of depression among Jewish men in epidemiological studies.

There have been suspicions that Jews may be more susceptible to bipolar disorder, which is highly heritable, than people from other ancestral groups, but this does not appear to be a major or robust effect, and references to it have largely disappeared from the scientific literature. Recently, however, as more genome-wide studies are being conducted, there is evidence that Ashkenazi Jews are more likely than others to possess genetic variations that may or may not predispose to heritable psychiatric syndromes such as bipolar disorder or schizophrenia. One example has been found in a cerebellar gene [8], but many others are likely to come to light. Their significance at present is difficult to assess. Ashkenazi Jews, because of inbreeding over the years, are more prone than the general population to a number of diseases.

I saw a striking example on a website [9] that was clearly anti-Semitic. A heading on this website stated "Jews have 112 genetic/hereditary diseases" followed by the assertion that "these are not rare diseases, most Jews have them". The list starts with AIDS, and sodomy, and includes [among other conditions] "DEPRESSION, NEUROSES Afflict Primarily Jews". The list is considerably shorter than 112 items [there are 18], and most of the conditions listed are not psychiatric, and the list is followed by the assertion that "most Jewish writings indicate that the author has what we call a superiority complex, combined with a persecution complex, sprinkled with paranoia".

Not all stereotypes of this kind are intentionally anti-Semitic. There is a stereotype among some mental health professionals – and, indeed, lay people – that Jews are more likely than others to suffer from OCD. The conviction underlying this stereotype is that people who are obliged to follow strict religious rules will be more prone to develop general obsessionality, to the point of illness. There are two hypotheses here. The first is that scrupulous religious observance will generalize to overall scrupulosity. And the second is that scrupulous religious observance will extend into daily life and become pathological. There is some support for the first hypothesis. Lewis [10], in an extensive review, concluded that while scrupulous religious observance is associated with scrupulosity, it is not associated with *clinical* levels of scrupulosity or obsessionality. This conclusion held true for different faith traditions including Judaism. The second hypothesis appears not to hold – the evidence is consistent with the possibility that more scrupulous individuals may be more religiously active. Also – perhaps more plausibly – scrupulous religious observance may encourage scrupulosity in other areas of behaviour, but it is not associated with obsessional *illness*.

The stereotype of scrupulous religiosity causing OCD is widespread. An Orthodox Jewish patient recently asked if I could help with his OCD. He said he believed this condition to be very prevalent in the Orthodox Jewish community. And I was telling a non-Jewish acquaintance that I was due to give a conference paper soon on mental illness in the OJ community – "Oh, OCD I expect" she said. The stereotype that religious activity may play a role in the development of OCD was tested [11] by asking research participants to read clinical vignettes depicting someone with obsessional behaviour. Some participants read a vignette which included a description of the person as religiously active, while others read a vignette which was otherwise identical but included a description of the person's interests which were not religious. The person's psychological symptoms were rated for severity. The religiously active individual was seen as more likely to suffer from obsessionality and overall psychological distress, compared to the non-religiously active individual. The effect was not one which extended to all psychological symptoms: the religious individual was not seen as more likely to suffer from sadness and tension. The specificity of this effect lends weight to the argument that there really is a stereotype linking Jews – at least observant Jews – with OCD.

Another stereotype is that of the Jewish American Princess [JAP]. Evelyn Torton Beck [12] considers this an issue that needs to be addressed when Jewish women come into psychotherapy. Beck argues that Jewish women shoulder the double burden of anti-Semitism and misogyny. An example is lawyer Shirley Frondorf's depiction of the successful defence of a husband who murdered his wife in the *Death of a Jewish American Princess: The True Story of a Victim on Trial* [13]. The defence consisted of the accused murderer's assertion that his late wife was a JAP – materialistic, addicted to shopping and spending and a constant nag who bothered him at work. Apparently, this extraordinary defence was successful: the [supposedly] nagging Jewish wife was found to "deserve to die".

The stereotype was notoriously perpetuated in a popular song by Zappa in 1979, referring to a "nasty little Jewish princess". He refused to retract anything, insisting that he "didn't make up the idea of a Jewish Princess. They exist, so I wrote a song about them". The stereotype appears to be current and prevalent – I obtained *six million* hits for the term Jewish American Princess in recent Google search.

While the JAP stereotype is often seen as light-hearted and comical, Beck points to similarities with anti-Semitic portraits of Jews in general. According to Beck, the stereotypical Jew, represented by Shakespeare's Shylock, is avaricious, calculating, manipulative, sexually perverse, materialistic and ugly. These qualities are combined with misogynist views to create the JAP stereotype. The JAP is allegedly avaricious, manipulative and calculating [after men's money], materialistic [focused on clothes, furniture and youthful looks, sporting flashy jewellery and designer clothes], sexually perverse [both promiscuous and frigid] and ugly [addicted to plastic surgery]. The JAP stereotype has been well documented [14] and, in Beck's view, needs to be taken seriously when graffiti saying "Kill JAPs" appear side by side with swastikas and traditional anti-Semitic slogans such as "Give Hitler a second chance" and "Kill Jews".

Simon Dein [15] has examined another stereotype: Jewish guilt. He examines recent work on anthropology and emotion, focusing on shame and guilt among Jews and psychoanalytic and theological theories about this association. He considers guilt a cultural stereotype that is linked with the caricature of the Jewish mother. Examples include the opening of Dein's article which quotes the joke, "What's Jewish Alzheimer's disease? It's when you forget everything but the guilt". The article continues by describing the popularization of the stereotype of Jewish guilt by Philip Roth in his classic *Portnoy's Complaint* [16], in which Alexander Portnoy, a young Jewish man brought up by highly neurotic parents, is preoccupied with sexual guilt. The notion of the overbearing and overly critical guilt-inducing Jewish mother is a popular theme in American cinema – e.g. in Woody Allen films.

Andrew Rosenheim in *The Secrets of Carriage H* [location 487] [17], in describing his experiences of a horrific rail disaster in which he was injured, says, "I have a Jewish father and a Yankee mother of old New England Puritan stock, so you might say my middle name is Guilt". Rosenheim goes on to discuss self-blame for the decisions he made, worrying that deaths and injuries were in some way the result of his decisions. He implies that guilt may be a culturally carried tradition, common to Jewish and Puritan traditions.

The rarity of eating disorders in Orthodox Jewish women is another stereotype. Here, the stereotype is that pious religious Jews are above consideration of bodily appearance, and hence young Orthodox Jewish women are not as preoccupied with slimness as their non-Jewish contemporaries [18]. This alleged comparative indifference to bodily shape – it is suggested – is exacerbated, or perhaps caused, by the lack of exposure of the Orthodox to the regular media – magazines, movies, aspects of the internet – which all promote slimness as an essential attribute of female beauty. In fact this alleged indifference to bodily shape and size does not seem to be in evidence. Many Jewish matchmakers have assured me that being overweight is a significant negative feature in young Jewish woman's marriageability. Many Jewish men – and many have told me so – do not want an overweight marriage partner. Eating disorders are common among young Jewish women, including the Orthodox.

It has been reported [19] that secular Jewish women report more eating disorder symptoms, more fear of being fat and more shame about appearance than Orthodox women, but other work [20] has not replicated these findings. A systematic review involving 22 studies of religion and spirituality in relation to disordered eating and body image concerns in several faith traditions [21] supports the conclusions that strong and internalized religious beliefs, coupled with a secure and satisfying relationship with God, are associated with comparatively low levels of disordered eating, psychopathology and body image concern. So, while religious Jewish girls may be relatively protected from eating disorders, it is probably not because of insulation from media but rather because of the quality of their religious beliefs.

It is difficult to ascribe anti-Semitism to all the illness stereotypes described above though occasionally the border between comedy and slander has been crossed. I conclude this section by referring to a fascinating article reflecting anti-Semitism embedded in American academia pre–World War II. A clearly anti-Semitic theme emerges from an extraordinary set of letters unearthed by Winston [22] and pertains to academic psychology. It is likely that similar ideas were current in universities and medical schools at this time. The letters are references by the distinguished head of the psychology department at Harvard, E.G. Boring, recommending graduating students for academic positions in universities. Winston describes how from the 1920s to the 1950s, Boring wrote letters of reference for Jewish students and colleagues in which he followed the common practice of identifying the students as Jews and assessing the degree to which they showed the "objectionable traits" believed to characterize Jews. Here are some samples of Boring's references:

> You would get a good and enthusiastic worker in X … but I most emphatically do not recommend him, because he has some of the personal unpleasantnesses that are usually associated with Jews.

> Y is a Jew, and his inferiority sometimes expresses itself in aggression

> [And a more favourable] Z is a Jew but doesn't show it much.

Diagnosis and Treatment

What effects might biases about Jewish proneness to particular disorders such as OCD [23] have on accuracy of diagnosis and effectiveness of treatment? I am not aware of any specific evidence on this point. There is some broader evidence, however, that religious behaviour among the culturally alien may be mislabelled as psychopathology. For example, religious enthusiasm among black minority groups in Britain has led to a misdiagnosis of psychiatric disorder [24]. This, in turn, can lead to unhelpful treatment – notably unnecessary hospitalization or medication. It is also likely that needed mental health treatment in tight-knit, closed ethnic and religious groups, such as Orthodox Jewry, is avoided for fear of being stereotyped and stigmatized [24].

Effect of Jewishness and Religiosity in Psychiatrists

Finally, I turn to a consideration of Jewishness and religiosity among psychiatrists and other mental health professionals, including the perception of the over-representation of Jews among psychiatrists. They have, in fact, been over-represented in Britain and the USA since the prelude to World War II when they were expelled from their posts in Germany, Austria and Eastern Europe. Psychiatry, a relatively new specialty at the time, had been relatively open to the Jews of Europe. I came across the stereotype of the Jewish psychiatrist in the 1970s when trying to introduce the teaching of an undergraduate course in psychodynamic theory. My head of department repeated the well-worn joke that a psychoanalyst is a Jewish doctor who can't stand the sight of blood. Witty? Perhaps, but it implies that psychoanalysts and Jews are not "proper" doctors practising serious medicine. Because they were seen in the interwar years in Europe as not practicing serious medicine may be why, in fact, they were allowed to practice at all and why so many subsequently fled to Britain and the USA.

What starts off as jokes can culminate in anti-Semitic documents such as those appearing in the *Renegade Tribune* (accessed 14 April 2019). I quote a brief excerpt from an article headed "Psychiatry is a Jewish-Communist weapon against White people", dated 3 December 2015 [25]. The article asserts that "The Jewish occupation governments of the West know the value of using the mental health system as a weapon against the people. During the reign of the Soviet Union mental asylums were used to destroy people who opposed Jewish communism… Psychiatry is a Jewish creation. It has no foundation in science whatsoever, being the most fraudulent part of the entire Jewish medical establishment. A psychiatrist can … detain someone under the Mental Health Act with no evidence whatsoever". Readers of this article are offered numerous examples of destructive Jewish practices offered under the psychiatry heading, with arguments reinforced by illustrative material characterised by the work of art which follows. It concludes with the warning that "… all Jewry's political opponents will be herded into mental institutions, given their de facto death sentence, and chemically lobotomized, shutting us all up forever" (Fig. 15.1).

This is an extreme example of what may be a widespread stereotype that psychiatry is a Jewish dominated profession, a stereotype that may, in turn, lead to reluctance of many to seek and accept psychiatric help.

It is possible that a salient problem of anti-Semitism in psychiatry today may not merely be stereotypes of the psychiatric problems of Jews but also of the stereotypes held of Jewish psychiatrists.

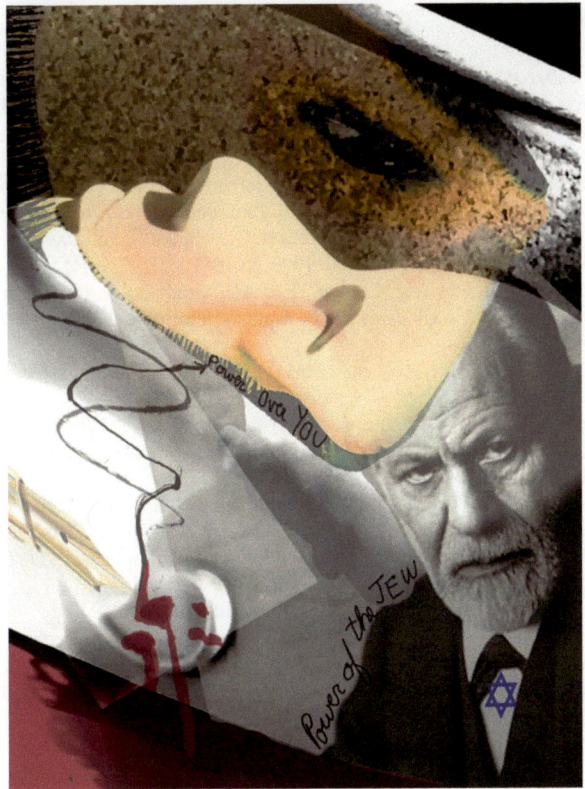

Fig. 15.1 A depiction of some anti-Semitic views on psychiatry, captured by artist Barry Marcus (barmar46@icloud.com)

This illustration was based particularly on the anti-Semitic material in the website consulted. We are unable to reproduce the illustrative material on that website, for copyright reasons, but this compelling illustration was composed by Barry Marcus to embody the frightening and sinister messages contained in the website

Barry's commentary on his depiction: Here we have the insidious Jewish psychiatrist invading the consciousness of an innocent white patient. Blood dripping down the patient's ear signifies the puncturing wounds caused by the malevolent weapon of words employed in therapy. The blood is also a product of the sharp-bladed pen coming from the lower left side of the image. The adjacent scrawl symbolizes a prescription and the power of the pill to stimulate, sedate and confuse. Dr. Freud looks out at the viewer with disdainful pride

Conclusions

This chapter reviewed some stereotypes of psychological and psychiatric issues attributed to Jews. Some have been scientifically investigated, while others are based on unfounded prejudice, sometimes clearly anti-Semitic. Even though most stereotypes are untrue, it is advisable for mental health professionals to be aware that they exist. The chapter also draws attention to the stereotype that the mental health profession as a whole is often perceived as "Jewish", a fact that may hinder help-seeking and treatment adherence.

References

1. Lam DCK, Salkovskis PM, Hogg LI. "Judging a book by its cover": An experimental study of the negative impact of a diagnosis of borderline personality disorder on clinicians' judgements of uncomplicated panic disorder. Br J Clin Psychol. 2016;55(3):253–68. https://doi.org/10.1111/bjc.12093.
2. Levav I, Levinson D. The epidemiology of affective disorders in Israel. In: Levav I, editor. Psychiatric and behavioural disorders in Israel. Jerusalem: Gefen; 2009. p. 186–99.
3. Loewenthal KM, Goldblatt V, Gorton T, Lubitsch G, Bicknell H, Fellowes D, et al. Gender and depression in Anglo-Jewry. Psychol Med. 1995;25:1051–63.
4. Loewenthal KM, MacLeod AK, Cook S, Lee MJ, Goldblatt V. Drowning your sorrows? Attitudes towards alcohol in UK Jews and Protestants: a thematic analysis. Int J Soc Psychiatry. 2003;49:204–15.
5. Levav I, Kohn R, Golding JM, Weissman MM. Vulnerability of Jews to affective disorders. Am J Psychiatry. 1997;154:941–7.
6. Loewenthal KM. The alcohol-depression hypothesis: gender and the prevalence of depression among Jews. In: Sher L, editor. Comorbidity of depression and alcohol use disorders. New York: Nova Science Publishers; 2009. p. 31–40.
7. Loewenthal KM, MacLeod AK, Cook S, Lee MJ, Goldblatt V. Tolerance for depression: are there cultural and gender differences? J Psychiatr Ment Health Nurs. 2002;9:681–8.
8. Todd L, Guha S, Darvasi A. Genome-wide association study implicates NDST3 in schizophrenia and bipolar disorder. Nat Commun. 2013;4:2739.
9. www.fathersmanifesto.net/jewdiseases.htm. Accessed 12 Apr 2019.
10. Lewis CA. Cleanliness is next to godliness: religiosity and obsessiveness. J Relig Health. 1998;37:49–61.
11. Yossifova M, Loewenthal KM. Religion and the judgement of obsessionality. Ment Health Relig Cult. 1999;2:145–52.
12. Beck ET. Therapy's double dilemma: anti-semitism and misogyny. In: Siegel RJ, Cole E, editors. Jewish women in therapy: seen but not heard. New York: Harrington Park Press; 1991.
13. Frondorf S. The death of a Jewish American princess: the true story of a victim on trial. New York: Random House; 1988.
14. Siegel RJ. Antisemitism and sexism in stereotypes of Jewish women. Women Ther. 1986;5(2/3):249–57.
15. Dein S. The origins of Jewish guilt: psychological, theological, and cultural perspectives. J Spiritual Ment Health. 2013;15(2):123–37. https://doi.org/10.1080/19349637.2012.737682.
16. Roth P. Portnoy's complaint. New York: Random House; 1969.
17. Rosenheim A. The secrets of carriage H. Kindle Single; 2014.
18. Loewenthal KM. Modest dress: the rules, the controversies and the experiences. Jewish Spiritualiy and Social Transformation Conference, Westchester, New York, July 2017.
19. Gluck ME, Geliebter A. Body image and eating behaviors in orthodox and secular Jewish women. J Gend Specif Med. 2002;5(1):19–24.
20. Pinhas L, Heinmaa M, Bryden P, Bradley S, Toner B. Disordered eating in Jewish adolescent girls. Can J Psychiatr. 2008;53(9):601–8. https://doi.org/10.1177/070674370805300907.
21. Akrawi D, Bartrop R, Potter U, Touyz S. Religiosity, spirituality in relation to disordered eating and body image concerns: a systematic review. J Eat Disord. 2015;3:29. https://doi.org/10.1186/s40337-015-0064-0.
22. Winston AS. The defects of his race: E. G. Boring and antisemitism in American psychology, 1923-1953. Hist Psychol. 1998;1(1):27–51. https://doi.org/10.1037/1093-4510.1.1.27.
23. Gartner J, Hermatz M, Hohmann A, Larson D. The effect of patient and clinician ideology on clinical judgement: a study of ideological counter transference. Psychotherapy. 1990;27:98–106.
24. Loewenthal KM. Spirituality and cultural psychiatry. In: Bhugra D, Bhui K, editors. Textbook of cultural psychiatry. 2nd ed. Cambridge: Cambridge University Press; 2017. p. 59–69.
25. Sinead. Psychiatry is a Jewish-Communist weapon against white people. Renegade Tribune, 3 Dec 2015. www.fathersmanifesto.net/jewdiseases.htm. Accessed 12 Apr 2019.

Anti-Semitic Transference and Countertransference Reactions

Neil Krishan Aggarwal

Introduction: Defining Anti-Semitism and Its Psychological Effects

This chapter addresses manifestations of anti-Semitism within health settings and how clinicians can transform challenging encounters into treatment opportunities. Anti-Semitism has been defined as "hostility to Jews as Jews (or for the reason that they are Jews)" [1, p. 471]. As recent as April 2019, the US Congress has debated whether the Boycott, Divest, and Sanction (BDS) movement to protest Israel's treatment of Palestinians represents a form of anti-Semitism or principled political action [2]. Anti-Semitic attitudes in Europe have tracked with public opinions on the Israeli-Palestinian conflict, leading to a disturbing increase in the number of attacks in 2018: France reported a 74% increase since 2017 to over 500 incidents, and Germany had a 10% increase to 1646 incidents [3]. These attacks have reverberated throughout society. According to a Pew Research Center study, 64% of 1503 Americans surveyed in March 2019 who were Jewish and non-Jewish agreed that Jews face some sort of discrimination, marking a 20% increase from 2016; the number of Americans who believed that Jews face "a lot" of discrimination has nearly doubled from 13% to 24% [4]. In 2018, out of 16,395 adults who self-identified as Jewish in 12 European Union member states, an astonishing 85% considered anti-Semitism to be their society's most pressing problem, and 89% agreed that anti-Semitic attitudes have worsened in the past 5 years; over 40% have worried about being the victim of a verbal or physical attack [5]. These statistics indicate that anti-Semitic thoughts, emotions, and behaviors are clearly ascendant. Experts trace this trend to three interrelated factors: (1) the resurgence of white, Christian nationalism in American and European politics, (2) the Internet's ability to unite

N. K. Aggarwal (✉)
Columbia University Medical Center, New York, NY, USA

New York State Psychiatric Institute, New York, NY, USA
e-mail: Neil.Aggarwal@nyspi.columbia.edu

© Springer Nature Switzerland AG 2020
H. S. Moffic et al. (eds.), *Anti-Semitism and Psychiatry*,
https://doi.org/10.1007/978-3-030-37745-8_16

fundamentalists beyond geographical restrictions, and (3) the success of far-right politicians in Israel who have dominated rather than negotiated with a weakened Palestinian leadership, polarizing views of Jews across the Muslim world [2, 6].

Mental health professionals have generated multiple hypotheses to explain anti-Semitism. After World War II, psychoanalysts formulated theories to explain the Holocaust through classical theories: as Nazis acting violently in a form of sibling rivalry between Jews and Christians, as an Oedipal reaction since Judaism can be seen as the "father" of Christianity, as an anxiety about the castration of Jewish men, or as a sadomasochistic response to perceptions of Jews being intellectually superior or a chosen people who regard themselves as victims of historical injustices [7]. Others speculate that the opinion of Jews as "Christ killers" has been circulated in the Christian Bible and transmitted across generations, leading to a form of "scapegoat prejudice" [8] and that Christians have projected their own ambivalence about adhering to religious practices onto Jews who are typically more observant [9]. In fact, psychoanalytical studies of anti-Semitism constitute a scholarship in their own right: an April 2019 search in the psychoanalytical database PEP-Web for the phrases "anti-Semitic" or "anti-Semitism" in the title produced 62 articles, with the first article by Sigmund Freud (who, for those who are not aware, was from a Jewish background himself), the founder of psychoanalysis, from 1938!

Social psychologists have conducted experiments to examine how anti-Semitic attitudes emerge in specific situations. Early work saw anti-Semitism as "the displacement of aggression"; in one novel experiment that divided 48 American college students into those who were "either high or low in anti-Semitism" and introduced a stimulus designed to anger them, investigators found that those with more anti-Semitic traits and prone to anger are less likely to restrain their impulses and express discriminatory behaviors [10]. Another study of 183 American college students showed that anti-Israeli attitudes were often a veil for anti-Jewish attitudes – as respondents demonstrated greater antipathy for Israeli human rights violations than those from the Indian or Russian governments – and that people tended not to disclose their true emotions unless they were concerned that they would be caught lying [11]. Notably, those in the United States with less education, income, direct personal contact with Jews, and a less favorable opinion of Israel were more likely to express anti-Semitic beliefs compared to those with higher education and direct personal contact with Jews [12]. Studies among Pakistani college students showed that those with greater anti-Semitic attitudes were more likely to join extremist groups that espouse violence, though students introduced to an educational intervention designed to dispel anti-Semitic stereotypes were less likely to join extremist groups compared to those without such exposure [13]. Surprisingly, there is scant literature on empirical studies with adults who are not in educational settings. In one notable exception, one study with employed adults in Malaysia confirmed that anti-Semitic attitudes track with anti-Israeli attitudes [14].

Nonetheless, these studies cannot explain the prevalence of anti-Semitism before the creation of the Jewish state of Israel in 1948, indicating that there are a variety of causes for prejudicial attitudes and discriminatory behaviors toward Jewish people. The spread of anti-Semitic attitudes in Europe and the United States suggests that practicing clinicians would benefit from understanding its manifestations, especially since Jews have traditionally been reluctant to access mental health services due to stigma and the perception that mental disorders stem from moral failings [15]. For hundreds of years, medical scholarship from the Middle Ages onward has perpetuated stereotypes that Jews are more prone to mental illnesses than other social groups, exacerbating the stigma of accessing mental health services [16]. Cultural psychiatrists strive to improve services for minority populations [17], including Jewish patients who live in societies that are now characterized by growing anti-Semitism. The next section describes common types of anti-Semitic transference and countertransference reactions for clinicians to understand and address [18].

Anti-Semitism in Transference and Countertransference Reactions

Anti-Semitism has been an active topic of discussion among psychiatrists. In an early case report that discussed treatment with a nurse whose parents migrated to Germany and expressed anti-Semitic sentiments during in-depth therapy, a Jewish psychiatrist speculated that his motives for continuing treatment rather than terminating stemmed from identifying with the aggressor as the more powerful member of the relationship [19]. One psychoanalyst offered three vignettes to show that anti-Semitic behaviors occur at critical junctures in psychotherapy, such as to help patients defend against erotic transferences, aggressive competition with their clinicians, and identification with a therapist who could victimize them like their parents [20].

This last article [20] referenced a paper that is now considered canonical within the field of cultural psychiatry and is worth analyzing in depth. In 1991, Lillian Comas-Diaz and Frederick Jacobsen suggested that identity traits such as culture, race, and ethnicity "can touch deep unconscious feelings in most individuals and may become targets for projection by both patient and therapist" [21, p. 392]. By taking a stand against a more traditional psychoanalytical orientation that saw patient remarks about cultural differences with clinicians as defensive deflections from underlying conflicts [22], Comas-Diaz and Jacobsen suggested that "by encouraging the elaboration of ethnoculturally-focused devaluing concepts and feelings, the therapist can offer patients a richer opportunity to know and resolve their own ethnocultural and racial conflicts" [21, pp. 392–393]. Consider the revolutionary nature of their clinical technique: Comas-Diaz and Jacobsen are suggesting that providers investigate conflicts around cultural differences as a way of investigating the patient's intrapsychic and interpersonal worlds, not shun conflicts. If a patient's statements about social differences related to race, ethnicity, religion, or culture are among the first signs of an emerging transference relationship [22], then we can also assume that the clinician's awareness of social differences with patients signifies the start of a countertransference relationship. Comas-Diaz and Jacobsen [21] described distinct types of ethnocultural transference and countertransference reactions through case vignettes, and this method is reproduced here to discuss anti-Semitism.

Transference Reactions

Denial of a Religious or Cultural Identity   In this reaction, patients refuse to self-identify as Jewish. This denial may come from a desire to avoid discrimination by concealing one's identity, especially with immigrants who come from host societies with strong anti-Semitism [23]. The following vignette illustrates this kind of transference:

> An 18-year-old woman presented to university student services for evaluation of acute depression. Her clinician, a Jewish woman psychiatrist, conducted the intake in the presence of psychiatric residents. She began with the DSM-5 Cultural Formulation Interview [CFI] before proceeding to the rest of the history. When the psychiatrist asked CFI Question #8 – "For you, what are the most important aspects of your background or identity?" – the patient replied, "I'm Russian-American." When asked if there were any aspects of her background or identity that have impacted her depression, the patient replied, "My parents are Orthodox Jews and don't believe in sex before marriage. I could never talk to them about drinking, partying, and trying to date guys. I don't see what being Jewish has ever done for them since they were always called '*zhid*' [an anti-Semitic term in Russian similar to 'Yid' in English] and hissed at when they went out for walks on Saturdays." When asked if there were other aspects of her background that have caused concerns for her, she answered, "A lot of students on campus want me to join Hillel, but that's just not me. I'm a cultural Jew. I go to Temple with my parents on the High Holy Days, but I don't need to market my identity."

The psychiatrist's intake revealed the patient's complicated understandings of herself and others. She saw herself in ethnic terms, not religious terms, because of the persecution her parents faced in Russia. Nonetheless, religious values anchored her family's beliefs around love, romance, and sex, and depression resulting from the unexpected end of a romantic relationship revealed an intergenerational rift in the family about her lifestyle.

Mistrust, Suspicion, and Hostility   Comas-Diaz and Jacobsen indicate this reaction occurs when patients doubt the clinician's intentions, which boils down to the fundamental question in every therapeutic relationship: "How can this person understand me?" [21, p. 394]. Patient mistrust can escalate into explicit aggression:

> The police brought a white Christian male in his thirties from a poor, underserved rural area after his girlfriend called 911. She relayed to the emergency dispatcher on the phone that her boyfriend made threats about wanting to kill her and himself after she took away his bottle of prescription opiates. Although he received the prescription months ago to treat lower back pain from a work-related construction injury, she grew alarmed at his increasing doses and doctor shopping to get high. After two shifts of observation and stabilization, the emergency room attending physician called the psychiatric consult-liaison service to conduct a violence risk assessment. A Jewish psychiatrist knocked on the door and introduced himself. The patient immediately noticed the psychiatrist's yarmulke. "Now I gotta please this guy to get outta here? These Hebrews run the world," he said disapprovingly to his girlfriend seated next to him.

The patient's self-image as a strong, independent laborer – along with no direct personal contacts with Jews – led him to viewing his Jewish psychiatrist as a despised outsider. The psychiatrist's yarmulke, a symbol of observance for many Jewish men, became the focus of hostility right from the first moment. In some types of anti-Semitism, people who cannot live up to ideological or personal ideals project a sense of "treachery" onto Jews rather than exercise personal responsibility [24]. The trope of Jews disproportionately wielding influence over worldly matters manifests in his statement about needing to please his psychiatrist whom he derides as a "Hebrew."

This example illustrates how mistrust, suspicion, and hostility can appear when patients and clinicians belong to different religions. However, a similar dynamic can occur even between patients and clinicians who belong to different sects of Judaism. In the United States, anti-Semitic quotas to restrict admission into medical school, residency programs, and hospitals were common from the 1920s to the 1960s, with two known attacks of Christians attacking Jews [25]. As a result, Jews established separate institutions. The next example demonstrates that the patient-clinician relationship can occasion reenactments of geopolitical conflicts even within historically Jewish medical institutions:

> An Orthodox woman in her late thirties presented for treatment of chronic bulimia to a hospital in Brooklyn with a long history of serving the Jewish community. The ethnic origins of the hospital staff gradually changed as newer immigrants from the Middle East resettled in Brooklyn. Her psychiatrist introduced herself as a Yemeni Jew who resettled in the United States about a decade ago. The patient glanced at her and muttered under her breath, "You're almost too slim and fair to be Sephardim. You don't support those Palestinians against us just because you're all Arabs, do you?"

The patient's hostile statements reflect long-standing challenges with her self-image along with the perception that her psychiatrist was beautiful. The erotic transference – she refers to her psychiatrist as "slim and fair" – leads to a physical idealization that heightens attention to her own perceived deficiencies. To compensate, she devalues her psychiatrist by banishing her from the ingroup of Ashkenazi Jews to which she and most of the hospital staff belong. The Israeli-Palestinian conflict replays as an intra-sectarian Ashkenazi-Sephardim dynamic.

Ambivalence   Comas-Diaz and Jacobsen describe this reaction as a patient's manifestation of simultaneous negative feelings and interpersonal attachments toward the clinician. Ambivalence can come either from a patient's lack of awareness about these mixed feelings or the patient's conscious awareness. This anecdote expresses a patient's ambivalence toward her clinician's religion:

> An African-American woman in her early forties had been attending treatment for postpartum depression at an academic medical center in New York City. She noticed her psychiatrist exiting the clinic after their appointment ended just moments before. There were two sets of elevators: one where people could select the floor they wished to reach and another that stopped on all floors for Jews who observe Sabbath rituals. The patient had already been standing before the first type of elevator and was surprised to see her psychia-

trist stand before the second elevator. "I didn't know you were one of them," she said with a puzzled look. "One of who?" asked her psychiatrist. "One of those Jews," the patient responded. "I've been coming to you for several years. I just assumed that because you were black like me and understood me so well, that you were Christian like me. I come in and talk to you about all of my feelings, but I guess I don't really know who you are."

Perceptions of physical resemblance led this patient to assume that she and her psychiatrist shared the same religion. The patient acknowledged her ambivalence by recognizing that they "understood each other so well" but that the psychiatrist was "one of those Jews." She possessed sufficient insight to appreciate that the asymmetric nature of the therapeutic relationship entailed that she would need to share information with her psychiatrist without expecting that the psychiatrist would disclose information about her personal life beyond what was in the patient's fiduciary interests.

Countertransference Reactions

Denial of Religious Differences Just like patients, clinicians can also deny their religious identity because of concerns about anti-Semitism. One reason may be that many clinicians like to see themselves as part of a healing profession that is divorced from cultural and political divisions in society [21]. The case below exemplifies this dynamic:

A Puerto Rican man in his fifties presented for treatment of generalized anxiety disorder to an outpatient clinic that works with Hispanics and is affiliated with a residency training program in Florida. His anxiety began after the stock market's crash in 2007 when he became homeless with his wife and two children upon not being able to make mortgage payments. Over time, he grew accustomed to the annual turnover of resident physicians each summer. At his appointment time, the resident physician, a Hispanic-American man in his mid-twenties, introduced himself as "Dr. Pedro Amiel." In an effort to establish familiarity, the patient smiled and said, "Amiel? That's an Iberian Jewish name, isn't it? I also have Jewish blood from my mother's side. We were crypto-Jews." Embarrassed that others in the waiting room could hear the exchange, the resident said, "I'd prefer to not talk about my religious background. Let's keep this conversation about you and your treatment needs once we go inside."

The resident psychiatrist, new to the outpatient setting and to long-term psychotherapy, felt discomfort at this perceived intrusion into his personal life, an attempt to ensnare him in disclosing personal information. Rather than respond positively or even neutrally to the patient's demonstration of strong affect, he sought to immediately establish professional boundaries and minimize discussion of his religious or cultural identity. That week in clinical supervision, a seasoned psychotherapist questioned whether the resident psychiatrist was trying to defend against his own anxieties around incompetence as a novice clinician treating a patient with chronic anxiety.

Aggression and Anger   This countertransference reaction can occur when clinicians overidentify with their patients to the extent of expressing antagonism. Clinicians unaccustomed to managing their emotions in real time can exhibit anger, as this example illustrates:

> A Muslim-American man in his forties presented to the faculty clinic of a prominent Ivy League medical center in New England to establish care for treatment of a personality disorder. He informed the intake coordinator on the phone that his wife threatened to leave him if he did not initiate therapy to treat his anger and malignant narcissism. The medical center staffed the clinic with faculty members who are looking to supplement their incomes because they do not receive 100% grant support as researchers. A middle-aged, Jewish psychiatrist, internationally renowned for his work on elucidating the biomarkers of psychotic disorders, was assigned to the case. "Hi," he said to the patient as they walked into the waiting room. The patient looked at the psychiatrist's phylacteries and said with a smirk, "You know in my country, they teach us that the Jews have really manipulated the media. That the Holocaust didn't kill as many people as the Jews claim and that there were others who were also killed by the Nazis that don't get so much attention." The psychiatrist turned to him and said coldly, "You don't know how incredibly offensive that is to me as someone who lost grandparents in the Holocaust. You really should see someone else if that's what you think. I'll get your case reassigned." The patient responded, "I didn't say that I think that, but it's good to know just how close minded you are. You can't help me."

This case shows that even experienced psychiatrists who do not maintain their skills in psychotherapy can identify with a patient's negative emotions to act out aggressively. Over the past decade, academic centers in North America have devoted fewer resources to psychodynamic psychotherapy and more to medication management, in line with insurance reimbursement models that value psychiatrists as prescribers rather than therapists [26, 27]. This psychiatrist's professional interests took him away from psychotherapy long ago, which made him a target for the patient's provocative statements about Holocaust denial. Rather than explore why the patient chose to express this sentiment at this particular time, as reflecting personal discomfort from a new conception of Jews as healers rather than as enemies, the psychiatrist chose to defend himself against any devaluing statements.

Ambivalence   Clinicians, like patients, may experience awareness of their mixed feelings. The following example illustrates this process:

> A woman who migrated from the Palestinian territories as a teenager after the 1967 war presented with her adult daughter to establish care at an outpatient geriatric clinic for the treatment of dementia. The psychologist, a secular Jewish male whose parents migrated from Israel to settle in New York City, conducted a detailed social history. The woman recounted her history of trauma at seeing her village occupied by the Israel Defense Forces [IDF]. A visa lottery through the United Nations helped her resettle in the United States. The psychologist, a self-identified "cultural Jew" who observed Jewish holidays more from a sense of community belonging than from any personal spirituality, found himself caught between his duty as a health provider and his loyalty to his family's legacy. The woman did not think to censor herself since the social history took only a few minutes out of an extensive neuropsychological evaluation. Nor did she pause to consider her clinician's religion.

After the evaluation, the psychologist debated whether he would be best suited to continue with the case and raised the possibility of transferring her care to someone else with his clinic's supervisor.

His supervisor said that she saw no direct reason to reassign the case to someone else. She asked why he identified so much with what the patient was saying. The psychologist acknowledged, "I think it's because my father had compulsory military service in the IDF as a young man. I know he didn't like it. He often talked about feeling guilty that ordinary Palestinians would be mistreated because of their community's leadership, but he also felt strongly about protecting Israel's security." His supervisor asked whether he was projecting his family's ambivalence into the dynamic with this patient, noting that the woman did not target him or Jews in general, but expressed legitimate concerns about her personal losses. If session could not be a safe place to express her vulnerabilities, then where could she go? The psychologist agreed that these dynamics could be at play and continued with the case, as his supervisor did not give him a choice. The patient and her family never mentioned their life in Palestine again as they were focused on addressing more immediate concerns related to her activities of daily living. The psychologist grew to develop a strong bond with the family over several years until she was admitted to an assisted care facility. At his final session with her, he realized just how much of a mistake it would have been to act rather than process the strong emotions from his initial session.

This vignette encapsulates why patients and clinicians cannot take each other's identities for granted. The Palestinian woman did not deliberately attempt to insult her psychologist and would not have answered questions about her 50-year migration history had the psychologist not been so thorough with his social history. The psychologist never thought that his personal background would manifest in a clinical setting since he saw himself as a cultural Jew who maintained a loose religious identity for predominantly social reasons. Nonetheless, her personal history activated latent concerns of anti-Semitism that his parents experienced during their migration from Israel. All the same, he appreciated his fiduciary duty to her as a health professional and considered referring her case to someone who could provide greater empathy.

Strategies to Work Through Anti-Semitic Transference and Countertransference

For over 80 years, mental health clinicians have recognized that anti-Semitic thoughts, emotions, and behaviors can manifest within the patient-clinician relationship. How can clinicians confront anti-Semitism in real time, while maintaining their fiduciary responsibility to do no harm to their patients? Cultural psychiatrists and psychologists have developed tools to work through such differences. The concept of "cultural humility" encourages clinicians to engage in self-reflection in order to reduce power imbalances so that disadvantaged racial and ethnic minority patients do not experience discrimination [28, 29]. The examples above reveal that anti-Semitism can create a power imbalance whether or not the patient or clinician expresses such discriminatory attitudes. To operationalize this tenet of self-evaluation, cultural psychiatrists have suggested three steps for clinicians to address differences in background or identity with patients: (1) allowing oneself to experience strong emotions rather than presuming a clinical stance of neutrality or objectivity, (2) processing the subsequent countertransference rather than reacting defensively, and (3) using countertransferential reactions to engage with patient narratives through curiosity, especially when empathy seems impossible [30, 31].

Each transference and countertransference reaction lends itself to these three steps. One way to systematically implement these steps is to use the DSM-5 Cultural Formulation Interview (CFI), a semi-structured interview that consists of 16 questions for clinicians to use with patients. DSM-5 specifies that the CFI can be used partially or in its entirety, especially in the following situations: difficulty in diagnostic assessment owing to significant differences in the cultural, religious, or socioeconomic backgrounds of clinician and the individual; uncertainty about the fit between culturally distinctive symptoms and diagnostic criteria; difficulty in judging illness severity or impairment; disagreement between the individual and clinician on the course of care; and limited engagement in and adherence to treatment by the individual [32, p. 751]. The final question in the CFI is intended to explicitly elicit concerns about patient-clinician cultural differences that could undermine goodwill, communication, or healthcare delivery: "Sometimes doctors and patients misunderstand each other because they come from different backgrounds or have different expectations. Have you been concerned about this and is there anything that we can do to provide you with the care you need?" [32, p. 754]. Although patients may not respond immediately, clinicians are signifying their openness to work through cultural differences by asking this question [33].

Clinicians may also find questions from the CFI supplementary module on the patient-clinician relationship to be helpful in self-reflection [34]. Key questions that clinicians can ask themselves include:

- How did I feel about my relationship with this patient? Did cultural similarities and differences influence my relationship? In what way?
- What was the quality of communication with the patient? Did cultural similarities and differences influence my communication? In what way?
- How do the patient's cultural background or identity, life situation, and/or social context influence my understanding of his/her problem and my diagnostic assessment?
- How do the patient's cultural background or identity, life situation, and/or social context influence my treatment plan or recommendations?
- Did the clinical encounter confirm or call into question any of my prior ideas about the cultural background or identity of the patient? If so, in what way?
- Are there aspects of my own identity that may influence my attitudes toward this patient?

This supplementary module on the patient-clinician relationships suggests that clinicians ask themselves such questions after the interview, but these questions may also be helpful in stimulating an internal dialogue during sessions. The ability to introspect in session by examining one's "reveries" such as self-absorptive states, ruminations, daydreams, and fantasies reflects the clinician's receptivity to the patient and constitutes an alternate form of unconscious data that clinicians can bring into conscious awareness [35]. Cultural psychiatrists understand transference and countertransference reactions as patients and clinicians responding to each other based on their backgrounds and identities, and clinicians can use cultural reveries to process their own countertransferential reactions [36]. Administrators and educators may also see this supplementary module as a way of providing clinical supervision to trainees who discuss cases, such as during psychotherapy training in residency or fellowship programs.

This supplementary module also includes questions that clinicians can ask during sessions for patients to process transferential reactions [36]. Such questions include:

- Have you had difficulties with clinicians in the past? What did you find difficult or unhelpful?
- Now let's talk about the help that you would like to get here. Some people prefer clinicians of a similar background (e.g., age, race, religion, or some other characteristic) because they think it may be easier to understand each other. Do you have any preference or ideas about what kind of clinician might understand you best?
- Sometimes differences among patients and clinicians make it difficult for them to understand each other. Do you have any concerns about this? If so, in what way?
- What patients expect from their clinicians is important. As we move forward in your care, how can we best work together?

Each question explores the patient's experiences through curiosity, not defensiveness. Just as the second question asks about, "What kind of clinician might understand you best?," we could also ask, "What kind of clinician might not understand you?" to elicit anti-Semitic thoughts and emotions. The goal of such questions is not to legitimize negative attitudes, but to model behaviors of interpersonal negotiation and broaden the capacity for self-reflection among patients and clinicians alike.

Conclusion

After defining and discussing anti-Semitism's harmful effects on mental health, this chapter has presented case vignettes on how anti-Semitism can manifest through common transferential and countertransferential reactions. Finally, the article has proposed the DSM-5 Cultural Formulation Interview and its supplementary module on the patient-clinician relationship as a way for clinicians to respond to challenging situations in a constructive manner. Three steps may help clinicians resolve these conflicts: (1) allowing themselves to experience strong emotions rather than presuming a stance of neutrality or objectivity, (2) processing their countertransference rather than reacting defensively, and (3) using countertransferential reactions to engage with patient narratives through genuine curiosity.

References

1. Klug B. Interrogating "new anti-Semitism". Ethn Racial Stud. 2013;36:468–82.
2. Reuters. U.S. House rebukes Trump on Saudi Arabia, backs measure to end Yemen involvement. New York Times. 4 April 2019.
3. Kingsley P. Anti-Semitism is back, from the left, right and Islamist extremes. Why? New York Times. 4 April 2019.
4. Pew Research Center. Sharp rise in the share of Americans saying Jews face discrimination. Washington, DC: Pew Research Center; 2019.
5. European Union Agency for Fundamental Rights. Experiences and perceptions of anti-Semitism: second survey on discrimination and hate crimes against Jews in the EU. Luxembourg: Publications Office of the European Union; 2018.
6. Nefes TS. Scrutinizing impacts of conspiracy theories on readers' political views: a rational choice perspective on anti-semitic rhetoric in Turkey. Br J Sociol. 2015;66:557–75.
7. Weill TL. Anti-Semitism: selected psychodynamic insights. Am J Psychoanal. 1981;41:139–48.
8. Rosenman S. A critique of classical psychoanalytic theories of anti-Semitism: a commentary on M. Ostrow's myth and madness: the psychodynamics of anti-Semitism. Am J Psychoanal. 1998;58:417–33.
9. Frosh S. Freud, psychoanalysis and anti-semitism. Psychoanal Rev. 2004;91:309–30.
10. Berkowitz L. Anti-semitism and the displacement of aggression. J Abnorm Soc Psychol. 1959;59:182–7.
11. Cohen F, Jussim L, Harber KD, Bhasin G. Modern anti-Semitism and anti-Israeli attitudes. J Pers Soc Psychol. 2009;97:290–306.
12. Rebhun U. Correlates of experiences and perceptions of anti-Semitism among Jews in the United States. Soc Sci Res. 2014;47:44–60.
13. Amjad N, Wood AM. Identifying and changing the normative beliefs about aggression which lead young Muslim adults to join extremist anti-Semitic groups in Pakistan. Aggress Behav. 2009;35(6):514–9.
14. Swami V. Social psychological origins of conspiracy theories: the case of the Jewish conspiracy theory in Malaysia. Front Psychol. 2012;3:280.
15. Loewenthal KM. Mental health and mental health care for Jews in the Diaspora, with particular reference to the U.K. Isr J Psychiatry Relat Sci. 2012;49:159–66.
16. Gilman SL. Jews and mental illness: medical metaphors, anti-Semitism, and the Jewish response. J Hist Behav Sci. 1984;20:150–9.
17. Kirmayer LJ. Cultural psychiatry in historical perspective. In: Bhugra D, Bhui K, editors. Textbook of cultural psychiatry. Cambridge: Cambridge University Press; 2007. p. 3–19.
18. Traub-Werner D. A note on counter-transference and anti-Semitism. Can J Psychiatry. 1979;24:547–8.
19. Knafo D. Anti-Semitism in the clinical setting: transference and countertransference dimensions. J Am Psychoanal Assoc. 1999;47:35–62.
20. Comas-Diaz L, Jacobsen FM. Ethnocultural transference and countertransference in the therapeutic dyad. Am J Orthopsychiatry. 1991;61:392–402.
21. Evans DA. Psychotherapy and black patients: problems of training, trainees, and trainers. Psychotherapy. 1985;22:457–60.
22. Varghese FTN. The racially different psychiatrist – implications for psychotherapy. Aust N Z J Psychiatry. 1983;17(4):329–33.
23. Tartakovsky E. Cultural identities of adolescent immigrants: a three-year longitudinal study including the pre-migration period. J Youth Adolesc. 2009;38:654–71.
24. Glasberg R. The treachery trope: anti-Semitism as indicative of a psycho-spiritual disease associated with the betrayal of cultural ideals and of the self. J Relig Health. 2018;57:311–27.
25. Halperin EC. "This is a Christian institution and we will tolerate no Jews here": the Brooklyn Medical Interns Hazings. Am J Med Sci. 2018;356:505–17.
26. Sudak DM, Goldberg DA. Trends in psychotherapy training: a national survey of psychiatry residency training. Acad Psychiatry. 2012;36:369–73.

27. Stovel LE, Felstrom A. A survey of psychotherapy training in Canadian psychiatry residency programs. Acad Psychiatry. 2013;37:431–2.
28. Tervalon M, Murray-García J. Cultural humility versus cultural competence: a critical distinction in defining physician training outcomes in multicultural education. J Health Care Poor Underserved. 1998;9:117–25.
29. Jenks AC. From "lists of traits" to "open-mindedness": emerging issues in cultural competence education. Cult Med Psychiatry. 2011;35:209–35.
30. Kirmayer LJ. Empathy and alterity in cultural psychiatry. Ethos. 2008;36:457–74.
31. Aggarwal NK. Challenges in treating undocumented immigrants. Am J Psychiatry. 2017;174:833–7.
32. American Psychiatric Association. Diagnostic and statistical manual of mental disorders. 5th ed. Washington, DC: American Psychiatric Publishing; 2013.
33. Aggarwal NK, Nicasio AV, DeSilva R, Boiler M, Lewis-Fernández R. Barriers to implementing the DSM-5 cultural formulation interview: a qualitative study. Cult Med Psychiatry. 2013;37:505–33.
34. American Psychiatric Association. Patient-clinician relationship. Supplementary modules to the core cultural formulation interview. 2017. Available at https://www.google.com/url?sa=t&rct=j&q=&esrc=s&source=web&cd=2&cad=rja&uact=8&ved=0ahUKEwjZjMqJuevWAhWLwYMKHdd2D5cQFgguMAE&url=https%3A%2F%2Fwww.psychiatry.org%2FFile%2520Library%2FPsychiatrists%2FPractice%2FDSM%2FAPA_DSM5_Cultural-Formulation-Interview-Supplementary-Modules.pdf&usg=AOvVaw1Viw3gk_WlBQVOsXRtQBfE. Accessed 12 Oct 2017.
35. Ogden T. The analytic third: working with intersubjective clinical facts. Int J Psychoanal. 1994;75:3–19.
36. Aggarwal NK. Intersubjectivity, transference, and the cultural third. Contemp Psychoanal. 2011;47:204–23.

Anti-Semitism, the Holocaust, and Intergenerational Transmission of Trauma

17

Mary V. Seeman

> *It happened, therefore it can happen again: this is the core of what we have to say. It can happen, and it can happen everywhere.*
> —*Primo Levi*

Introduction

Anti-Semitism in its many different forms existed for centuries before the Holocaust, the World War II attempt to annihilate the Jewish population of Europe. Because it is impossible in one chapter to cover the determinants and effects of anti-Semitism as they apply to different European communities before the war, I will focus on my ancestral hometown, Zgierz, situated in central Poland, just north of the large industrial city of Łódź (Lodz).

Since the thirteenth century, Jews had found sanctuary in many regions of Poland. The town of Zgierz is first mentioned in the historical record in the year 1231, but Jewish presence in Zgierz is recorded only after 1815. This is when Congress Poland came into being, so designated by the Congress of Vienna, the pact that redrew the map of Europe at the end of the Napoleonic Wars. In the beginning, 3.3 million people lived within the borders of Congress Poland. Seventy-five percent were ethnic Poles; 10% were Jews; all were subservient to the Russian Czar but constitutionally governed by Polish rather than Russian law [1].

M. V. Seeman (✉)
Department of Psychiatry, University of Toronto, Toronto, ON, Canada
e-mail: mary.seeman@utoronto.ca

© Springer Nature Switzerland AG 2020
H. S. Moffic et al. (eds.), *Anti-Semitism and Psychiatry*,
https://doi.org/10.1007/978-3-030-37745-8_17

The Beginning of Anti-Semitism in Poland

Prior to 1815, during the long period of the Polish-Lithuanian Commonwealth (1386–1795), Jews on Polish soil were treated with great respect because of (or in spite of) the quaintness of their customs and the curious nature of their religious observances, diet, dress, and language. They were referred to as "Old Believers." With the birth of Congress Poland, however, Polish nationalists began to urge Old Believers to abandon their orthodox traditions and embrace modernity. The Jewish religion per se was not a problem; Poland was home to a variety of religious rites that co-existed with the Roman Catholic state religion. The problem, as viewed by Polish nationalists, was the stubbornness of the Jewish community in keeping to its idiosyncratic ways. This tenaciousness became the target not only of anti-Semitic feelings but also of anti-Semitic policies in the new Poland. While the *Haskalah* (Jewish enlightenment movement) in Poland encouraged Jews to integrate with the society in which they lived, it also promoted Jewish identity. The result, for most Jews, fell far short of full assimilation, as a result of which rumors began to circulate that they owed little allegiance to their Polish homeland and that they belonged, so the suspicion went, to a secret conspiracy whose eventual aim was world dominance [2].

To counter this imaginary threat, a Polish government official, Gerard Witkowski, proposed asking the Czar to set aside a remote area of land in Russia to which Polish Jews could be exiled [1]. This suggestion was never acted on; the new parliament, however, passed a constitution that granted civil rights only to Christians. Non-Christians were required to petition the government for privileges, but the granting of such petitions depended on the abandonment of traditional Jewish dress, forsaking Yiddish as the everyday language of communication, and using Roman rather than Hebrew characters when writing. As an example, in Zgierz, Jews were only permitted to live in a restricted area, a ghetto. However, if the men shaved off their beards, abandoned their *kapotas* (long black coats), could prove they had sufficient money, could demonstrate their Polish reading and writing abilities, and expressed willingness to enroll their sons in Polish schools (instead of *cheders* or Jewish schools), an exemption from residential restrictions could be arranged [3].

Box 17.1

My great-grandfather came to Zgierz in 1843. He was an iron merchant and was relatively well off. He was, however, unable to write Polish. He petitioned several times to be given permission to live outside the congested Jewish area and was several times refused. At one of the hearings, he appeared with a bandaged right hand saying that he could indeed write in Polish but was unfortunately unable to do so because of his injuries [4]. This subterfuge did not work.

The liquor trade was also forbidden to Jews, but there seemed to have been ways around this [5]. Family lore is that my great-grandmother, after whom I was named and whom I apparently resembled, ran a successful underground distillery in Zgierz.

In June 1862, the Czar abolished Jewish residential restrictions on Jews through-out Congress Poland (but kept the restrictions on liquor). After 1862, Polish Jews were allowed to enter professions such as law and medicine. They began to enjoy far greater privileges than did Jews living in the Russian Pale of Settlement, the large geographic area east of Congress Poland governed by Russian law, with the result that masses of Russian Jews migrated westward and settled in Warsaw and Lodz.

This occurred during the prelude to the Russian revolution. The Polish Catholic Church perceived the new immigrants as atheists, communists, and potential sowers of political unrest [6]. To add to the discontent of the Polish public, the new immigrants proved successful in business, and their children outsmarted their classmates in school. As a consequence, what is still referred to as Jewish emancipation in Poland had unfortunate unforeseen consequences. It led indirectly to a mixture of mounting fear, suspicion, resentment, and envy on the part of the majority Polish population. A *pogrom* (anti-Jewish violence) took place in Warsaw on Christmas Day, 1881. It started in a crowded church. Would-be pickpockets apparently yelled "fire," which set off a stampede that left 29 persons dead. Someone spread the rumor that the pickpockets were Jews. A mob began to attack Jewish stores, businesses, and homes near the church; riots continued in Warsaw for 3 days. A total of 2600 people were arrested. Two persons died in the riots and two were injured. One thousand Jewish families lost their homes and their businesses. In retrospect, it is possible that the *pogrom* was instigated by the Russian authorities in an attempt to drive a wedge between Jews and Poles [7]. The 1906 *pogrom* in Siedlce, in east central Poland, was organized by the Russian secret police in order to quell the rise of revolutionary factions. Siedlce inhabitants were 60% Jewish. On August 26, a socialist party activist, disguised as a Jew, assassinated a Russian police captain. The retaliation, which was systematically organized, took place in early September. Perpetrators were Russian soldiers who fired guns in the town square, set fires, and looted Jewish stores. Private Jewish homes were broken into. Thirty-four Jews were killed, and hundreds were injured. One thousand people were arrested. Poles, for the most part, did not participate; they, in fact, helped to shelter Jews from the Russians. Polish public opinion condemned the *pogrom*, and the Polish press unanimously denounced the violence [8].

Box 17.2
During World War I, many Polish Jews were transformed into loyal Polish nationalists. My father, for instance, ran away from home to serve in General Piłsudski's Polish legions to fight against the Soviets and to champion Polish independence.

Numerous instances of Jewish loyalty to Poland did not prevent the right-wing factions in Poland from scapegoating Jews, holding them responsible for wartime food shortages and calling for Jewish business boycotts. The Treaty of Versailles at the end of the war enshrined Polish independence from Russia, and the Polish

Minority Treaty became a model for other nations. The new Polish Constitution prohibited all discrimination on religious, racial, or national grounds. Polish right-wing parties, however, saw the requirements of the minority treaty as interference with Poland's autonomy and attributed their imposition to Jewish plotting. In direct contrast to the treaty, the actual policy of interwar Polish governments was to promote Polish ethnicity at the expense of minority rights [9].

Interwar Polish-Jewish Relations

According to contemporary accounts, the three distinct ethnic populations in Zgierz – Christian Poles, Poles of German origin known as *Volksdeutsche* [10], and Polish Jews – lived in relative harmony during the interwar period (M. Gruszewska, personal communication, Leokadia Leniart, Marianna and Kazimierz Królikowski, and Wojciech Bryszewski in conversation with Mazenna Gruszewska, 2014). Nonetheless, even in this small town, the Jewish cemetery was desecrated in 1919 – tombstones were destroyed, and the fencing was torn down. Unemployment compensation in some companies was deliberately handed out on the Jewish Sabbath (Saturday), which meant that religious Jews were unable to obtain it. Polish workers opposed the employment of Jews in Zgierz factories and went on strike for 5 weeks demanding their dismissal. In May 1920, there was an anti-Semitic riot over an incident involving Jewish children marching in a parade. In 1932, a railway station near Zgierz posted a placard, which read, "Jews are forbidden to get off here!" [11]. Polish-Jewish relations were far worse in the bigger cities, especially so during the latter half of the 1930s [12]. This was a time of radical anti-Jewish propaganda in Poland, of anti-Semitic brawls, and of discrimination against Jews in all spheres of life, part of a general tendency in an increasingly nationalistic Europe.

I will describe two important Polish-Jewish controversies that surfaced during that period, both of which pertain to university teaching and medical training.

Ghetto Benches

Concerned with the expanding proportion of Jews in Polish institutions of higher learning, most Polish universities by 1939 had implemented a *numerus clausus*, setting the percentage of admission of Jewish students at 10%, to reflect the percentage of Jews in the Polish population. Jewish competition in academia was said to be unfair; Jews were too studious. Psychoanalyst Sandor Gilman has since explored the many unfortunate historical consequences of attributing superior book learning abilities to the "People of the Book" [13].

To distance themselves from the contamination of Jewish proximity, university students throughout the country began a campaign of segregation, demanding that Jewish students sit on the left of the classroom in what became known as "ghetto benches." Jewish students refused to sit in the designated seats but stood, instead, at the back of the room. Some Polish professors stood with them, in solidarity. The situation degenerated; in March 1936, 50 Jewish students were injured, 2 seriously, in a confrontation over refusal to sit in the ghetto benches. In an attempt to put an end to the unrest, university authorities in much of Poland yielded to the wishes of the majority and officially endorsed and authorized ghetto bench seating [14].

Cadavers

The second issue was cadavers for medical students. In 1921, 30% of students in Polish medical schools were Jewish. Cadavers were needed for anatomy class. The rabbinical interpretation of Jewish law dictated that Jewish bodies needed to be buried within 24 hours of death and could not, therefore, be available for dissection. Christian students protested the fact that all the bodies used in anatomy class were Christian bodies. They interpreted the rabbinical rationale to mean that Jews considered Jewish corpses too holy to desecrate but had no such scruples with regard to Christian corpses [15, 16].

Fights and rioting broke out over this issue. Jewish students were blocked by force from entering dissecting rooms. As a result, they failed their anatomy exams and brought their complaints to the notice of university authorities. Universities made a Solomonic decision: Jewish students could not be locked out of dissecting rooms; on the other hand, neither could they dissect Christian bodies. After lengthy negotiations, Warsaw rabbis agreed to provide corpses of Jews who died in hospital and whose bodies were not claimed by relatives within 48 hours of death. The number of available bodies, however, remained insufficient. In 1935, all Jewish medical students at the University of Warsaw lost credit for one semester of study because, for want of corpses, they had not completed their anatomy course. No one could have known at the time that the problem of insufficient Jewish corpses would soon disappear [17].

Holocaust in Zgierz

The population of Western Poland, which included Zgierz, was the first to experience the brutality of Nazi occupation [18].

The Nazi goal was to Germanize the whole of Western Poland, to assimilate the territory politically, culturally, and economically, chase out the Jews, and bring in German settlers. Town and street names were Germanized and property expropriated. Lodz became *Litzmannstadt*; Zgierz became *Görnau*.

As *Wehrmacht* units began moving across Poland, special paramilitary death squads, the *SS Einsatzgruppen*, deliberately singled out Jews for humiliation, abuse, and massacre [19]. Atrocities occurred within hours of occupation. In the first 6 weeks of the war, 16,336 Polish civilians were murdered by the Germans, at least 5000 of whom were Jews [20].

Approximately 4800 Jews, 16–18% of the total population, lived in Zgierz when the German air bombardment began on September 3, 1939. The bombs lasted for

3 days in Zgierz [21]. Townspeople fled in all directions. On September 7 at 10 AM, German armed forces entered the town. En route, they had already cornered and murdered five Jewish men. On September 8, the German army started rounding up all the Jewish men in the town. For 3 days, they kept them imprisoned in the Catholic Church, where the men were starved and beaten and where their beards, or half their beards by some accounts, were burned off.

Several prominent Zgierz Jews took their own lives. Local *Volksdeutsch* took over the administration of the town and issued various anti-Semitic decrees. A curfew was set for Jews between 5 PM and 8 AM. The synagogue and prayer houses were closed, and all forms of Jewish prayer were forbidden. Severe punishment, even death, was the official sanction for anyone who disobeyed. A central bureau was established to register ethnicity – Polish, German, Jewish. Jewish stores were pillaged and destroyed; their owners were beaten [11].

A series of searches in Jewish homes began on September 10; money, jewelry, food, clothing, linens, and furniture were taken away. German commissars were appointed for Jewish factories. Jews were required to register their gold, silver, jewelry, and furs. They were permitted to keep only a small amount of cash, the rest to be deposited in a "spare account." New taxes were imposed on all Jewish citizens.

Jews were conscripted for hard labor, beaten, tortured, and shamed. The women were told to wash the floors of the German barracks using their clothes for rags. They were forced to clean latrines with their hands. Jews who refused to work were tormented and sometimes shot.

On September 21, Reinhard Heydrich, who, in January 1942, was to chair the Wannsee Conference where plans for the "Final Solution" would be finalized, started arrangements to make Western Poland *judenrein* (free of Jews). In October, Himmler ordered 100,000 Jews to be expelled from Western Poland or *Wartheland*, now considered German territory, between November 1939 and February 1940 [18].

In November, well off Zgierz Jews as well as the Polish intelligentsia of Zgierz – teachers, local and state bureaucrats, social and political activists, and artists – were sent to the Radogoszcz concentration camp in Lodz. After a perfunctory trial, most were sentenced to death and executed. Their bodies were buried in the forests surrounding Lodz.

The Germans posted placards, slogans, and derogatory caricatures of Jews in the streets of Zgierz, spreading "fake news" to turn Poles against Jews, e.g., "The Jews are our enemies," "The Jews are war mongers."

Religious Jews were coerced into washing floors, trash bins, and lavatories with their prayer shawls. Pages of holy books were desecrated, torn, and burnt in the market square. On Sundays, the *Volksdeutsche* and *Wehrmacht* soldiers organized entertainment. They forced Jews to put on *tallises* (prayer shawls) and *tefillin* (small black leather boxes containing verses from the Torah and worn during morning prayer) or dress in women's clothing wearing silly hats or wigs or wave Chinese lanterns or brooms. Jews were forced to sing and shout slogans such as "All Jews are swine," "We Jews are responsible for the war." Hundreds of Jews were made to perform gymnastics, jump, dance, crawl on the ground, and dance on makeshift stages to the accompaniment of the jeers of the crowd.

On October 27, 1939, Germans attempted to burn down the synagogue and the religious study hall. Local residents successfully put out the fire and saved the Torah scrolls, which were buried in the Jewish cemetery. A Jewish resident was blamed for the fire and spent 6 weeks in jail. One month later, on November 24, the synagogue and study hall were burned to the ground. The rabbi was told that the community owed 250 *złoty* as payment for the intervention of the fire department. Witnesses relate that pressure was put on the rabbi to admit that Jews themselves had set the synagogue on fire.

On November 1939, Jews were ordered to wear a yellow band on their sleeve for purposes of identification. A month later, the order was changed to a yellow Star of David worn on the chest. On December 29, the majority of Zgierz Jews (about 2500) were evicted from the town (Figs. 17.1 and 17.2).

Box 17.3

My grandfather, 80 years old, was spared eviction. He had died the day before when his house and beloved library were entered and ransacked. My aunt, who lived with him, and her small son were sent east to the town of Głowno. They were rounded up at 7 AM in the Zgierz sports arena and given a baggage limit of 25 kg and a cash limit of 50 *złoty* for the trip.

From Głowno, my aunt and cousin made their way to Warsaw and from there to the Warsaw ghetto, where they died from hunger 2 years later. Had they lived, they would have been transported with the other inhabitants of the Warsaw ghetto to the Treblinka death camp in the summer of 1942.

My immediate family lived in Lodz. On the first day of the war, my father left with the Polish army. The Russians captured his unit, but he escaped, managed to get to France, and sent us French visas, which allowed us to leave Poland in January 1940. From France, thanks to the heroic Portuguese consul, Aristide Sousa Mendes [22], we crossed through Spain into neutral Portugal and, in the spring of 1941, came to Canada, where, eventually, I became a physician. Perhaps to better understand what makes people do the incomprehensible things they do, I subsequently trained in psychiatry.

There was a small group of Jews left in Zgierz after the expulsion – people whose skills the Germans needed. On January 12, 1942, those who remained were transported to the Lodz ghetto. In August 1944, the last surviving Jews from the Lodz ghetto were murdered in the gas chambers of Auschwitz.

In total, approximately 350 Zgierz Jews were still alive after the war. A few had managed to flee the country. A few had survived German concentration camps and labor camps. A few survived in Siberia. A few survived the war pretending to be "Aryan" (pure blooded – i.e., not Jewish). Sixty Jews returned briefly to Zgierz at the end of the war (Fig. 17.3).

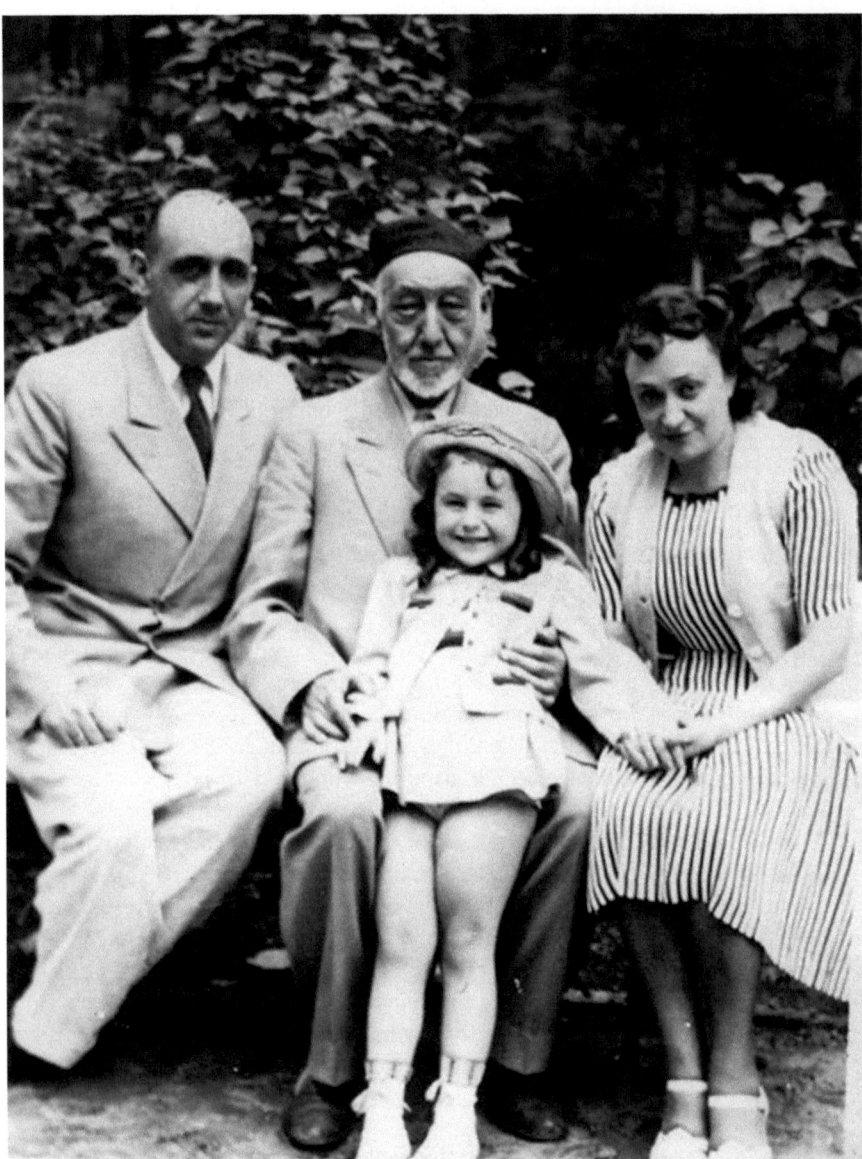

Fig. 17.1 The author with her parents and grandfather, 1938, in Zgierz

Since Germany and the Soviet Union had initially divided the country between them, eastern Poland, until 1941, was under Soviet occupation. Polish Jews in the east, hearing of the atrocities carried out by the Germans, identified with the less evil aggressor and became Russophiles. Russian soldiers treated both Christians and Jews badly, but they treated them equally. The relative accommodation of Jews to Russian rule resulted in Christian Poles accusing them of collaboration, of being *quislings* (traitors) [23]. The Soviets, for their part, deliberately exploited ethnic tensions between Christians and Jews.

Fig. 17.2 The author's cousin, Rysio, who died of hunger in the Warsaw ghetto. (Photo taken in Zgierz, early 1939)

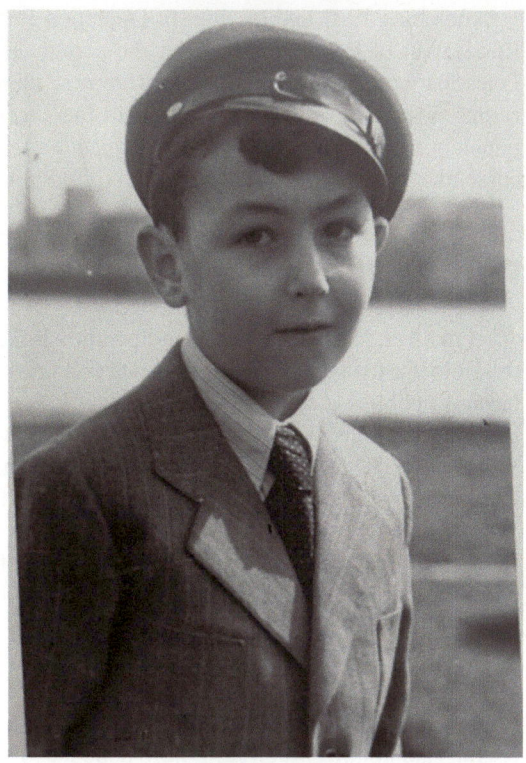

Fig. 17.3 In Memoriam

In Eternal Memory of the community of Zgierz who were exterminated in the years 5699-5705 (1939-1945)

May their souls be bound in the bonds of life and may their memory remain a blessing forever

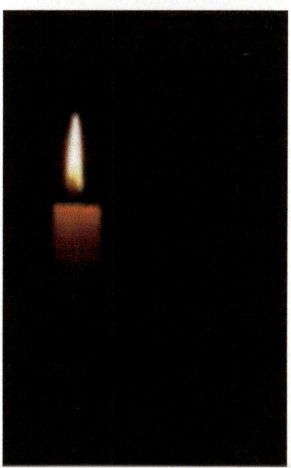

After June 1941 and the start of Operation Barbarossa (the German invasion of Russia), all of Poland came under the command of the German Reich. Ordinary Poles lost contact with Jews, who were now either in ghettos or in concentration camps or passing as Aryan or dead. In the absence of actual contact, the Polish population began to believe Nazi propaganda that Jews were diseased, spreaders of epidemics, dangerous profiteers, traitors, Russian spies, and war mongers.

Postwar Polish Anti-Semitism

After the war, in Soviet-ruled, post-liberation Poland, the fate of Polish Jews during the Holocaust was well known. Despite this knowledge, the anti-government press began to publish a series of anti-Jewish articles that accused Jews of being secret communist agents on a mission to destroy Catholic Poland [24–26].

The hatred that Poles felt for their Soviets war lords was redirected toward an easy target – returning Jews who had survived Russian exile or labor camps and who were attempting to regain ownership of the properties they had left behind. Returning Jews were met with strong anti-Semitic sentiment and, often enough, with violence. In total, 1500 Polish Jews were killed during this period [27] and 46, including an uncle who had survived Siberia, in the 1946 Kielce *pogrom* [28].

Matters further deteriorated when Jews began to occupy relatively powerful posts in the new communist regime in Poland. The fiercely anti-communist Catholic Church condemned all violence but did not take a stand against stigmatization. The church said nothing when Jews were denounced as immoral, freethinking, godless, Bolshevik, swindlers, usurers, and pornographers [2, 29].

In the twenty-first century, Poland has abandoned "old-fashioned" anti-Semitic beliefs such as holding Jews responsible for the death of Jesus or believing that Jews use Christian blood for ritual purposes. Nevertheless, a fair number of Poles still believe in a Jewish conspiracy ("Jews secretly want to influence world economy"; "they want to rule the world"; "they control international banking") [30].

A friend recently visited a souvenir shop in restored old Warsaw. To her horror, she saw refrigerator magnets and figurines that looked as if they belonged in Nazi Germany – caricatures of Jews with beards, *payot* (sideburns), *tzitzit* (tassels), black hats, and disproportionally large noses holding money sacs and gold coins as if they were, indeed, "controlling international banking." Poles say that these are talismans, good luck charms, akin to lucky leprechauns. Owning them is supposed to make you as lucky financially as Jews are purported to be. According to Wikipedia (https://en.wikipedia.org/wiki/Jew_with_a_coin), 19% of Poles keep "Jew with a coin" statuettes in their homes. The saying in Polish goes: "Jew in the hall, coin in your pocket." These amulets have been described as Jungian "old man" archetypes, semi-sacred objects that ensure financial prosperity [31]. Figures 17.4 and 17.5, more than a thousand words can ever do, symbolize the complicated attitude toward Jews in present day Poland.

Today's Poles also believe that Jews make too much of their victim status ("they want to make the world feel guilty"; "they keep wanting more reparations") [32]. Such prejudices are expressions of stereotypic anti-Semitic beliefs, but they are not necessarily evidence of animosity toward Jews.

Fig. 17.4 Refrigerator magnet. (Photo taken in Warsaw by Joan Cohen, July, 2019)

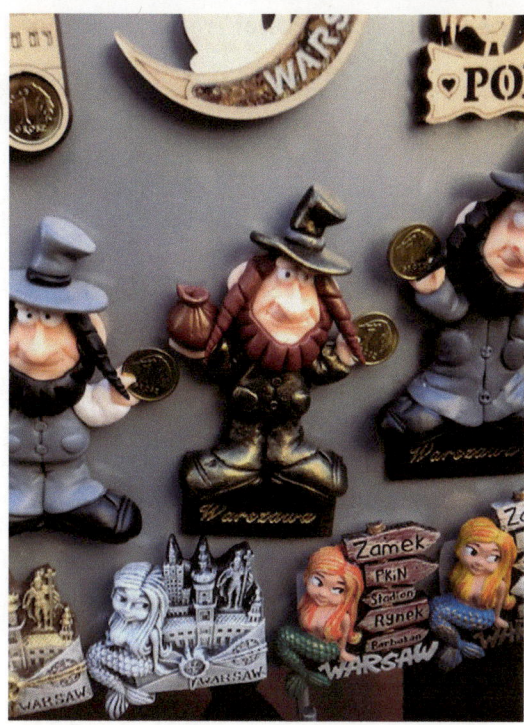

Fig. 17.5 Jew with a coin statuette. (Photo taken in Warsaw by Joan Cohen, July, 2019)

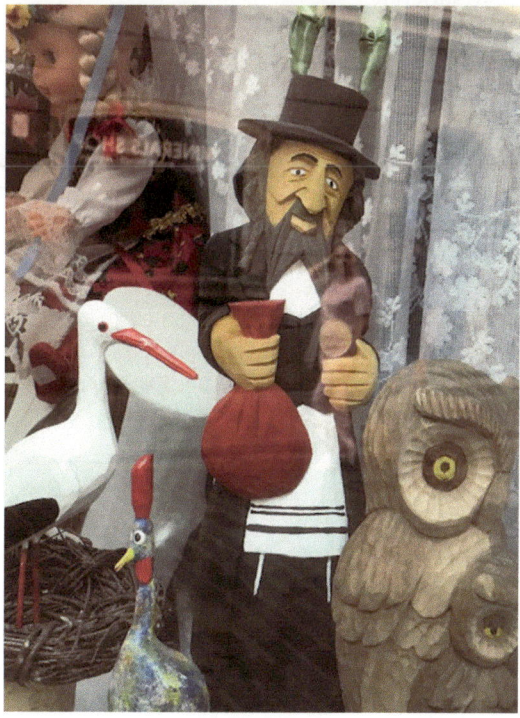

The Intergenerational Transmission of Trauma

Can the trauma of events such as the Holocaust leave its mark on the generations that follow? It is probably not coincidence that several of my Zgierz grandfather's descendants have gone into the helping professions, especially psychology and psychiatry. Even more have devoted their lives to advocating for peace between Palestinians and Jews in the Middle East, a form of solidarity among the children of Shem.

Children of survivors are all defined by the Holocaust, but in different ways.

> **Box 17.4**
>
> One of my ex-patients, both of whose parents were Holocaust survivors, despised her parents and blamed them for her disastrous childhood. She blamed them for all the physical, psychological, academic, occupational, and relationship problems that she experienced as a young adult. She ended up hating all things Jewish. When she decided to enter psychoanalysis, she chose a German analyst, the son of a Nazi officer, and her parents paid for the analysis.

Canadian psychiatrist and scholar, Vivian Rakoff, in 1966 first observed the paradox that, among the families he was treating in Montreal, the generation that had survived the Holocaust was doing relatively well but their children, born in Canada, were suffering [33].

This was the start of psychiatric research into intergenerational effects among second-generation survivors, who have turned out to be a very heterogeneous group. Both they and their parents underwent substantially different experiences at different ages and stages of life. Each person responded to these experiences differently, according to their diverse personalities and backgrounds and capabilities [34]. The parenting style of Holocaust survivors has been described as distant, uncommunicative, and irritable [35]. Second-generation survivors have been characterized as struggling with separation-individuation, being prone to anxiety and posttraumatic stress and vulnerable to depression [36], but these generalizations are mainly based on samples who have sought psychiatric help. The duration of trauma symptoms in the parents and the quality of parenting depend, to a large degree, not only on what individuals went through during the war but also on their post-Holocaust experiences [37], which help to explain the wide range of reactions in subsequent generations.

> **Box 17.5**
>
> The characterization of survivors of the Holocaust into first, second, and third generations is problematic. I am first generation in that I was there, remember the shame of wearing the yellow star, and remember the terror of having a

Nazi officer billeted in our apartment. I remember the panic when Polish neighbors tried to drive us out of our apartment, as well as an immense gratitude when the Nazi officer chased them away. As a result of these early experiences, I am probably more risk averse than I would otherwise be. I am also a second-generation survivor in that I grew up with parents who had lost so much. As a result, I am more protective of my children (and probably also of my patients) than I ought to be. And I am a third-generation survivor because I identify with my scholarly grandfather who died in a vain attempt to prevent his precious books from falling into evil hands. As a result, I am overly bookish.

Epigenetics

The vulnerability of children of Holocaust survivors to personality problems and to psychopathology has been attributed to defects in parenting or to parents unconsciously modeling anxiety and fearfulness. More recently, Nathan Kellerman points out that the indelible marks left by the Holocaust on descendants, reminders of the tattooed numbers on their parents' forearms, may be epigenetic chemical coatings on their DNA that represent a biological memory of their parents' experience [38]. Children are influenced by their parents via different pathways – they share half of each parent's genes, which, from birth, makes it easy to follow in their parents' footsteps. They learn from early on to imitate their parents by watching them, by listening to their stories, and by taking to heart parental warnings, corrections, and rewards. Methylation of DNA, modification of the histone framework of DNA, and changes to noncoding RNA are all newly discovered mechanisms that are responsive to the environment, especially at critical time periods early in life. They either allow the expression of existing genes or they work to silence their expression [39]. In other words, only some of our genes are ever expressed; some lie dormant, but they can sometimes be roused into action by appropriate stimuli. The good news is that epigenetic marks, if they silence beneficial genes or rouse harmful genes, can, at least theoretically, be reversed [40].

Rachel Yehuda has done important work on the intergenerational transmission of Holocaust trauma and trauma in general. Her work has led to the current understanding that physical or mental stress experienced by parents prior to conception, at conception, during pregnancy, or during the early postnatal period can be transmitted to offspring via enduring epigenetic modifications [41]. Parental stress can result in structural brain changes in offspring; it can shape children's personalities and their cognitive functioning and can serve as the root of physical and mental illnesses.

One hypothesis for transfer of stress vulnerability is via placental transfer from mother to fetus of high levels of stress hormones [42]. The role of transplacental passage of other body chemicals that can affect the fetus, such as immune factors or the hormone, oxytocin, has also been considered [43]. But most recent work stresses epigenetic influences, investigates both maternal and paternal transfer [44, 45], and addresses differential effects on male and female offspring [46]. The field is relatively new and therefore complex, but it is rapidly adding to our understanding of generational effects [47].

Conclusion

What I have learned in writing this chapter is that anti-Semitism existed for centuries before the Holocaust and continues to exist and to periodically prosper, especially in times of widespread stress and deprivation. Fear and ostracism of the "other" appear to be natural human phenomena – natural but irrational. Jews have been vilified as unpatriotic world citizens and, at the same time, as insular isolationists; as freethinkers and, at the same time, as mystic; and as weak and sickly while, at the same time, cunning, sly, and militaristic. They are excoriated as rabid communists and, at the same time, as greedy, grasping capitalists, simultaneously as left-wing socialists and right-wing imperialists. The specific stereotype changes from one era to another, from one location to another [48]. I have learned that anti-Semites have no identifying characteristics and that the expression of stigmatizing clichés about Jews does not necessarily mean animosity. Very often, it is outside parties, for political or economic reasons of their own, who incite anti-Semitic aggression. I have also learned how much the trauma of discrimination, of being excluded, dismissed, and disrespected, hurts, how often the hurt is passed on, and how it can last and exert its influence for generations.

References

1. Dynner G, Wodziński M. The kingdom of Poland and her Jews: an introduction. In: Dynner G, Polonsky A, Wodziński M, editors. Jews in the Kingdom of Poland 1815-1918. Polin: studies in Polish Jewry, vol. 27. Oxford/Portland: The Littman Library of Jewish Civilization; 2015. p. 3–44.
2. Kofta M, Sedek M. Conspiracy stereotypes of Jews during systemic transformation in Poland. Int J Sociol. 2005;35:40–64.
3. Jagodzińska A. Overcoming the signs of the "other". Visual aspects of the acculturation of Jews in the Kingdom of Poland in the nineteenth century. Polin. 2011;24:71–83.
4. Wolf-Yasni A. Jews in Zgierz until 1862. In: Landau J, translator. Shtockfish D, Kanc S, Fisher Z, editors. Memorial book of Zgierz, Poland. Tel Aviv: Zgierz Society; 1975–86. p. 82–93.
5. Dynner G. Legal fictions: the survival of rural Jewish tavern keeping in the Kingdom of Poland. Jew Soc Stud. 2010;16(2):28–66.
6. Gerrits A. Antisemitism and anti-communism: the myth of "Judeo-Communism" in eastern Europe. East Eur Jew Aff. 1995;25(1):49–72.
7. Friedrich A. The image of the Warsaw Pogrom of 1881 in late nineteenth-century Polish literature. East Eur Jew Aff. 2010;40(2):145–57.
8. Rudnicki S. The Siedlce Pogrom. Jew Hist Quart. 2010;233(1):18–39.
9. Janowsky OI. The Jews and minority rights. New York: Columbia University Press; 1933.
10. Wynot ED Jr. The Polish Germans, 1919-1939: national minority in a multinational state. Pol Rev. 1972;17(1):23–64.

11. Gradel M. "Zgierz" – encyclopedia of Jewish communities in Poland, Vol I (Poland). Pinkas Hakehillot Polin. Wirth M. (project coordinator). Jerusalem: Yad Vashem Publications; 1976. p. 106–11.
12. Wynot ED Jr. "A necessary cruelty": the emergence of official anti-Semitism in Poland, 1936-39. Am Hist Rev. 1971;76(4):1035–58.
13. Gilman SL. Smart Jews: the construction of the image of Jewish superior intelligence. Lincoln: University Nebraska Press; 1996.
14. Rabinowicz H. The battle of the ghetto benches. Jew Quart Rev. 1964;55(2):151–9.
15. Aleksiun N. Christian corpses for Christians!: dissecting the anti-Semitism behind the cadaver affair in the second Polish Republic. East Eur Polit Soc. 2011;25(3):393–409.
16. Aleksiun N. Jewish students and Christian corpses in interwar Poland: playing with the language of blood libel. Jew Hist. 2012;26:327–42.
17. Seeman MV. Cadavers for dissection. Hektoen Int. 2016;8:1. http://hekint.org/2017/01/22/cadavers-for-dissection/.
18. Pentlin SL. The Holocaust experience in western Poland. J Ecumenical Stud. 2011;46(4):557–66.
19. Gilbert M. The Holocaust: a history of the Jews of Europe during the Second World War. New York: Henry Holt and Co; 1985. p. 85.
20. Vinen RA. History in fragments: Europe in the twentieth century. Cambridge: Da Capo; 2001. p. 200.
21. Dąbrowska D, Wein A. Jews of Zgierz under the German occupation of terror. In: Landau J, translator. Shtockfish D, Kanc S, Fisher Z, editors. Memorial book of Zgierz. Tel Aviv: Zgierz Society; 1975–86. p. 537–551.
22. Afonso R, Koifman F. Sousa Mendes, Souza Dantas, and the flight of Polish refugees from France. Pol Rev. 2015;60(3):21–42.
23. Smolar A. Jews as a Polish problem. Daedalus. 1987;116(2):31–73.
24. Blatman D. The encounter between Jews and Poles in Lublin district after liberation, 1944-1945. East Eur Polit Soc. 2006;20(4):598–621.
25. Engel D. Patterns of anti-Jewish violence in Poland, 1944–1946. Yad Vashem Stud. 1998;26:43–85.
26. Michlic-Coren J. Anti-Jewish violence in Poland, 1918–1939 and 1945–1947. Polin Stud Pol Jew. 2000;13:34–61.
27. Gross JT. After Auschwitz: the reality and meaning of postwar antisemitism in Poland, dark times, dire decisions, Jews and communism. Stud Contemp Jew. 2004;20:214–5.
28. Kirsten K. The pogrom of Jews in Kielce on July 4, 1946. Acta Pol Hist. 1997;76:197–212.
29. Harris LT, Fiske ST. Social neuroscience evidence for dehumanized perception. Eur Rev Soc Psychol. 2009;20:192–231.
30. Hassian M Jr. Understanding the power of conspiratorial rhetoric: a case study of the protocols of the elders of Zion. Commun Stud. 1997;48(3):195–214.
31. Naraniecki A. Poland's "lucky Jew" statues: between philosemitic idolatry and anti-Semitic demonology. 21 Aug 2012. https://ejewishphilanthropy.com/polands-lucky-jew-statues/.
32. Bilewicz M, Winiewski M, Kofta M, Wójcik A. Harmful ideas, the structure and consequences of anti-Semitic beliefs in Poland. Pol Psychol. 2013;34(6):821–39.
33. Rakoff V. A long term effect of the concentration camp experience. Viewpoints. 1966;1:17–22.
34. Kellermann NPF. Transmitted Holocaust trauma: curse or legacy? The aggravating and mitigating factors of Holocaust transmission. Isr J Psychiatry Relat Sci. 2008;45:263–71.
35. Barel E, Van Ijzendoorn MH, Sagi-Schwartz A, Bakermans-Kranenburg MJ. Surviving the Holocaust: a meta-analysis of the long-term sequelae of a genocide. Psychol Bull. 2010;136:677–98.
36. Kellermann NPF. Psychopathology in children of Holocaust survivors: a review of the research literature. Isr J Psychiatry Relat Sci. 2001;38:36–47.
37. Greenblatt Kimron L, Marai I, Lorber A, Cohen M. The long-term effects of early-life trauma on psychological, physical and physiological health among the elderly: the study of Holocaust survivors. Aging Ment Health. 2019;10:1340–49.

38. Kellerman NPF. Epigenetic transmission of Holocaust trauma: can nightmares be inherited? Isr J Psychiatry Relat Sci. 2013;50:33–9.
39. Perez MF, Lehner B. Intergenerational and transgenerational epigenetic inheritance in animals. Nat Cell Biol. 2019;21:143–51.
40. Aoued HS, Sannigrahi S, Doshi N, Morrison FG, Linsenbaum H, Hunter SC, et al. Reversing behavioral, neuroanatomical, and germline influences of intergenerational stress. Biol Psychiatry. 2019;85:248–2.
41. Yehuda R, Bierer LM. The relevance of epigenetics to PTSD: implications for the DSM-V. J Trauma Stress. 2009;22:427–34.
42. Moog NK, Buss C, Entringer S, Shahbaba B, Gillen DL, Hobel CJ, et al. Maternal exposure to childhood trauma is associated during pregnancy with placental-fetal stress physiology. Biol Psychiatry. 2016;79:831–9.
43. Toepfer P, Heim C, Entringer S, Binder E, Wadhwa P, Buss C. Oxytocin pathways in the intergenerational transmission of maternal early life stress. Neurosci Biobehav Rev. 2017;73:293–308.
44. Bohacek J, Mansuy IM. Molecular insights into transgenerational non-genetic inheritance of acquired behaviours. Nat Rev Genet. 2015;16:641–52.
45. Rando OJ. Daddy issues: paternal effects on phenotype. Cell. 2012;151:702–8.
46. Carpenter T, Grecian S, Reynolds R. Sex differences in early-life programming of the hypothalamic-pituitary-adrenal axis in humans suggest increased vulnerability in females: a systematic review. J Dev Orig Health Dis. 2017;8:244–55.
47. Yehuda R, Lehrner A. Intergenerational transmission of trauma effects: putative role of epigenetic mechanisms. World Psychiatry. 2018;17:243–57.
48. Cohen F, Jussim L, Harber KD, Bhasin G. Modern anti-Semitism and anti-Israeli attitudes. J Pers Soc Psychol. 2009;97:290–306.

Part IV

Social Psychiatric Implications

Community Resilience and the Pittsburgh Synagogue Shooting

Suzanne Vogel-Scibilia

> That which does not kill us, makes us stronger. – Friedrich Nietzsche in *Twilight of the Idols*, 1888.

Introduction

Shortly before 10 am on Shabbat (Jewish Sabbath) morning, October 27, 2018, Robert Bowers entered the Tree of Life building in the quiet Pittsburgh neighborhood of Squirrel Hill where three separate congregations, Dor Hadash, New Light, and Tree of Life, worship. Carrying four firearms including an AR-15-style assault rifle and shouting anti-Semitic slurs, he killed eleven individuals and injured four responding police officers and two other congregants [1]. Less than 1 year before, Robert Bowers opened an account on Gab, a site known to allow controversial speech [2, 3]. In the month before the shooting, written comments from that account addressed HIAS (Hebrew Immigrant Aid Society), a Jewish nonprofit organization that assists refugees from many areas of the world: "Why hello there HIAS! You like to bring in hostile invaders to dwell among us?" [2]. Shortly before the shooter entered the Tree of Life building, another message was posted from that account: "HIAS likes to bring invaders in that kill our people. I can't sit by and watch my people get slaughtered. Screw your optics, I'm going in" [2].

Robert Bowers was wounded during the police response. One of the cantors from a Tree of Life congregation stated that police intercepted Bowers as he exited the building, and later police expressed their concern that Bowers was leaving the synagogue at the time to go to another synagogue about 4 minutes away. The rapid police response is credited with saving lives and preventing further injury. At the

S. Vogel-Scibilia (✉)
Chatham University, Pittsburgh, PA, USA
e-mail: svs2u@hotmail.com

© Springer Nature Switzerland AG 2020
H. S. Moffic et al. (eds.), *Anti-Semitism and Psychiatry*,
https://doi.org/10.1007/978-3-030-37745-8_18

time of this publication, Robert Bowers is awaiting trial on 29 federal criminal counts including firearm charges during commission of murder and hate crime designated obstructing the free exercise of religious beliefs. He also faces 11 counts of criminal homicide, 6 counts of aggravated assault, and 13 counts of ethnic intimidation which are state-level charges [2]. Bowers was brought back to court in February 2019 to face 19 further counts; he acknowledged reading the indictment and was aware that the prosecution was seeking the death penalty [4, 5]. This shooting was the largest mass murder against Jews in US history [6]. Robert Bowers had no prior criminal record.

Killed in the Pittsburgh shooting were 11 faithful individuals described by all as the mainstays of their congregations [7]. The youngest were two brothers, David (aged 54) and Cecil (aged 59) Rosenthal who had developmental disabilities but lived independently. They were weekly Tree of Life worshipers. Jeffrey Solomon, another lifelong Tree of Life congregant related to the brothers by marriage, recalled "they were what we call "shomerim," people who guard the religion even for the rest of us who don't go all the time" [7].

The rest of the victims from Tree of Life congregation included Irving Younger (aged 69) who was a retired real estate agent and former little league coach [8], Sylvan (aged 86) and Bernice Simon (aged 84) who died in the same synagogue where they married over 60 years ago, and Joyce Feinberg (aged 75), a grandmother and retired University of Pittsburgh researcher [9]. The oldest member killed that day, Rose Mallinger (aged 97), had survived the Holocaust and enjoyed life and her family. Her daughter, Andrea Wedner (aged 61), was wounded in the attack [10].

Killed among the worshipers at New Light Congregation were Daniel Stein (aged 70), a substitute teacher who had just welcomed a new grandson in that sanctuary [11], Dr. Richard Gottfried (aged 65) who was a beloved dentist assisting immigrants and refugees, and the always joking Melvin Wax (aged 88) who loved his grandson, the synagogue, and the Pittsburgh Pirates [12].

Fatally injured Congregation Dor Hadash member, Dr. Jerry Rabinowitz (aged 66), was a well-loved, respected family physician to many generations. He was also one of the first physicians treating Pittsburghers who had AIDS in the 1980s [13]. Daniel Leger (aged 70), a surviving Congregation Dor Hadash member and a University of Pittsburgh chaplain, was shot in the torso [9, 14].

Recent Increase in Anti-Semitic Incidents

Numerous articles in both academic and journalistic publications describe a recent rise in North America and Europe of anti-Semitic statements, demonstrations, and acts of violence [15–18]. The Anti-Defamation League in its 2017 Audit of Anti-Semitic Incidents in the United States describes a clear rise in overall incidents of harassment, vandalism, and assaults from 941 in 2015 to 1267 in 2016 and 1986 in 2017 [19]. The largest percentage increase from 2016 to 2017 was an 86% increase in vandalism and an 89% increase in college and university-related events [19]. Increases in vandalism are worrisome because the perpetrators are more secure advancing from harassment to breaking existing laws [19].

Current anti-Semitic rhetoric spues from such odd bedfellows as the alt-right, parts of radical left as well as Islamic extremists [20]. These groups often justify these statements by wrapping their commentary in an anti-Zionist message [21, 22]. One faction of US citizens often identifying from the radical left currently supports the Boycott, Divestment, and Sanctions (BDS) strategy [23]. This Palestinian-led movement urges boycotts and sanctions against Israel and its supporters until Israel accepts the conditions of (1) withdrawal from occupied territory, (2) removal of separation for West Bank residents, and (3) acknowledgment of the rights of Palestinian refugees for returning their homes and properties in current Israeli areas [24].

At the core of BDS strategy is associating Israel with an apartheid-type policy while advocating for a one-state model for resolution [24]. The other perspective argues that BDS is inherently anti-Zionist and that apartheid does not apply to the Palestinian situation since Muslims and Jews live together today within Israel; BDS requirements would jeopardize the safety of Israeli inhabitants [25]. Others argue that the BDS movement is a weapon in the attempt to delegitimize Israel and its Jewish inhabitants and remove their ability for self-determination [26]. Many critics of BDS further assert that its purpose is anti-Semitism cloaked in an anti-Zionist message [27].

An increase in economic uncertainty and societal upheaval coincides with increased anti-Semitic rhetoric. History supports these social changes as a precursor to anti-Semitic surges [28]. Even more troubling is the increased visibility and acceptance of such speech in the mainstream media by prominent politicians [29].

Though not necessarily related to the rise of BDS, there is a simultaneous proliferation of nationalistic sentiments and anti-immigrant policies in North America and Europe. Robert Bower's comments on Gab suggest that part of his targeting of the Tree of Life congregations may have come from a warped association on his part about refugees and Judaism. His verbalized slurs at the time of the shooting suggest he also had internalized anti-Semitic beliefs.

Interviews for this Chapter Within the Pittsburgh Jewish Community

Ten Jewish individuals from Pittsburgh participated in interviews for this chapter with open-ended discussion where spontaneous themes were noted and tallied about anti-Semitism and resilience – two interviews were only ½ hour; others lasted 2 or 3 hours. Seven out of ten interviewees allowed me to tape the interviews for accuracy of comments. Releases were obtained for five people who discussed their personal experiences. Others discussed a more narrow focus involving anti-Semitism in Pittsburgh, past and present, and reactions to the Pittsburgh shooting or providing support to the Jewish community, including family members who lost loved ones or the survivors. The sample, though small, was diverse – spanning millenials to octogenarians, survivors at the building that day to survivors of the Holocaust, and therapists/administrators involved in the post-incident counseling to religious leaders in the community – all connected to the three congregations worshipping at the Tree of Life building.

Resurgence of Anti-Semitism and Anti-Zionist Rhetoric in Recent Years

Several respondents described a belief prior to the recent events that anti-Semitism did not exist in Pittsburgh as it did in the twentieth century. They discussed how Jewish individuals were more integrated and accepted in American society. But after the recent US surge in hate crimes and racism followed by the recent synagogue shootings in Pittsburgh and then the 2019 attack at the Chabad of Poway, California, people described feeling more vulnerable. One therapist stated: "We used to say it could not happen here, but now we don't say that. We say it has happened and it could happen (again). That is something we are still trying to wrap our heads around."

Even antiquated anti-Semitic fearmongering about a Judeo-Bolshevism network of financial control and antidemocratic intrigue common in the mid-twentieth century has resurfaced in the current US milieu [30, 31]. Interviewees almost universally commented on these developments as unsettling. One older individual who was a Holocaust survivor likened some of these developments to propaganda campaigns during the early days of Nazi rule.

There were worries verbalized by two individuals that Holocaust deniers will become more vocal since Holocaust survivors are passing away or becoming more frail. One Rabbi stated: "Every day we lose more Holocaust survivors and that brings more strength to the deniers." In many areas of Europe where Jewish life is almost completely obliterated, Holocaust deniers now accuse the Jewish people of attempting to benefit from memorials or symbols in these areas that reflect the losses from the Holocaust. Those who deface Jewish synagogues and cemeteries present another form of anti-Semitism that seeks to negate the human suffering involved. Every one of the Holocaust survivors interviewed emphasized the importance of Shoah testimony (describing in detail one's personal experience of the Holocaust in permanent form) to address this. Several have already participated.

Societal Response of Non-Jews to Anti-Semitism

In environments where anti-Semitism is overt, society-wide denial, acceptance of marginalization, and even discrimination are unfortunate common responses from the non-Jewish populations. The degree of moral resistance, both transparent and discrete, from the non-Jewish population often is a factor in preventing escalation of anti-Semitic actions. While the individuals whose views are on the extremes are often vocal participants in advancing or mitigating anti-Semitic rhetoric, there is much to be said for people in the middle of the political spectrum speaking up and demonstrating that anti-Semitic behavior is unacceptable.

Pennsylvania Supreme Court Judge David Wecht publically discussed anti-Semitism after the Pittsburgh shooting. He noted this tragedy at the synagogue where he was married and previously worshipped: "For a time after the Holocaust, the sheer horror and magnitude of the slaughter tended to tamp down the most vocal anti-Semites. But something's changed both on the right and the left. People are increasingly willing to voice anti-Semitic sentiments. And when people, particularly leaders, don't publically oppose anti-Jewish speech, hatred against Jews festers and grows. And that's why I think this is a critical time in America" [32].

Historically, speaking out against anti-Semitism can be fraught with great risk when the government involved in these actions represses human rights of all individuals. An example is the outcome of the White Rose passive resistance by medical personnel and students in Munich, Germany, in 1943 [33]. Governmental policies and legislation vigorously addressing anti-Semitism along with grassroots community support from a consortium of non-Jewish and Jewish citizens can restrict the propagation of anti-Semitic culture in societies at risk.

Responses from Members of the Jewish Communities in Pittsburgh

Many interviewed members of the Pittsburgh Jewish community commented on the shock that such a thing could happen within an area of Pittsburgh known as a safe neighborhood for all individuals. Interviewees identified Squirrel Hill as both the historic and current center of the region's Jewish life. This is verified by 2017 Pittsburgh Jewish Community Study describing the greatest concentration of Jewish households in the Squirrel Hill section of Pittsburgh, including 48% of the Jewish children under the age of 18 [34].

At the same time, many of these same interviewees referenced the long history of oppression, violence, and discrimination that Jewish people have experienced even within those civilizations where they had the appearance of cordial relations with the non-Jewish majority. Despite this uncertainty, the interviews show uniform themes of resilience and survival, partially due to an understanding of Jewish historical adversity. One therapist described a "Judaism 101" class provided by their Jewish counseling agency to non-Jewish employees, where an encapsulation of the Jewish holidays was summed up as: "They tried to kill us; we prevailed; let's go eat." The repetitive theme portrayed is living in a disadvantaged place in society, being attacked, struggling, and surviving with celebration.

Interviewees verbalized uniform understanding of the persistent anti-Semitism that Jewish people have experienced which transcends any one area, time, or culture. They also noted the precarious status of the Jewish people as minorities within most countries where they have lived throughout recorded time and the constant cycle of relative societal acceptance followed by increased restrictions and discrimination, even pogroms. The creation of the word pogrom supports this belief. Of Russian/Yiddish origin about 1882, pogrom first described the violence and murder perpetrated on Russian Jews after Tsar Alexander II's assassination by a non-Jewish individual [35].

Elaborating on the nature of anti-Semitism historically, many identified societal acceptance of Jewish people as being fragile. This echoes the comments from an earlier discussion in this chapter that anti-Semitism could become more mainstream within a culture experiencing change in the controlling government regime or the general level of prosperity or security of the country they lived in. Three interviewees commented on the knowledge not just within the Jewish people but within non-Jewish of the meaning of the word "pogrom" as evidence of a common realization of longitudinal historical violence and discrimination based on being of Jewish religion.

Respondents from the Pittsburgh Jewish community could relate many historical examples of past violence or repression referenced first in the Torah, continuing in the following centuries, transitioning to earlier European pogroms, and then spending more time discussing the twentieth-century Holocaust. Their individualized comments had a striking similarity suggesting that many Jewish people in Pittsburgh if not in a broader sample have learned in a culturally ingrained manner that the historical dangerousness of being Jewish is an ongoing risk. Follow-up questions led to the interviewees describing their families, elders, and religious educators as being instrumental in this perspective as well as further self-guided reading and learning on the subject.

Individual Responses to Anti-Semitism

Another area of the interviews focused on individual experiences of anti-Semitism in Pittsburgh both past and present, how individuals coped, and what coping skills were utilized. Again, interviewees described experiences of anti-Semitism as being more overt and accepted within the greater society at earlier periods of the twentieth century. Common examples given by the interviewees included personalized stories of the use of limiting quotas for graduate education, restriction of home ownership to certain areas, employment discrimination, and barring of individuals from membership in professional societies, guilds, swimming pools, or country clubs. They also cited problems when Jewish friends attempted to marry outside their religion.

Possibly because this author identified herself as a native Pittsburgh physician, three interviewees gave the example of the restriction banning Jewish physicians from having medical privileges at a major academic hospital in Pittsburgh for a large portion of the twentieth century. This led to the Jewish community building an equally large and esteemed hospital, Montefiore, on the next block which functioned with a separate medical staff, medical records system, and residency program until merging with the other hospital in 1990. This author was a Montefiore house staff member for a transitional internal medicine year in 1985–1986 and was impressed by the strong competition between the two hospitals in recruiting well-qualified University of Pittsburgh medical students who rotate through both programs.

When describing these specific personal experiences of anti-Semitism, multiple respondents described these events as part of the historical culture of being Jewish. They identified this as a barrier that they and their ancestors had triumphed over and would continue to do in the future. Many discussed these actions as being due to character defects in the aggressors, not something the Jewish people have brought upon themselves. One person referenced the Jewish valued principles of family, education, and altruism directed in the Torah as drawing jealousy from others.

Others talked about the association of family life as integral to the Jewish religion, providing a sense of strength and resiliency for themselves. They provided examples of Kosher food preparation, celebrating High Holy Days with home-based meals, lighting candles at home during Shabbat, funeral or marriage rituals, and specific instructions in Torah about the importance of marriage and family life as providing a sense of interpersonal strength and support for their human as well as Jewish identity.

Two respondents referenced their distinct Jewish culture, dress, and language along with possible legal statutes that restricted where Jewish people lived or worked as aiding identification as a recognizable minority subgroup within the larger population, making Jews a convenient target for societal anger and frustration. One therapist described Jewish individuals as having had their feelings of safety in their Jewishness being compromised by the Pittsburgh shooting. Then the Poway, California, synagogue shooting "amplified the feeling that they were being targeted. Their personal history of anti-Semitism and any family history of the Holocaust were brought front and center."

One therapist interviewed described how since the shooting many loosely observant Jewish people have expressed a desire or a need to be more active in the synagogue and share their religion with family members by increasing family time, lighting Sabbath candles, saying kiddush over wine, or giving parental blessings to the children. Several people noted the marked general increase in synagogue worship not just for Holy Days but for weekly Shabbat services. One therapist noted the importance of community in worship and gave as an example the minyan or need to have ten people over the age of 13 to conduct public Jewish worship. This trend of increased interest in religious observance, inside and outside of a synagogue, has been sustained for almost a year at the time of this manuscript submission.

There is a perception from many interviewees that the shooting brought members of the Jewish community closer together. One person commented that the shooter wanted to impede the Jewish religion, incite terror, and kill the Jewish people, but despite the loss of 11 devout members, Judaism in Pittsburgh has been unbroken and possibly more ardently practiced since the tragedy. Rabbi Jeffrey Myers from the Tree of Life congregation wrote in an Ideas Op-ed in *Time Magazine*: "Yet my deep abiding faith grew even greater. I turn to God daily for support, guidance and inspiration. It was apparent from the beginning that my being spared had to lead to action, that the 11 must not have died in vain" [36]. Another interviewee echoed those sentiments "when you survive a violent event because of your religion, your faith means more to you."

Four people also described feeling closer to their non-Jewish neighbors who presented a groundswell of support for the Jewish community after the massacre. Over 3000 Pittsburghers congregated later on the day of the shooting for an interfaith prayer vigil organized by Taylor Allderdice High School students which began across from the Jewish Community Center, at the Sixth Presbyterian Church. Sixth Presbyterian's Reverend Vincent Kolb was direct about the community response to this attack: "We gather because we are heartbroken but also to show zero tolerance for anti-Semitic speech, anti-Semitic behavior and anti-Semitic violence" [37]. Rabbi Keren Gorban of Squirrel Hill's Temple Sinai taught the crowd a Hebrew phrase that translates into English: "May you spread your shelter of peace over us" [37].

Many additional gatherings were designed to help the community heal and address the feelings of grief, vulnerability, and uncertainty [38–40]. Messages of zero tolerance for anti-Semitism and ending hate crimes were also prominent. Members of the Jewish community met with other US victims of religious hate crimes as well as survivors of other mass murder incidents [41, 42]. Ultimately the topic changed to how can people affected by this violence heal and how can incidents like this be prevented in the future?

The Role of Social Media and the Internet in Anti-Semitic Behavior

Many disparate groups have identified the Internet as changing the face of political and social discourse, but the Internet's anonymity and open access can create havens for people promoting hate speech. While the Pittsburgh shooter used Gab for his comments, 8chan, a message board on the Internet which is a bastion of the alt-right community, also offered anonymity and no supervision [43].

8chan has been involved in postings by the shooter in three other recent mass murders: a mosque in New Zealand; the synagogue in Poway, California; and a Walmart that serves many Hispanic residents in El Paso, Texas. The pattern has been to post manifestos or political commentary, and then shortly before the crime, the shooter places an announcement of his intent and asks others to promote his actions. After the August 2019 massacre in the El Paso Walmart, 8chan promoted a vile, virulent thread celebrating the deaths of so many victims as well as the motives of the shooter. One response by another contributor urged 8chan participants to develop memes and original content (OC) to facilitate easy distribution of the "heroic" shooter's perspective throughout the Internet: "You know what to do!!! Make OC; Spread OC; Share OC; Inspire OC. Make the world a better place" [44].

Another problem with hate-filled sites is that they can radicalize people who otherwise would not be exposed to this ideology. The suspected murderer at the synagogue, Chabad of Poway, shooting in April 2019 wrote on 8chan before the attack that he'd been visiting 8chan for "a year and a half, yet what I've learned here is priceless. It's been an honor" [45].

Ms. Joan Donovan, the director of the Technology and Social Change Research Project at Harvard University's Shorenstein Center, describes how mass shooters have learned to send out messages online before the shooting to enhance the focus and the dissemination of their views [45]. Donovan further elaborates: "Mass shooters can control the public conversation about their motives, while at the same time provide the public with a clear explanation for their actions" [45].

After three mass shootings in 6 months were publicized by the alleged murderers, 8chan's decision to continue the site with nonexistent supervision created pressure against other companies who supported 8chan's presence on the web. Cloudflare, the Internet security and infrastructure company which prevents 8chan from being shut down due to distributed denial-of-service attacks by activists, first defended the presence of 8chan and then bowed to pressure and refused services to the message board. 8chan quickly announced it was transferring services to a smaller Canadian company, BitMitigate.

Two years ago, Cloudflare under similar pressure had cut loose a neo-Nazi site, Daily Stormer. Thus, Daily Stormer migrated to BitMitigate where Gab, the social network site used by Robert Bowers prior to the Pittsburgh shooting, was also hosted. Very quickly, Alex Stamos, a Stanford University researcher noted publically that BitMitigate's parent company, Epik, uses servers from another company, Voxility [46]. This public shaming of Voxility caused the lights to go off recently for both Daily Stormer and 8chan when Voxility removed Epik's access to their servers [47]. Tucows, another Internet service which assists in the registry of Internet addresses for 8chan, also removed its tech support [48].

In the immediate days after the shutdown, online messages suggest that both sites are trying to re-enter the Internet; there is also commentary suggesting that 8chan has moved over to the dark web [49]. The dark web is difficult for law enforcement to monitor and can only be accessed by specialized servers which are not easy to obtain. This presents a conflict. While access to 8chan's members' viewpoint will be more difficult and less people will be radicalized, the membership will be harder to monitor [49]. This represents the extreme difficulty in monitoring or eliminating social media sites that allow hate speech.

Ultimately monitoring and addressing hate speech and actions for domestic perpetrators in a way that allows government authorities more latitude particularly on the dark web could be helpful. It is not unexpected that the rise of domestic terrorism toward many groups has an eerie parallel to other terrorist organizations such as Islamic State, which has successfully used social media sites like 8chan and then progressed to the dark web for messaging and recruitment [50].

Characteristics of Anti-Semitic Trauma Compared to Other Violence-Related Trauma

Traumatic events are one of the most important environmental etiologies of mental illness. Lenore Terr identified four basic characteristics of childhood trauma symptoms which can continue into adulthood: (1) repeatedly perceived memories of the event, (2) repetitive behaviors, (3) trauma-specific fears, and (4) changed attitudes about life, people, and the future [51]. Terr also differentiated type I trauma which involved misperceptions and full, detailed memories from type II trauma that includes denial, numbing, dissociation, and rage [51].

Research on types of reminiscences involving Holocaust survivors in Israel documented three areas: self-positive (adaptive), self-negative (detrimental), and prosocial with common themes of horror, resilience, generativity, and gratitude [52]. An integrated review of 23 articles on life review or reminiscence functions in Holocaust survivors found that positive life events determined well-being, that using reminiscence positively was related to health, and that resilience and efforts to integrate the past into one's life review were ongoing [53].

While the experience of trauma from any source has universal manifestations and remedies, some aspects of trauma responses occurring from anti-Semitism are specific. Post-traumatic stress disorder (PTSD) is known to be more likely with man-made traumas, with man-made PTSD episodes being of longer duration and necessitating extended time for symptom recovery [54].

One therapist working with Jewish community members in Pittsburgh commented that with other types of trauma, the response of the individual is often based on their personal trauma history in unique ways. With anti-Semitic trauma, the responses of people are very similar and centered around their safety as it relates to their Jewishness. Interviews with people who are aware of the Jewish community response in Pittsburgh concur. One religious leader described people continuing to receive therapy and are on a trajectory toward feeling better – they are in the process of "allowing themselves to cope." Rabbi Myers echoes that sentiment as a nonlinear process: "Healing is not a constant upward line on a graph, but more like the peaks and valleys of an oscilloscope" [36] One interviewee had concern that Robert Bower's trial with the death penalty attached "may be like ripping the bandage off quickly when the scab is attached."

Antonovsky – while studying female Holocaust survivors as a subgroup of other women in Israel – found that 29% identified their health as good [55]. This led Antonovsky to change his focus from identifying pathology to searching for what is termed "salutogenesis," or discerning what leads to health and well-being in Holocaust survivors [55]. He found that coping well with stress and trauma was correlated to a "sense of coherence" defined as:

> a global orientation that expresses the extent to which one has a pervasive, enduring, though dynamic feeling of confidence that (1) the stimuli from one's internal and external environments in the course of living are structured, predictable, and explicable; (2) the resources are available to one to meet the demands posed by these stimuli; and (3) these demands are challenges, worthy of investment and engagement [56].

Two Holocaust survivors interviewed for this article did verbalize features of this viewpoint:

1. Seeing what has happened to the Jewish people over many generations as expected, though not deserved, and explained by others' character defects.
2. There is help and support particularly from their Jewish community as well as with non-Jews who have helped them heal. One Holocaust survivor described a previously little known relative who helped her immensely when she immigrated to the United States after World War II. Then she received the support of the Jewish communities within the United States where she lived. Both mentioned that these resources have been present now and for their ancestors.
3. They and their ancestors have addressed anti-Semitism, including the Holocaust and the Pittsburgh shooting, with resilience.
4. Despite the trauma and pain, it is their duty to live a good life and survive for all those who were lost.

The Nature of Resilience to Anti-Semitism

Many risk factors decrease resilience in the face of trauma. Issues such as the overall health of the individual, presence of cognitive impairment, and current level of stress at the time of trauma are not circumstances easily changed. The presence of past traumas including developmental trauma is a risk which cannot be changed but instead should be addressed.

One controversial risk is the concept of intergenerational trauma transmission. Epigenetic changes can be transmitted between generations either by DNA methylation, small noncoding RNA sequences, or histone posttranslational modifications and are recent avenues of research interest involving stress tolerance and PTSD risk [57, 58]. Methodological challenges and a dearth of extensive human studies of epigenetic mechanisms are limitations which should be remediated by future research efforts.

This chapter's focus on promoting resilience involves aspects that respond to therapeutic intervention and utilizes individuals' innate coping skills.

Resilience of Pittsburgh Jewish Individuals and Their Communities

The themes that support personal resilience by the Pittsburgh interviewees involved four areas: (1) identity, both personal and group, (2) mindfulness, (3) social integration, and (4) altruism.

Identity

Over half of the respondents spontaneously described a clear personal identity that embraced resilience themes – often fostered by their parents or extended family. This identity facilitated resilience behaviors in times of adversity. One respondent, a Holocaust survivor, described his mother's bravery and intellectual talents that allowed him to survive a concentration camp experience as a child, giving him a sense that she was able to control the arbitrary violence and frequent deaths that occurred around him. Another interviewee described an upbringing where parents and older siblings modeled a pattern of not backing down toward anti-Semitic intimidation or adversity. Other comments included the value of support from the broader Jewish community as mitigating negative emotional effects from anti-Semitism. The experience of anti-Semitism appeared to be acknowledged as wrong but something that people rose above. Multiple interviewees cited older relatives who modeled appropriate ways to address anti-Semitism when the Jewish interviewees were developing their personal identity as children or young adults that made coping more manageable. One respondent stated: "You see your parents and grandparents deal with it - you know what to do."

Mindfulness

It is not surprising given the body of evidence endorsing mindfulness as helping manage stress, anxiety, and adversity that anti-Semitic-based trauma improves when using mindfulness strategies. Several respondents talked about using mindfulness after anti-Semitic violence to help ground individuals in reality and allow the healing process to start. One respondent recalled being released from medical treatment after liberation from a concentration camp and seeking a walk on the beach, feeling the sand between her toes, and associating this with a return to a normal existence. She felt this experience facilitated the process of her recovery. Another respondent described using instrumental music to focus on positive ideas and to destress after the Pittsburgh shooting.

Social Integration

Resilience is enhanced by having strong community support and daily activities involving others who normalize everyday functioning after anti-Semitic trauma. Many interviewees discussed as positive events the community vigils, spontaneous gatherings, and religious services that occurred after the shooting in Pittsburgh. Much as the rituals surrounding funerals and mourning serve to assist the grieving, the nature of feeling welcomed by friends and neighbors helps integrate the traumatic event into a personal recovery narrative. All the people interviewed mentioned the community support and outreach in the aftermath of the shooting as helping individuals focus on positive concepts and resilience themes.

Altruism

Several respondents described altruism as being a healing component of their recovery. One interviewee described the process of focusing on a greater good as assuaging the feelings of personal pain or uncertainty in the aftermath of the shooting.

Synthesizing the Resilience Themes from the Pittsburgh Interviews into a Psycho-Developmental Framework

These four themes related by the interviewees support the concept described by Antonovsky earlier in this chapter as a "sense of coherence" that promotes positive coping skills for stress and trauma. The value of constructing an integrated life narrative echoes the psychological concept of life review often associated with Erikson's later stages of human development [59]. Prior publications by this author also discuss the similarities between the concept of resilience and recovery from another traumatic experience, severe mental illness, and the human developmental model posited by Erik Erikson [60].

Based on the themes from the Pittsburgh interviews, how humans cope with developmental life trauma especially in later Eriksonian stages appears to parallel the process of resilience from anti-Semitic trauma. Erikson's seventh stage of generativity versus stagnation has similarities to the interview themes of empowerment, identity, and altruism, while an integrative life narrative represents a successful positive resolution to Erikson's eighth stage of integrity versus despair. One striking observation from the interviews is that while aware that the focus of the interview was to be about anti-Semitism, the mass murder at Tree of Life, and resilience, all the older interviewees proceeded in the unstructured interview by recounting their views in the form of a longitudinal life narrative that started well before the Tree of Life shooting, often in childhood. Even with the focus of discussion being redirected to the more recent events, older interviewees had a common tendency to return to a sequential life narrative format. Often the interviews would extend well beyond the estimated 1-hour duration. This tendency was not observed in the interviewees younger than 40 years – though the sample size was very small. This small interview sample suggests that especially older individuals would benefit from open, unstructured life review therapeutic techniques that allow time to process anti-Semitic trauma into a coherent life narrative.

Where to Go from Here?

Dennis Prager and Joseph Telushkin posit that "Jew-haters begin with Jews but never end with them, as anti-Semitism is ultimately a hatred of higher standards..... Whoever sees anti-Semitism as only some aberrational hatred on the part of an otherwise morally acceptable group does not understand anti-Semitism" [61]. These authors also note that "It has gradually become clear that a hatred of Israel is a moral indicator of some precision. As the Christians of Lebanon, who have suffered far more from Muslim hatred than the Jews of Israel, have learned. Arab leaders who call for wars to annihilate Zionism are not otherwise tolerant, democracy loving gentleman (Syria's Assad, Iran's Khomeini, Libya's Gadhafi, Iraq's Hussein and Osama bin Laden are five examples given)" [62].

Anti-Semitism has been the most global, long-standing, and societally sanctioned hatred in history, with further evidence that hatred of the Jews is "the lightening rod for evil in every culture in which it lived" [63]. Despite this clear data, many societies experiencing any form of anti-Semitism often excuse incidents as being a "Jewish problem." It behooves non-Jews in any society to address anti-Semitic actions quickly and thoroughly to avoid escalation of sanctioned hate certainly for Jews but also for all members of that society.

Jewish Community Federation and Endowment Fund's website described suggestions for coping with anti-Semitic actions in ways that foster resilience [64]:

1. Find solidarity at a local synagogue.
2. Find solidarity outside the synagogue; you could become involved with Hillel or join/start a Moishe House. Moishe House's website states "Seeking out young professional or graduate students between the ages of 22 and 30, to live together and create their ideal Jewish community" [65].

One participant in Europe gave a testimonial about the Moishe program:

Since being involved with Moishe House, I really understand what it means to meet Shabbat in a "home" setting. And it is so inspiring! And now I understand that I can gather my friends from the community and help them feel inspired and comfortable in a Jewish home, sharing the atmosphere, knowledge and tradition with them. Alexandra Gorbataya, Moishe House Chisinau (Moldova) Resident [65].

3. Attend Shabbat at OneTable event.
4. Celebrate Jewish learning and living.
5. Pursue social justice or Tikkun olam described as acts of kindness meant to repair the world, while connecting with peers [66].
6. Show your solidarity online.
7. Support those affected by the shooting.
8. Support organizations combating hate and violence.
9. Receive help for trauma, fear, and anxiety.
10. Access resources to help have conversations with children and adolescents.

Aftermath

In the wake of the shooting, Tim Hindes developed a symbol by changing one of the three diamonds in the Pittsburgh Steeler logo into a Star of David and attaching the words – Stronger than Hate. Apparel using this symbol sold very briskly, while social media uploads occurred frequently [67].

The Tree of Life building has not reopened as of December 2019. The three congregations are worshipping at other locations in Pittsburgh [69]. As mentioned previously, clergy from the synagogues who were interviewed for this chapter state attendance has increased in the congregations affected by the shooting.

Administrators of the Pittsburgh Tree of Life synagogue building asked teenage artists to submit "original, uplifting works that express messages of peace, love, community, hope, healing and resilience" that will be placed in fencing outside the building to strengthen the community feelings of support [68].

There is visible evidence that Robert Bower's intent to wound HIAS has been unsuccessful. After the Pittsburgh shooting, the Hebrew Immigrant Aid Society, a national organization founded in 1881 and serving people immigrating to the United States from all countries and of all religious backgrounds, reported increased visibility and donations [69].

On August 17, 2019, members from two of the three congregations worshipping at the Tree of Life building, Dor Hadash, and New Light wrote letters asking for a plea deal for life in prison without parole for Robert Bowers [70]. The groups arguing against the death penalty cite religious reasons and avoiding the need of testimony which would be traumatic for surviving victims and their families. The justice department has rejected this request as discussed earlier and is proceeding with a death penalty case against Robert Bowers.

Members from Uganda's Tree of Life synagogue visited Pittsburgh on August 19, 2019 in order to foster greater connections between the two congregations. The leaders of the Ugandan synagogue adopted the Tree of Life name with the Pittsburgh congregation's approval after the October 2018 attack. Rabbi Jeffrey Myers commented that the Pittsburgh congregation will be sending prayer books to Kampala, Uganda, and stated "it's a dream one day to bring a Torah scroll to the Kampala congregation" [71].

Pittsburgh's newspaper, the *Post-Gazette*, won the 2019 Pulitzer Prize for breaking-news reporting of the Tree of Life shooting. In April 2019, the newspaper donated the $15,000 prize to the Tree of Life synagogue [72].

Several members belonging to Tree of Life (L'Simcha) congregation toured the Calvary Episcopal Church in Shadyside on September 9, 2019, to familiarize themselves with this location where they would celebrate the High Holy Days of Rosh Hashanah and Yom Kippur in 2019. The membership has been worshipping since the 2018 attack at Rodef Shalom Congregation in Shadyside but accepted the offer from the neighboring church. During the visit they used a ram's horn or shofar to test the acoustics for the typical Jewish new year greeting [73].

Rabbi Cheryl Klein from Congregation Dor Hadash found that her quote from the post-shooting vigil – "We will never let hatred be the victor" – was transcribed onto a Squirrel Hill street. Just as a shooter's comment can be virally dispersed over social media, Rabbi Klein's quote on the sidewalk was photographed by another individual and disseminated widely over the Internet [74].

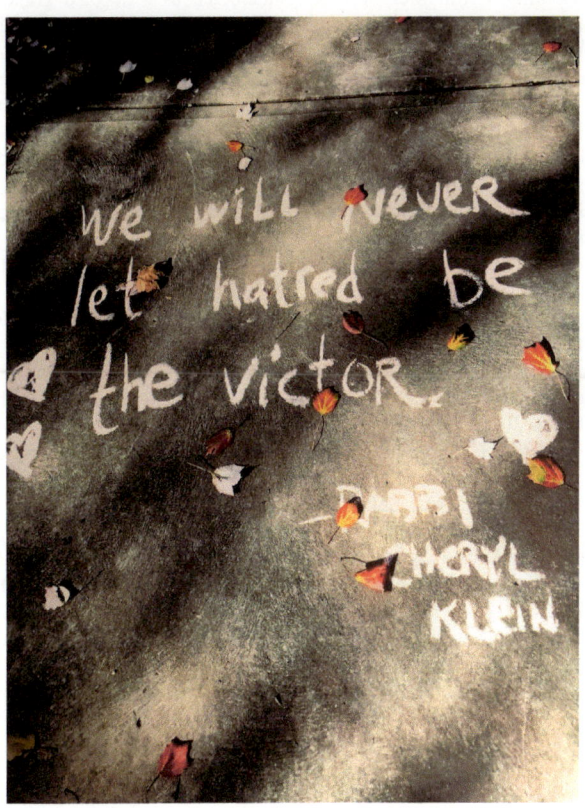

References

1. Pittsburgh's darkest day: a minute-by-minute account of the mass shootings at Tree of Life Synagogue. Cato J. www.archive.triblive.com. 2018 November 3.
2. Robertson C, Mele C, Tavernese S. 11 killed in synagogue massacre; suspect charged with 29 counts. The New York Times. 2018 October 27.
3. Hess A. The far right has a new digital safe space. The New York Times. 2016 November 30.
4. Fox News – The Daily Briefing. Pittsburgh synagogue shooting suspect pleads not guilty to charges in new indictment. Perino, Dana. 2019 Feb 11. https://video.foxnews.com/v/6000950687001/#sp=show-clip.
5. Justice department to seek death for Tree of Life suspect Robert Bowers. Ove, Torsten. Pittsburgh Post-Gazette. 2019, August 26.
6. Anti-Defamation League. Deadly Shooting at Tree of Life Synagogue. www.adl.org/educator/education-resources.
7. Romero S, Medina J, Williams T. Tree of Life synagogue victims remembered as guardians of their faith. The New York Times. 2018 October 28.
8. Irving Younger, 69, remembered as devout father, grandpa, "beautiful soul". Lindstrom, Natasha. TRIB Live, Allegheny. 2018, October 28.
9. Names of deceased victims in Squirrel Hill massacre released. Pittsburgh Post-Gazette 2018 October 28.
10. Sostek A, Ward R. Synagogue victim Rose Mallinger was a young 97. Pittsburgh Post Gazette. 2018 October 28.
11. Daniel Stein shot in sanctuary where grandson was welcomed to Jewish community. www.forward.com. Pink Aiden. 2018 October 28.
12. Pittsburgh shooting victim Melvin Wax remembered as a devoted grandfather and selfless community member. Kaplan, Arielle and Sales, Ben. Jewish Telegraphic Agency. .2018,October 31.
13. CNN-go.com; downloaded 4-29-18.
14. Survivor of synagogue shooting, Daniel Leger, discharged from hospital. TribLive; Tuesday Nov 27, 2018. www.archive.triblive.com. Downloaded 4-27-19.
15. Anti-Semitism Today and Tomorrow: Global Perspectives on the Many Faces of AntiSemitism. Shainkman, Michael. Academic Studies Press, 2018. ISBN:978-1618117441.
16. Violent anti-Semitic Incidents Rose 13% Worldwide Last Year, Report Says. Tamkin Emily. The Washington Post. 2019 May 1.
17. Staggering Rise in anti-Semitic Attacks in New York in 2018, Reports ADL Ziri, Danielle. HAARETZ. 2019 May 1. Downloaded 8-5-19.
18. Surge in anti-Semitic Attacks Has Caused a "Sense of Emergency' Among Jews Worldwide, New Report Says. Roache, Madeline. Time. 2019 May 2.
19. Audit of Anti-Semitic Incidents: Year in Review 2017. Anti-Defamation League.
20. Anti-Semitism is back, from the left, right and islamic extremes. Why? Kingsley P. The New York Times. 2019 April 4.
21. Liskowski, Sidney. U.N. Resolution on Zionism. American Jewish yearbook. vol. 77; 1977. p. 109. Editors: Fine, Morris and Himmelfarb, Milton.
22. Anti-Zionism is Anti Semitism. Sufi, Sherry. The Jerusalem Post. 2019, June 25. https://www.jpost.com/Opinion/Anti-Zionism-is-antisemitism-593635.
23. What is BDS? BDS website. https://bdsmovement.net/what-is-bds. Downloaded 8/23/2019.
24. The Power and the People. Tripp, Charles. Paths of Resistance in the Middle East. Cambridge University Press. p. 125–6. ISBN 978-0-521-80965-8.
25. Israel isn't and will never be an apartheid state Los Angeles Times Staff. LA Times. 17 May 2014.
26. The Reut Institute. Contending with BDS and the Assault on Israel's Legitimacy. 2015, June 25. reut-institute.org/en/Publication.aspx?PublicationId=4224.
27. Is BDS Hate speech? The Jewish Daily Forward 14 Feb 2013 19 August 2019.

28. Anti-Semitism in Medieval Europe. Encyclopedia Britannica. Berenbaum, Michael. 2019 June 21. https://www.britannica.com/topic/anti-Semitism/Anti-Semitism-in-medieval-Europe.
29. Democrats Need to Oust Rep. Ilhan Omar from the Foreign Affairs Committee. Baron, Seth and Miller, Judith. The New York Post, 2019, March 5.
30. Hanebrink P. A specter haunting Europe: the myth of Judeo-Bolshevism: Harvard University Press; Boston, MA; 2018. p. 11–45.
31. The Death and Life of the Jewish Century. Balthaser, Benjamen. Boston Review. 2019 March 20.
32. Pennsylvania Judge David N. Wecht talks about anti-Semitism. Cohen, Joel. Pittsburgh Jewish Chronicle. 2019, April 12.
33. 75 years since the White Rose siblings were killed for resisting Hitler. Haswell, Julius. The Local, Germany. 2018 February 22. https://www.thelocal.de/20180222/feb-22nd-the-day-the-white-rose-were-killed-for-resisting-hitler.
34. Boxer M, Brookner M, Aronson J, Saxe L. 2017 Pittsburgh Jewish Community Study. 2018, Brandeis University, Steinhardt Social Research Institute. Figure 2.4, Page 19, Table 2.9, Page 20. www.brandeis.edu/ssri. Downloaded 8-2-19.
35. Dictionary.com Unabridged, based on Random House Unabridged Dictionary, @ RandomHouseInc 2019. Downloaded 8-1-19.
36. I Am the Rabbi of Tree of Life Synagogue. Here Is a Simple Thing We Can all do to Help Stop the Next Christchurch. Myers, Jeffrey. Time Magazine. 2019 April 2.
37. Thousands Gather for Vigil HonoringVictims in Squirrel Hill. 2018 October 27. Pitz, Marylynn and Smith, Peter. Pittsburgh Post-Gazette. https://www.post-gazette.com/local/city/2018/10/27/Two-vigils-planned-pittsburgh-mass-shooting-tree-of-life-synagogue/stories/201810270084.
38. Community, Religious Leaders Say Pittsburgh Synagogue Shooting 'Will Not Break Us' At Vigil. Gajanan, Mahita. Time. 2018 October 29. https://time.com/5437299/pittsburgh-tree-of-life-shooting-vigil/.
39. The Latest: Vigil at Tree of Life after California shooting. AP News staff. AP News. 2019, April 27. https://www.apnews.com/873c777008e347dea01588ce5fb5db40.
40. 'We'll all struggle together for answers': One week after synagogue shooting, Pittsburgh tries to heal. Stanglin, Doug. USA Today. 2018, November 3. https://www.usatoday.com/story/news/2018/11/03/pittsburgh-synagogue-shooting-shabat-service-vigils-tree-life/1871835002/.
41. Parkland survivors visit Tree of Life to help community find voice. Guza, Megan. Trib Live. 2019, April 5th. https://triblive.com/local/pittsburgh-allegheny/parkland-survivors-visit-tree-of-life-to-help-community-find-voice/.
42. Tree of Life Survivors Meet With South Carolina Church Shooting Survivors. CBS Pittsburgh Staff. CBS Pittsburgh. 2019, January 21. https://pittsburgh.cbslocal.com/2019/01/21/tree-of-life-synagogue-emanuel-ame-church-shooting-survivors-meet/.
43. The Weird Dark History of 8chan. McLaughlin, Timothy. Wired. 2019, August 6. https://wired.com/story/the-weird-dark-history-8chan/ downloaded 2019, August 21.
44. After several mass shootings this year, 8chan's founder calls this site a terrorist refuge. Harwell, Drew, Pittsburgh Post-Gazette Aug 5 2019. https://www.post-gazette.com/business/tech-news/2019/08/04/El-Paso-8chan-founder-mass-shooting/stories/201908040204.
45. Three mass shootings this year began with a hateful screed on 8chan. Its founder calls it a terrorist refuge in plain sight. Harwell, Drew. The Washington Post. 2019, August 4. https://www.washingtonpost.com/technology/2019/08/04/three-mass-shootings-this-year-began-with-hateful-screed-chan-its-founder-calls-it-terrorist-refuge-plain-sight/?utm_term=.954705f235cb.
46. 8chan said it was coming back online. Now another internet company appears to have blocked it. Kates, Graham. CBS News. 2019, August 5. https://www.cbsnews.com/news/8chan-down-forum-tried-to-get-back-online-bitmitigate-but-voxility-appears-to-have-blocked-it/.
47. 8chan, the infamous message board linked to the El Paso shooting, was briefly back up before getting taken down again by another service provider. Leskin, Paige. Business Insider. 2019, August 5. https://www.businessinsider.com/8chan-el-paso-shooting-daily-stormer-cloudflare-bitmitigate-voxility-2019-8.

48. Inside the Dark Web Scramble to Get 8chan Back on Line, Led by Tech Companies Hiding in the Shadows. Conger K and Popper N. https://independent.co.uk. 2019, Aug 6.
49. 8chan struggles to stay online after links to mass shootings. CBS News. 2019, August 6. Kates, Graham. https://www.cbsnews.com/news/8chan-struggles-to-stay-online-after-links-to-mass-shootings/.
50. White Terrorism Shows 'Stunning' Parallels to Islamic State's Rise. Fisher, Max. The New York Times. 2019 August 5. https://www.nytimes.com/2019/08/05/world/americas/terrorism-white-nationalist-supremacy-isis.html?searchResultPosition=2.
51. Terr LC. Childhood traumas: an outline and overview. Am J Psychiatr. 1991;148(1):10–20.
52. O'Rourke N, Canham S, et al. Holocaust survivors' memories of past trauma and the functions of reminiscence. Gerontologist. 2016;56(4):743–52. https://doi.org/10.1093/geront/gnu168. Epub 2015 Feb 11.
53. Zimmerman S, Forstmeier S. From fragments to identity: reminiscence, life review and well-being of holocaust survivors. An integrative review. Aging Mental Health. 2018:1–25. https://doi.org/10.1080/13607863.2018.1525608. [Epub ahead of print].
54. Kessler RC, Aguilar-Gaxiola S, Alonso J, Benjet C, Bromet EJ, Cardoso G, Koenen KC. Trauma and PTSD in the WHO World Mental Health surveys. Eur J Psychotraumatol. 2017;8(sup5):1353383.
55. Antonovsky A. The sense of coherence: Development of a research instrument. Newsletter Research Report. Schwartz Research Center for Behavioral Medicine, Tel Aviv University, vol. 1; 1983. p. 11–22.
56. Antonovsky A. Unraveling the Mystery of Health. How people manage stress and stay well. San Francisco: Jossey-Bass; 1987. p. 19.
57. Rodgers AB, Bale TL. Germ cell origins of PTSD risk: the trans- generational impact of parental stress experience. Biol Psychiatry. 2015;78(5):307–14. Pub online 2015 Mar 23. https://doi.org/10.1016/j.biopsych.2015.03.018.
58. Cunliffe VT. The epigenetic impacts of social stress: How does social adversity become biologically embedded? Epigenomics. 2016;8(12):1653–69.
59. The Erik Erikson Reader. Erik Erikson, W. W. Norton and Company, March 17, 2001, ISBN-13 978-0393320916.
60. Vogel-Scibilia SE, et al. The recovery process utilizing Erikson's stages of human development. Community Mental Health J. 2009;45:405–14. https://doi.org/10.1007/s10597-009-9189-4.
61. Prager D, Telushin J. Why the Jews? The reason for Anti-Semitism, the most accurate predictor of human evil: Simon and Schuster; Boston, MA; 2016. p. 191.
62. Prager D, Telushin J. Why the Jews? The reason for Anti-Semitism, the most accurate predictor of human evil: Simon and Schuster; Boston, MA; 2016. p. 196.
63. Prager D, Telushin J. Why the Jews? The reason for Anti-Semitism, the most accurate predictor of human evil: Simon and Schuster; Boston, MA; 2016. p. 20.
64. https://jewishfed.org. Downloaded August 10, 2019.
65. https://moishehouse.org. Downloaded August 10, 2019.
66. The Pittsburgh Attack Inspired Calls for Tikkun OLam. What to Know About the Evolution of an Influential Jewish Idea. Lawrence Fine. TIME. https://time.com. 2019 February 25. Downloaded 2019, August 24.
67. The man behind the Tree of Life 'Stronger Than Hate' image says every posting is 'a WIN for love'. Pittsburgh Post-Gazette. Sciullo, Maria. October 28, 2018. https://www.post-gazette.com/new/crime-courts/2018/10/28/Stronger-Than-Hate.
68. Grieving Pittsburgh Synagogue Calls on Young Artists to Help Beautify Building. Carol Kuruvilla, Huffington Post. https://m.huffpost.com. 2019 April 16. Downloaded 2019, August 24.
69. After the Pittsburgh Shooting, the Hebrew Immigrant Aid Society Receives an Outpouring of Support. Masha Gessen. New Yorker Magazine. 2018 October 31. https://newyorker.com/new/our-columnists/our-conversation-with-the-head-of-hias/.

70. Rabbi, other survivors urge no death penalty for synagogue killer. Peter Smith, Pittsburgh Post Gazette. 2019 Aug 17. https://post-gazette.com.
71. Uganda's Tree of Life leaders visit Pittsburgh namesake. Peter Smith. Pittsburgh Post – Gazette. 2019, August 19. https://post-gazette.com. Downloaded 2019, August 26.
72. 'Pittsburgh Post-Gazette' Donates Pulitzer Money to Tree of Life Synagogue. The Algemeiner, by JNS.org. September 9, 2019. https://algemeiner.com/2019/09/09/pittsburgh-post-gazette-donates-pulitzer-prize-money-to-tree-of-life-synagogue/.
73. Shadyside church to host Tree of Life's High Hold Day services. Peter Smith. Pittsburgh Post-Gazette. September 9, 2019. post-gazette.com/news/faith-religious/2019/09/09/Tree-of-Life-Calvary-Episcopal-Rosh-Hashana-Yom-Kippur/stories/201909090141.
74. Photo provided by Rabbi Klein.

Anti-Semitism and the Deep South: A Psychiatrist's Perspective

19

Elizabeth C. Henderson

In the mid-1960s, Rabbi Perry Nussbaum of the Beth Israel Congregation in Jackson, MS, had a dilemma. He had moved to Mississippi as the new rabbi for the congregation in 1954, just following the Brown v. Board of Education decision. He felt strongly as a Jew that it was his obligation to speak up about the injustice of racial discrimination. But many members of the congregation were strongly opposed. For more than two centuries, Jews settling in Mississippi did their best to assimilate into local culture and avoid controversy that might ignite the latent anti-Semitism that was a continuous but usually covert presence. The implicit threats of retaliation were real and were both physical and economic. There was no room in white Mississippi society for dissension. It was better to keep silent. But Rabbi Nussbaum did speak out about civil rights and took actions to support Northern activists to the extent that he could. The synagogue was bombed in September of 1967, causing severe damage to the place that the rabbi customarily used for study in the evenings. He was, providentially, not there that night. His house was bombed a month later [1, 2].

Understanding Jewish life and anti-Semitism in the Deep South is not possible without understanding the nuances of its culture and history. The Deep South states include Mississippi, Alabama, Louisiana, and South Carolina. These states were distinguished by their cotton production and had many large and small plantations that were dependent on black slaves to do the work. Mississippi is considered by many to be the "deepest" of the Deep South states, and much of the focus of this chapter is on Mississippi.

Mississippians often use an indirect style of communication, especially when discussing other people, problems, and things that are upsetting. Being upset is acceptable. Being angry is unacceptable, to the degree that some Mississippians are unable to accurately identify feelings of anger. Face-to-face confrontation is

E. C. Henderson (✉)
Henderson Clinic & Consulting, Hickory, MS, USA
e-mail: hendersonclinic@gmail.com

© Springer Nature Switzerland AG 2020
H. S. Moffic et al. (eds.), *Anti-Semitism and Psychiatry*,
https://doi.org/10.1007/978-3-030-37745-8_19

avoided, but the issue is sent on a roundabout route, through church, family, and friends until the appropriate person (mother, sibling, father, etc.) broaches the topic as something "they" are saying.

These qualities of communication are important when considering the way the Jewish community has adapted to local culture. Mississippians are accustomed to presenting a superficial veneer of pleasant acceptance, with no hint of what's underneath. Anti-Semitism in Mississippi is often subtle and easy to overlook, especially given the cultural prohibition against saying anything "ugly" about someone in public. Subtlety, however, belies undercurrents of anti-Semitism that continue. Some Jewish families have been in Mississippi for two centuries or more, but are still not fully accepted [3]. The sense of exclusion and alienation from the larger white, Protestant culture of Jackson Mississippi in the 1950s is a recurring theme in Edward Cohen's memoir, *The Peddler's Grandson – Growing up Jewish in Mississippi* [4].

Caste and Class

The persistent importance of caste and class divisions leads to a cliquishness that is not seen outside of the South. An Australian immigrant once commented to me, regarding Northeast Jackson society, that "it is positively tribal."

Family ties are important in the South. The extended family and its social position determine one's place in society. But outsiders remain outsiders, no matter how long they have lived in Mississippi. I learned quickly, when asked where I'm from, not to just say "I'm from New York" (true and to the point) since this was invariably followed by a cautious pause and then, "Oh. You're a Yankee." It was much better to start with "I was raised up north but my mother's family is from North Carolina and Tennessee" (also true). This got a positive response and often the follow up question, "Are you kin to…?"

Mississippi's population is becoming more diverse, but since the early 1800s, there have been only three major ethnic groups. Jews are considered to be white and are included in the group of Anglo-Saxon whites with origins in England, Scotland, and Ireland. African Americans in Mississippi were slaves or the descendants of slaves. Native Americans, mostly Choctaws, were set apart and have had little interaction with the other two groups. Race is the still immutable variable that determines caste. Recent data finds that 59.2% of the Mississippi population are white and 37.8% are black [5].

Within each caste are the more fluid class divisions. The white upper class aristocracy initially consisted of the plantation owners, professionals, and wealthy merchants. Jews were identified as white, and Jewish planters, professionals, and wealthy merchants were considered to belong to the aristocracy. Many of these families still exist and their descendants are born into this class. Today, there are large farms and large-scale food-processing plants, whose owners belong to the upper class. In the 1800s, the white middle class included merchants, tradesmen, and business owners living in towns and cities. The middle class has grown and includes employees of industry and paraprofessionals. The lower classes included the independent farmers or yeomen and the poor whites. Small self-sufficient farms no longer exist, and most of their descendants have moved into the middle class. The poor white class is made up of scions of the yeoman farmers and rural families that lack job opportunities [6].

The lowest white class was considered by whites to be above any of the black classes. White supremacist hate groups persist in this belief, but they have become isolated and small in number. There has been similar stratification in the black community in Mississippi. Since the early 1800s, a distinction was made between house slaves and those working in the field. The house slaves considered themselves to be a class above the field workers. Prior to the Civil War, all blacks in Mississippi were considered by the Mississippi government to be slaves, regardless of their status elsewhere where manumission (setting slaves free) was allowed. Following emancipation, thousands of blacks left Mississippi and settled in Northern industrial states, and Northern blacks came South with their capital to buy land or start businesses. At present, nationwide, black class divisions more closely resemble the white class divisions. W.E.B. DuBois identified three black classes in the South. The first was middle to upper class, including members of free black families prior to emancipation; the working class; and the poor including the "vicious and criminal" [7]. In recent decades black professionals, political leaders, and business managers have increased in numbers and in acceptance by whites, but in Mississippi, these social distinctions, though muted, remain.

Religion

Religion has been and still is at the heart of politics, culture, and day-to-day life in Mississippi. Churches are divided along racial lines. Protestant Christian denominations make up the majority of black and white churches, and 83% of Mississippians are Christian [8]. Black Protestant churches largely share the theology and values of the white Protestant churches. The Southern Baptist Church is the largest denomination, and the Southern Baptist Convention issues opinions on ethical issues. Conservative, evangelical Christian dogma influences Mississippians' attitudes about Jews.

Early settlers held Jews in high esteem for their role in preserving scripture and being chosen by God. But this sentiment shifted by the early 1800s. The Southern Baptist Church espouses active evangelism to bring Jews to salvation, and although not officially acknowledged, their beliefs about Jews are in tune with common anti-Semitic dogma. Jews have never made up more than 1% of the population, and most Mississippians have never met a Jew or know anything about Judaism. Evangelical Christians believe that, since Christ's crucifixion, there is one way only to get to heaven, that is, belief in Jesus Christ as lord and savior. Jews are seen as being under an old covenant with God that was cancelled out by Christ. They believe that Christ's crucifixion paid the price for each individual's sin and that the slate is wiped clean when the believer accepts Christ. Therefore, Judaism is perceived as a hopeless struggle that will forever keep Jews from reconciliation with God unless there is a profession of belief in Christ. Jews are also seen as only being interested in the welfare of other Jews and responsible for the killing of Christ. And ultimately this means that Jews who do not acknowledge the divinity of Christ will go to hell [9].

Evangelical Christians also believe that their mission is to bring non-believers to Christ, and they are encouraged to "witness" to Jews about the way to salvation. Jews who feel socially isolated in a majority Christian community may be approached by Christians only to find that there is a hidden agenda. The overt message of love and acceptance belies the undercurrent of doctrinal anti-Semitism. The covert message becomes the only message – that the Jew is socially unacceptable as is, as a Jew. This is especially confusing for Jewish children. The importance to children of a supportive Jewish community is clearly illustrated in Edward Cohen's memoir, noted above [4, 10].

Evangelical Christians are also strong supporters of the state of Israel, but this support is conditional. The return of Jews to Israel and the construction of the third temple, by Jews, are two of the prophecies that Christians believe must be fulfilled in Israel, by Jews, before the second coming of Christ. They believe that during the tribulation before the second coming, Jews, even those who are religious and observant, will be subject to eternal damnation with a remnant converting to Christianity before it is too late. Pastors Robert Jeffress and John Hagee, chosen by President Trump to speak at the opening of the American Embassy in Jerusalem, espouse these same beliefs. Their support of Israel is conditional and tied to the second coming of Christ and Israel becoming the Christian center of the world. There is a curious unawareness of the impact this message has on Jews [11].

The psychological impact of proselytizing depends upon how the message is delivered. Some have opined that the "convert or burn in hell" message is probably ineffective, much as the health warnings on cigarette packs have little impact on smokers. But this message also has a gut-wrenching similarity to the Holocaust, and to historical eras of forced conversions such as the Spanish Inquisition. In my work with patients with addictive disease, I have treated many patients who either return to or convert to Christianity. Their rationale for return to or conversion to Christianity has been based on what the individual gains by conversion, in this case, social support, sobriety, and recovery. Avoiding condemnation has not been a major motivator in their return to religious practice. Similarly, this approach tends to result in distancing rather than productive discussion of beliefs.

"Bringing people to Christ" is referred to by Evangelical Christians as the "Great Commission" and often involves outreach to members of the community. This includes establishing a relationship, manifesting Christian love, and, if needed, provision of material help – all in the service of facilitating conversion. But confident refusal to consider conversion may then result in loss of the relationship.

The History of Jews in the Deep South

Jewish roots in the South run deep. The first Jewish immigrants arrived in the South in the late 1600s. The Jewish community flourished in Charleston, South Carolina, during the early colonial period and beyond. Charleston's first congregation, Kahal

Kadosh Beth Elohim, was formed in the mid-1700s and followed Sephardic Orthodox tradition. Eventually Beth Elohim changed its constitution and welcomed members who had adopted the Reform style of worship while accommodating those who continued to observe Orthodox traditions [12].

Jews first settled in Mississippi in the late 1600s, in Spanish Gulf Coast colonies and the French Colony of Natchez. Following acquisition by the USA, the Mississippi territory was opened for settlement in the late 1700s. Some early Jewish settlers, such as Chapman Levy, had the means to purchase large tracts of land and operate large plantations using slave labor. But since many Jewish settlers were prohibited from owning land in their native countries, their skills and experience were more suited to commercial occupations. Many started out as itinerant merchants supplying a regional circuit with needed goods. As they accumulated capital, they would open a store and settle in town [13, 14]. The plantation owners readily accepted Jewish plantation owners into the upper class, from which the planters had considerable political influence. One Jewish planter, Judah Benjamin, was a New Orleans attorney and owned a large plantation with many slaves. He was a driving force in the secession movement and was second in command in the government of the Confederacy. There is ample evidence that Mississippi Jews of that period were not averse to the use of slaves and that one out of four Jewish adults owned slaves [15, 16].

In the towns where they settled, Jewish merchants took pains to assimilate into Gentile society by participating in civic activities and cultivating Gentile friendships. Efforts were also made to continue active contact with Jews in other parts of the state and elsewhere, with an emphasis on providing opportunities for their children to develop friendships and participate in Jewish education. These gatherings of Jews from the region also provided an opportunity for young adults to get to know each other and, as hoped, choose a Jewish spouse. Despite these efforts, intermarriage with Gentiles was common as was conversion of their children to Christianity [10]. Observance of Shabbat was another obstacle, especially for merchants. There was heavy traffic in stores on Saturdays, and again, observance of the laws of Shabbat proved to be a barrier in the quest for acceptance by Gentile society. Many Jews, even some who were Orthodox, opted to keep their businesses open on Saturdays [12, 17].

The Civil War Era

During the Civil War, the brisk cotton market continued despite military operations, and the Union's military orders included protection and facilitation of cotton trading and the use of the Mississippi River for commerce. Although the Jewish merchants were a small minority of those involved in these activities, they became the target of accusations that they were providing "shoddy" merchandise. Bunker and Appel, in their examination of these accusations, also describe two conditions that incite the popular expression of anti-Semitism, both of which were present at that time. First, the public must accept the rationale that the Jews are responsible for their distress and anxiety. Second, those who are in positions of power must endorse this rationale. Indeed, escalations in the publication and expression of anti-Semitic beliefs from the Civil War era to the present day meet these criteria. Jews were also accused by the Confederates and the Union alike of engaging in subversive activities and profiteering [18].

The media circulated provocative statements and illustrations of Jewish merchants as the embodiment of evil, as monsters, and subject to tar and feathering or hanging. The Union army also banned Jews from serving as chaplains. While responsible for operations that included Mississippi, General Grant issued the controversial "Order 11" that mandated the removal of all Jews from his area of operation in Mississippi within 24 hours of the issuance of the order. President Lincoln vacated the order as soon as it was brought to his attention, but scores of Jews were displaced from their homes and sent to Kentucky and elsewhere. Grant later claimed that Order 11 was issued as an impulsive reaction to the annoyances of the cotton trade. But the order's wording applied to any Jews, not simply those participating in the cotton trade. This order gave official sanction to the belief that when there were problems, the Jews were responsible. Jews involved in the cotton trade were, in fact, small in number and minor in their impact on this so-called orgy of corruption [19].

Known in Mississippi as the War of Northern Aggression, the Civil War ravaged the state. Crops were stripped and farm animals were confiscated by the Confederacy and the Union. Plantations continued cotton production but with disruption of their slave population as the war progressed. Support for secession and the Confederacy, especially among the yeoman class, was ambivalent at best, but, over time, morale plummeted and desertions escalated. Resentment flared with the passage of the Twenty Negro Law that provided an exemption from military service in the Confederacy for the planter class, exempting one white male per 20 slaves. At the same time, yeoman, already struggling to continue farming, were conscripted at gunpoint, leaving their families to fend for themselves. This atmosphere of anger and despair carried over to the Reconstruction, and blaming the Jews mitigated some of the widespread feelings of helplessness [20].

Reconstruction and the Rise in Anti-Semitism

The Reconstruction years brought a marked shift in political power. The election of black politicians in Mississippi and passage of laws guaranteeing rights regardless of race threatened to displace the Mississippi aristocracy. The postwar Mississippi legislature passed a series of laws in 1865 and 1866, known as the "Black Codes," that were meant to constrain the activities of freed slaves. Since federal law would not permit Mississippi to suspend voting rights for blacks, other methods such as literacy tests, poll taxes, intimidation, and violence kept many blacks away from the polling place. The Ku Klux Klan was initially established as a means to stem the influence of freed blacks and carpetbaggers from the North and to enforce the Black Codes [21, 22].

The popular demand for the Black Codes is important because it illustrates the capacity in the Deep South to rank citizens by their value, and this continues to the present day. There is a portion of the society that matters and a portion that does not matter. As a people under a disintegrating level of stress, white Mississippians could externalize feelings of anger, distrust, and powerlessness by uniting around white, Protestant Christianity as emblematic of what is right in the world. Although considered to be white, Jews served as scapegoats, a ready repository for these feelings and a focal point for cohesion.

During Reconstruction, Jews were seen as taking unfair advantage of the struggling farmers after the war. Some merchants, Gentile and Jewish, extended credit to the struggling yeomen who were later unable to pay this back. These merchants accepted land as payment of the debt, and the land was then leased to black sharecroppers. Some whites saw this as a Jewish conspiracy, even though the more numerous Gentile merchants also handled bad debt in a similar fashion. A Jewish merchant in Summit, Mississippi, eventually left the state after a group of whites burned 27 tenant houses on his properties that were leased to blacks [3].

From the late 1800s forward, national anti-Semitic sentiment continued and worsened. Waves of immigration of Jews from Eastern Europe inflamed the xenophobia of the South. Jews were increasingly restricted from resorts, clubs, and residential districts. Admission quotas were applied to limit Jewish students at universities, and Jews faced employment discrimination. Toward the turn of the century, commonplace characterizations described Jews as the murderers of Christ, as demonic beings who kidnapped and killed children and used their blood to make matzoh and as part of an economic conspiracy to control the world and its people [23].

Throughout the 1800s into the mid-twentieth century, eugenics, a theory that control of reproduction could result in a superior race of human beings, became increasingly popular. Researchers contended that each race shared distinguishing biometric values such as the volume of the skull and facial features, and these were correlated with physical and mental attributes. Proposals of the use of birth control and involuntary sterilization of the "feeble minded" and others deemed genetically inferior were introduced in the 1920s and gained acceptance in Europe and the USA as a means to improve the quality of the population over time by eliminating defective genes. Eugenic theories also espoused the classification of Jews by race. Early Jewish settlers had assimilated well into the Gentile society. But with the advent of larger numbers of Jewish immigrants from Eastern Europe through the turn of the nineteenth century, there was increased interest in the racial classification of Jews. One school of thought was that Jews and Italians were "invisible blacks," having a light complexion but distinguishing black features. A basic assumption of the eugenics movement was the superiority of the white race, specifically those of white Anglo-Saxon and Germanic descent, which provided a facile justification of white supremacy. Eugenic theories, however, resulted in a very slippery slope. Adolf Hitler was a strong proponent of eugenics and identified the "Aryan" race as superior. At the bottom of this slippery slope were the unspeakable actions taken during the Holocaust to pursue the doctrine of racial purity and superiority as practiced in the Third Reich [24, 25].

The 1913 trial and lynching of Leo Frank reflected this virulent rise of anti-Semitism. Leo Frank was an Atlanta factory manager raised in Brooklyn and educated at Cornell. He was accused of the rape and murder of a 13-year-old female employee. There was no evidence to support this charge except the testimony of a man who claimed that he helped Frank to dispose of the body. The fact that Frank was a Jew became the focus of sensational and highly anti-Semitic reporting that elicited murderous rage and became the catalyst for the cohesion of a violent mob mentality. Frank was convicted and sentenced to death by a clearly biased court. The death sentence was later commuted by a newly elected governor, based on a review of the facts of the case. But the mob violently wrested Frank away from prison and hanged him. The mob's conviction that he was guilty was built on nothing more than the fact he was Jewish [26, 27].

The Bolshevik revolution in Russia prior to World War I and reports of Jewish support for Marxist ideology were added to the anti-Semites' arsenal. Jews were seen not only as demonic and condemned but also as demonic, condemned communists. In the 1920s the anti-Semitic industrialist, Henry Ford, publicized a controversial treatise known as the Protocols of the Elders of Zion. This was a completely fictional account written by a Russian official in the Czar's secret police that accused Jews of a worldwide conspiracy to enslave non-Jews and govern the world. Although thoroughly debunked, it is still considered to be factual by anti-Israel, anti-Semitic, and terrorist groups such as Hamas [28].

In the 1930s and 1940s, a two-term Mississippi governor and three-term US senator was the openly racist and crude Theodore Bilbo. During a Democrat filibuster of the Fair Employment Practices bill, Bilbo maligned supporters of the bill, especially the blacks, and accused the New York Jews of conspiring to push forward bills such as these. Then he went on to state that, on the other hand, Mississippi Jews were "exemplary citizens." A Vicksburg rabbi wrote a letter to the editor challenging Bilbo's claim that Mississippi Jews supported him. In response, Bilbo went further, characterizing Mississippi Jews as "in thorough sympathy with the ideals and principles of the South and not negro-lovers – Jews who believe in the white race and white supremacy – Jews who are not Communists as many in New York are." One can only speculate as to Bilbo's motives in ending a racist, anti-Semitic diatribe with praise for the Jews in Mississippi, but making sure to stroke a segment of his constituency may well have been at the top of the list. The Vicksburg rabbi was taken to task by the synagogue board for provoking public controversy and decided not to pursue the matter further [29, 30].

This incident is noteworthy because it reflects the duality of Jewish life in Mississippi. The incessant undercurrent of anti-Semitism led Mississippi Jews to take pains not to become involved in controversies. The practice of Judaism and the welfare of the synagogue and fellow Jews continued unabated, but were thought to be conditioned on keeping their opinions on controversial topics to themselves. Northern Jews coming South to advocate for black civil rights had difficulty understanding this balancing act [29]. In a 1970 essay, Leonard Dinnerstein commented on the prevalence of anti-Semitic attitudes in the South and their hidden nature and notes the sentiment of one Southern Jew that he is not accepted but he is tolerated.

Adaptation to the Gentile culture and participation in civic activities and philanthropy diminished the local perception of Jews as alien, but had little effect on the anti-Semitic beliefs of the larger society [31].

The Civil Rights Movement

Blacks had long identified their struggle for freedom with the exodus of the Jews from Egypt. As the civil rights movement gained momentum, a strong alliance developed between blacks and Jews who supported their struggle for social justice. Northern Jews were also active in organizations that supported and defended the civil rights activists. Southern Jews tried to dissociate themselves from obvious sympathy for the civil rights movement and from support of the Northern Jews seen by the whites as malicious meddlers. But in spite of this balancing act, many whites in the Deep South considered Southern and Northern Jews together as liberal, communist, subversive, and degenerate [32].

The civil rights movement was a broadside attack on the presumed power and position of the Southern whites, with animus as fierce as that which led to secession. This was the atmosphere in Jackson when Perry Nussbaum, Beth Israel's new rabbi, encountered opposition to his support for the civil rights activists, his efforts to bring black and white pastors together, and his welcoming blacks to events at synagogue. The congregation was not so much opposed to his opinions as to their public display. Jewish business owners were also concerned about social and economic ostracism should they be connected with any aspect of the civil rights movement. Rabbi Nussbaum's candor and the participation of Northern Jewish activists threatened to destroy the good will they had so carefully cultivated. Their prescient warning to Rabbi Nussbaum went unheeded, and the newly constructed synagogue in Jackson was bombed by Ku Klux Klan operatives in September of 1967. Rabbi Nussbaum's home was bombed a month later. The same two KKK operatives bombed the Meridian synagogue in May of 1968. Meridian Jews had been outspoken about the burning of Mississippi black churches. A plan to bomb the home of a leader in the congregation was uncovered by an informant, and the bombers were intercepted at the scene. A hit list for the assassination of Jewish business owners in Meridian was also uncovered in the course of the investigation and subsequent arrest of the Ku Klux Klan members involved. It is important to note, however, that leaders in the white community, while opposed to (Northern) Jewish activism, were appalled by the bombings [2].

Where We Are Now

As it stands now in Mississippi, the children of the children of the Jews who lived through the civil rights era have moved on, many settling in areas with a larger Jewish community and some marrying out of the faith and converting to Christianity. The tension between blacks and whites has softened, and blacks have assumed positions of leadership in Mississippi. The mayors of both Jackson and Meridian are black. In Meridian, whites and blacks have been working together to rejuvenate the downtown area, and the black middle and upper middle classes are growing.

But the Jewish population in Mississippi is dwindling. There are, at present, 1500 Jews, 8 Reform synagogues, 3 Hillel Houses, and 1 Chabad House in Mississippi. Seventy percent of the Jews in Mississippi live in Jackson, and Beth Israel in Jackson is the largest synagogue in the state. Congregation B'nai Israel in Columbus, MS, is still healthy and active and also serves Starkville and Hillel at Mississippi State University. But in Meridian, the Beth Israel congregation is aging with few, if any, newcomers. Synagogues throughout the state are also facing similar challenges.

While there has been a chilling increase in anti-Semitism in the USA in recent years, Mississippi was cited in 2017 as one of the five states with no record of anti-Semitic incidents in 2016 and 2017 [33]. The increase in the diversity of the Mississippi population, increased acceptance of diversity, and the influx of new industry have damped down the level of white supremacist ideology in the general population. Black and white Christian values are still important, as touted by every politician running for office in Mississippi, but their primacy in day-to-day life has decreased, making room for improved relationships with those of other faiths without proselytizing. Triggers for the escalation of anti-Semitism in Mississippi are few [34].

Psychiatric Treatment of Jews in the Deep South

Cultural competency in treating Jewish patients in the Deep South should start with an understanding of the history and experiences of Southern Jews. There is very little, if any, literature to consult. My experience over 30+ years of practice in Mississippi includes the treatment of one Jewish patient, a college student adapting to early adulthood and college life. Anti-Semitism was not an issue for her. There are some Jewish faculty members at the University of Mississippi Department of Psychiatry and Human Behavior in Jackson. There was one Jewish psychiatrist in my call group when I started my private practice but he has since passed away. The only other Jewish psychiatrist I have encountered was a gentleman who came to interview for a position at the local psychiatric hospital. I attended a lunch for him where they served pork. He didn't come back.

Many of my patients, however, have asked if I'm Christian, usually during the first session. Their concern stems in part from conservative Christian views that mental health problems are spiritual in nature, and in part from the fear that psychiatric treatment will undermine their faith. They see the psychiatric community as hostile to religious beliefs and promoting a secular-humanist orientation that denies the existence or relevance of God. There is also the belief, as voiced by one elderly woman, that Freud and his cohorts were "godless Jews" who had Marxist political views. Coming to the Deep South to practice psychiatry requires the ability to adeptly and empathically address these concerns. Self-disclosure with further discussion and clarification often suffices. Alternatively, one could approach this issue by exploring further the reason why this is an issue for the patient. No matter how one handles this issue, it will come up frequently in this culture. Psychiatrists with a Jewish background should develop a working knowledge of the range of Christian beliefs, from the liberal denominations to the conservative stance of denominations such as the Southern Baptist church. Similarly, for psychiatrists who are locally trained and not Jewish, a working knowledge of the practice of Judaism is also necessary. For example, many Christians in the South believe that anyone who is religious should be at church any time the doors are open, and the converse - that those skipping services are seen as less religious and, possibly, not "saved". But it is important to note that many religious Jews do not attend services regularly but maintain their beliefs and their membership in a synagogue.

It is doubtful that Jews will ever be fully accepted in the Deep South, short of conversion to Christianity. But it is worth noting that there are now places of worship in Jackson for Muslims, Buddhists, Hindus, and Unitarians, and at least in Jackson, having a lifestyle that evinces adherence to evangelical, Protestant doctrine is less important.

While serving its purpose of adaptation to local culture, the focus by Jews on assimilation has led to the loss of many Jews to conversion and intermarriage. Similarly, the children of Southern Jewish families frequently move away to settle in areas with a larger Jewish community. Jews are not moving into rural areas of the Deep South, so losses in synagogue membership will continue. But there are also new opportunities to reach out to the Gentile community and help them understand real Judaism not the Judaism that is described in the New Testament and in entrenched cultural misapprehension.

References

1. Zola GP (Center for S of SC. Perry Nussbaum (1908–1987) [Internet]. Mississippi Encyclopedia. 2018 [cited 2019 May 8]. Available from: https://mississippiencyclopedia.org/entries/nussbaum-perry/.
2. Nelson J. Terror in the night. New York: Simon and Schuster; 1993.
3. Dinnerstein L. A neglected aspect of Southern Jewish. Am Jew Hist Q [Internet]. 1971;61(1):52–68. Available from: https://www.jstor.org/stable/23877842.
4. Cohen E. The Peddler's grandson - growing up Jewish in Mississippi. Jackson: University Press of Mississippi; 1999.
5. U.S. Census Bureau QuickFacts Mississippi [Internet]. U.S. Department of Commerce. 2018 [cited 2019 Dec 3]. Available from: https://www.census.gov/quickfacts/MS.
6. Moore WE, Williams RM. Stratification in the Ante-Bellum South. Am Sociol Rev [Internet]. 1942;7(3):343–51. Available from: https://www.jstor.org/stable/2085363.
7. Gates HL. Black America and the Class Divide NY Times. New York Times [Internet]. 2016 Feb 1; Available from: https://www.nytimes.com/2016/02/07/education/edlife/black-america-and-the-class-divide.html.
8. Pew Research Center. Religious composition of adults in Mississippi. Pew Res Cent [Internet]. 2016; Available from: http://www.pewforum.org/religious-landscape-study/state/michigan/.
9. Mohler RA. Do Jews really need Christ? Controversy over Jewish Evangelism [Internet]. 2009. Available from: https://albertmohler.com/2009/07/16/do-jews-really-need-christ-controversy-over-jewish-evangelism/.

10. Goldwasser T. The last rural Jew. The Washington Post [Internet]. 1985 Aug 25; Available from: https://www.washingtonpost.com/archive/lifestyle/magazine/1985/08/25/the-last-rural-jew/502d30d6-b232-4ee4-80ae-b3b11b711eaa/?utm_term=.7e9a397ef5c4.

11. Haag M. Robert Jeffress, Pastor who said Jews are going to hell, led prayer at Jerusalem Embassy. New York Times [Internet]. 2018 May 14; Available from: https://www.nytimes.com/2018/05/14/world/middleeast/robert-jeffress-embassy-jerusalem-us.html.

12. Encyclopedia of Southern Jewish Communities – [Internet]. Encyclopedia of Southern Jewish Communities, South Carolina. 2019. Available from: https://www.isjl.org/south-carolina-charleston-encyclopedia.html.

13. Lowery C. The Great Migration to the Mississippi Territory, 1798–1819 [Internet]. Vol. 2010, Mississippi History Now: an online publication of the Mississippi Historical Society. 2000. Available from: http://www.mshistorynow.mdah.ms.gov/articles/169/the-great-migration-to-the-mississippi-territory-1798-1819.

14. Marcus JR. United States Jewry, 1775–1985, Volume II, The Germanic Period. Wayne State University Press; Loc. p. 1181–240.

15. Pearsall M. Cultures of the American South. Anthropol Q [Internet]. 1966;39(2):128–41. Available from: https://www.jstor.org/stable/3316783.

16. Korn BW. Jews and Negro slavery in the old South, 1789–1865: address of the president. Publ Am Jewish Hist Soc. 2019;50(3):151–201.

17. Encyclopedia of Southern Jewish Communities – Meridian, Mississippi [Internet]. Institute of Southern Jewish Life. 2019. Available from: https://www.isjl.org/mississippi-meridian-encyclopedia.html.

18. Bunker GL, Appel J. "Shoddy," Anti-Semitism and the Civil War. Am Jew Hist [Internet]. 82(1/4):43–71. Available from: https://www.museum.msu.edu/wp-content/uploads/2018/05/Shoddy-Anti-Semitism-and-the-Civil-War.pdf.

19. Ash SV. Civil war exodus: the Jews and Grant's general order no. 11. History [Internet]. 1982;44(11):505–23. Available from: https://www.jstor.org/stable/24446261.

20. Jenkins S, Stauffer J. The free state of Jones. 1st ed: Doubleday; New York. 2009. p. 117–92.

21. Baudouin R. Ku Klux Klan: a history of racism and violence 6th edition [internet]. Klanwatch Project 2011. Available from: https://www.splcenter.org/sites/default/files/Ku-Klux-Klan-A-History-of-Racism.pdf.

22. Bigelow M. Public opinion and the passage of the Mississippi black CODES. Negro Hist Bull [Internet]. 1970;33(1):11–6. Available from: https://www.jstor.org/stable/24766779.

23. Rockaway R, Gutfeld A. Demonic images of the Jew in the nineteenth century United States. Am Jew Hist [Internet]. 2019;89(4):355–81. Available from: https://www.jstor.org/stabe/23886447.

24. Rogoff L. Is the Jew White?: The Racial Place of the Southern Jew. Am Jewish Hist. 2019;85(3):195–230. Special Issue: Directions in Southern Jewish History, Part One (September 1997), pp. 195–230 Published by: T.

25. Garland EA. The misuse of biological hierarchies: the AMERICAN eugenics movement , 1900–1940. Hist Philos Life Sci. 1983;5(2):105–28.

26. Moseley C. The case of Leo M. Frank, 1913–1915. Ga Hist Q [Internet]. 1967;51(1):42–62. Available from: https://www.jstor.org/stable/40578874.

27. Genzlinger N. Reverberations of a trial and its shocking aftermath. The New York Times [Internet]. 2009 Nov 1; Available from: https://www.nytimes.com/2009/11/02/arts/television/02frank.html.

28. Sion B. Protocols of the elders of Zion contents of the protocols – the lie that would not die [Internet]. My Jewish Learning. Available from: https://www.myjewishlearning.com/article/protocols-of-the-elders-of-zion/.

29. Brav SR. Mississippi incident. Am Jew Arch [Internet]. 1952:59–64. Available from: http://americanjewisharchives.org/publications/journal/PDF/1952_04_02_00_brav.pdf.

30. Rabinowitz HN. Nativism, bigotry and anti-Semitism in the South. Am Jew Hist [Internet]. 1988;77(3):437–51. Available from: https://www.jstor.org/stable/23883316.

31. Dinnerstein L. A note on southern attitudes toward Jews. Jew Soc Stud [Internet]. 1970;32(1):43–9. Available from: http://www.jstor.org/stable/4466553.

32. Webb C. Closing ranks: Montgomery Jews and civil rights, 1954–1960. J Am Stud. 1998;32(3):463–81.
33. Pink A. Which states had the fewest anti-Semitic incidents? The answer may surprise you [Internet]. Forward. 2017 [cited 2019 Sep 8]. Available from: https://forward.com/fast-forward/429227/white-supremacist-murder-charlottesville/.
34. Canter B. Jewish (and safe) In "Redneck Country" on finding a welcoming home in the small-town South [Internet]. My Jewish Learning. 2019. Available from: https://www.myjewishlearning.com/southern-and-jewish/jewish-and-safe-in-redneck-country/.

Anti-Semitism and Anti-Zionism in the Field of Psychiatry

Jessica M. Rabbany and Jacob L. Freedman

Anti-Semitism and Anti-Zionism: A Background History

Anti-Semitism is prejudice and violence against individuals and communities who identify as Jewish. Free speech is when negative opinions about Israel are legitimate criticism of Israeli policy. It is perfectly possible to argue the rights and wrongs of international politics without hate speech [1]. However, anti-Zionism, blanket criticism of Israel, may be a cover for anti-Semitism [2].

A useful objective measure to determine when sentiment crosses into anti-Semitic hate speech is former Israeli member of Knesset, Natan Sharansky's 3D test of Anti-Semitism: originally published in the *Jewish Political Studies Review* in 2004 [3]. The three *D*s stand for *Delegitimization* of Israel, *Demonization* of Israel, and subjection of Israel to *Double standards*. This test has been used by the US State Department for identifying when criticism of Israel is in fact anti-Semitic [4]. Delegitimization of Israel refers to denying Israel's right to existence [3]. Demonization of Israel is often seen through comparisons made between Israel and Nazis or between Auschwitz and Palestinian refugee camps [3]. Lastly, subjection of Israel to double standards consists of singling Israel out for human rights abuses at the United Nations while being more lenient with human rights abuses in other countries [3].

Even after controlling for numerous confounding factors, hate crime experts, such as Kaplan and Small, have found that anti-Israel sentiment consistently predicts the probability that an individual is anti-Semitic, with the likelihood of measured anti-Semitism increasing with the extent of anti-Israel sentiment observed [5].

J. M. Rabbany (✉)
Sackler School of Medicine – NY State/American Program, New York, NY, USA
e-mail: jessicarabbany@gmail.com

J. L. Freedman
Tufts University School of Medicine, Boston, MA, USA
e-mail: doctor@drjacoblfreedman.com

© Springer Nature Switzerland AG 2020
H. S. Moffic et al. (eds.), *Anti-Semitism and Psychiatry*,
https://doi.org/10.1007/978-3-030-37745-8_20

Thus, anti-Israel sentiment that is not necessarily anti-Semitic, per say, is nonetheless serious. However, the linkage between anti-Israel sentiment and anti-Semitism is often contested by anti-Israel activists, especially in the United States, where most Americans support the State of Israel while simultaneously questioning aspects of its policies toward the Palestinians [6].

Because the connection between anti-Israel speech and anti-Semitism remains somewhat disputed in certain circles, addressing it can be controversial. Since anti-Zionist and anti-Israel rhetoric qualify as protected speech under the First Amendment in the United States, they are permissible in certain forums in spite of their offensiveness. What then is the best response for a psychiatrist when faced with anti-Israel rhetoric? Experts in law and history—such as Bernstein and Alterman—advocate for educating the public to "see that [anti-Zionist rhetoric] is not helping the cause of peace" rather than publicly condemning these types of speech [7]. Other experts—such as Professor Alan Dershowitz, a distinguished law school professor at Harvard University and scholar of the US constitution—encourage aggressive pro-active discourse to ensure that pro-Israel voices are not silenced in the face of increasingly vocal anti-Israel and anti-Semitic critics [8]. As academics and proponents of maintaining open and honest discourse, this is most certainly relevant in the field of psychiatry.

Given the history of Jewish persecution, the recent resurgence of general xenophobia makes a robust response to such speech essential [9]. The Jews are no exception to xenophobia. In fact, although the Jewish people have lived in various "host nations" for about 2000 years—following the Roman exile from the Land of Israel—majority of the populations have continually perceived and treated the Jews in the diaspora as *different* and *less-than*.

One such example can be seen in pre-Enlightenment Europe, where anti-Semitic treatment often included pogroms, blood libels, social restrictions, occupation marginalization, ghettoization, forced conversions, and expulsions [10]. Following the Western Enlightenment of the nineteenth century, Jews were given the option of emancipation and full integration into European society only on the condition that they identify fully as a religious group and strip away any national aspects of their peoplehood [4]. Despite the fact that many Jews did so (creating in the process the various modern religious streams of Judaism that still exist today in the West) [11], the deeply embedded anti-Semitic feelings toward Jews persisted, eventually culminating in the twentieth century with the Holocaust. This tragedy is notable as the largest genocide in the world's history. It also coincided with the expulsion of close to 1 million Jews of Sephardic heritage from Northern Africa, Iran, and the Greater Middle East [12]. Here there is clear evidence that "there was collusion among the Arab nations to persecute and exploit their Jewish populations" [12].

In the twenty-first century, there has been an increase in anti-Semitic attacks; the number of severe and violent incidents worldwide had reached almost 400 in 2018—a 13% increase from the previous year. Additionally, in 2018, the world witnessed the largest number in decades of Jews murdered for being Jewish in a single year. Western European countries accounted for the largest increase in violent anti-Semitism. One example is Germany that documented a 70% increase in violent attacks against Jews compared to the previous year. However, the country with the highest number of total incidents of major violent attacks against Jews was the United States, with over 100 cases (making up more than 25% of cases worldwide) [13]. Each one of these is significant as it holds the potential to lead to consequences for the victims, ranging from humiliation and shame to death [14].

Physicians are not immune to anti-Semitism. In a particularly troubling incident that occurred at one of Sweden's most prestigious teaching hospitals affiliated with the Karolinska Institute in November of 2018, a senior surgeon was observed bullying Jewish colleagues [15]. He insulted Jewish staff members and put obstacles in the way of their professional success [16]. Jewish staff members were denied the chance to attend international conferences and to perform specific surgical procedures. Despite being equally qualified, they received lower wages than their colleagues [16]. The surgeon's remarks included "there goes the Jewish ghetto" when walking past a Jewish colleague in the hospital [16]. The management at the Karolinska Institute knew about the "obvious and open anti-Semitism" since February of that year, but the complaints were "ignored" [15]. Eventually, the surgeon was placed on a paid "time-out" [17] and the manager left for "A combination of personal reasons, but also because he has not handled the situation [efficiently] enough" [15].

Anti-Semitism and Anti-Zionism: Clinicians' Attitudes Toward Patients

Despite the fact that the American Medical Association revised the Code of Medical Ethics in 2001 to include the statement that "a physician shall support access to medical care for all people" [18], stories of physicians discriminating against specific patients are not rare.

One of the more publicized cases occurred in September of 2018, when the Cleveland Clinic fired Dr. Lara Kollab, a first-year medical resident. She had tweeted, "I'll purposely give all the [Jews] the wrong meds" in 2012 [19]. Following her dismissal, it was revealed that Dr. Kollab had a history of expressing anti-Israel sentiment, which could be seen in her social media posts. It should be noted that Dr. Kollab received her D.O. (Doctor of Osteopathic Medicine) degree from Touro College, a New York City–based Jewish college that is "rooted in Jewish tradition, built on Jewish values" [20]. Touro College enjoys extensive collaboration with Israeli academics and students and even has overseas offices in Israel, and this may have contributed to and/or exacerbated Dr. Kollab's anti-Israel sentiment.

Another prominent case was reported in Antwerp in July of 2014 when a Belgian physician refused to treat an elderly female patient named Bertha Klein. She had fractured a rib and the physician told her son, "Send her to Gaza for a few hours, then she'll get rid of the pain." When questioned about it, the doctor confirmed that he had made that statement and explained it as an "emotional reaction" [21].

Case 1

Eyal is an American-Israeli male with dual citizenship, born in Northern Israel and raised in Miami, USA. After graduating from high school, he enlisted in the Israeli military where he followed in his father's footsteps and served as an army tank driver for 3 years. He was injured during a training accident and was subsequently honorably discharged. Shortly upon his discharge, he developed symptoms of post-traumatic stress disorder (PTSD) and decided to return to America to be with his family. Eyal's family encouraged him to seek psychiatric care for his low mood, insomnia, and frustration. Eyal went to his local academic mental health center. When the treating psychiatrist, who was of Irish descent, took note of his having served in the Israeli Defense Force, he asked Eyal if he felt that, "He was on the right side or the wrong side." Eyal responded that he felt he was doing the "right thing serving in the Israeli Defense Force and protecting the Jewish people." The treating psychiatrist suppressed a laugh and said, "I think you mean the Israeli Offensive Forces." Eyal left and refused further treatment. His family filed a formal complaint against the psychiatrist, the department, and the hospital.

Incidents such as this threaten the well-being of patients by driving them away from psychiatric care and indirectly endangering their lives. It should be explicitly noted that the hospital's ethics board found the family's complaint to be worthy of further investigation. The associated psychiatrist was later dismissed from the hospital for what was referred to as "disciplinary reasons." Eyal himself was able to find a clinician in the outpatient setting with expertise in treating veterans and sensitive to both his clinical and cultural needs.

Patients' Attitudes Toward Clinicians and BDS (Boycott, Divestment, and Sanctions)

Not only are Jewish and/or Israeli patients on the potential receiving end of anti-Semitism and anti-Zionism but so are Jewish and Israeli physicians.

One of the most blatant examples of anti-Semitism and anti-Zionism is the BDS movement (Boycott, Divestment, and Sanctions). BDS is a global smear campaign that promotes various forms of boycott against Israel on a personal, institutional, and governmental level. The campaign claims its goal is to use various forms of non-violent punitive measures against Israel until it complies with "Its obligations under international law" [22]. However, its methods include libeling, demonizing, and viciously attacking the Jewish state, often equating Israel with Nazi Germany, an analogy that the European Union has defined as anti-Semitic [23]. BDS's co-founder Omar Barghouti has said, "We oppose a Jewish state in any part of Palestine … Ending the occupation doesn't mean anything if it doesn't mean upending the Jewish state itself" [24]. The BDS movement has seen its greatest success at American universities. This is in spite of the fact that by calling for a boycott of Israeli universities, they are fundamentally stifling the very open discourse which characterizes progressive modern academics. Its supporters organize demonstrations and protests on campuses and pass resolutions at meetings of student governments calling on their universities to divest from Israeli companies.

The movement on university campuses has been linked to several cases of anti-Semitism. In December of 2018, the Bronfman Center for Jewish Life at New York University was forced to temporarily shut its doors due to a security threat. They were made aware of several public online postings by an NYU student just days after NYU's student government passed a resolution in support of the BDS movement. This ruling was made despite warnings by Jewish students that BDS has led to an "Unsafe environment for students ... [who are] being targeted just because they support Israel" [25]. The student posted on Twitter that his account was suspended because, "I expressed my desire for Zionists to die [sic]" [25]. Another post applauded Hitler, and a third read, "Remember to spit on Zionists, it's proper etiquette [sic]" [25].

Similarly, in May 2019, a few weeks after the University of Oregon's student government passed a resolution in favor of boycotting and divesting from Israel, a welcome sign on the campus Hillel [*an international campus organization for Jewish university students*] was vandalized with graffiti that read "free Palestine you f**ks" and other racist slogans [25].

A team of professors at Brandeis University conducted an extensive study across 50 campuses and found that Jewish students reported increased campus harassment, intimidation, and hostility with rising BDS activity. BDS student leaders have been known to post on social media messages such as: "Every time I read about Hitler, I fall in love all over again" and "Let's stuff some Jews in the oven." BDS supporters on campuses are also known to regularly heckle and even shut down Israel-related events organized by Jewish student groups [26].

The AMCHA Initiative, a California-based campus watchdog, has claimed a direct correlation between anti-Israel and anti-Semitic activity on campuses. Their report, released in August 2018, revealed that "Israel-related incidents are ... more likely to contribute to a hostile environment for Jewish students" [25]. According to the study, there were 578 anti-Semitic incidents on more than 142 US campuses in 2018, which included being targeted, harassed, and physically threatened in blatantly discriminatory ways [24]. This is up from 204 anti-Semitic incidents on US campuses in 2017 (a more than 280% increase), as reported by the Anti-Defamation League [25].

Case 2

Dr. Simcha is a resident physician at a prominent teaching hospital in Chicago. Having done exceptionally in her first 3 years of the program, she was selected as the Chief Resident in Psychopharmacology. She was very excited to pursue her career in academic psychiatry. With an impeccable record and a unique idea for a research project focusing on post-traumatic stress disorder (PTSD), Dr. Simcha applied for an overseas grant to travel to Israel and work as a Primary Investigator in an ongoing study about secondary PTSD in family members of terror victims. Dr. Simcha's grant proposal was initially accepted and she was offered 1-month award, funded by a number of sources, in order to participate in this research project. Conducting research abroad was common practice, with the previous year's Chief Resident having traveled to Peru to work with an indigenous population and her fellow classmate and Co-Chief Resident planning to travel to do a public health project in Jordan. Dr. Simcha was therefore quite surprised when she was told by her Program Director that she would be unable to travel to Israel. When she discussed it with him, it became clear that this decision was not because of her obligations as Chief Resident, nor was her presence needed in the psychopharmacology clinic, but, rather, it was because he had "concerns about maintaining academic relationships with an Apartheid State." Dr. Simcha filed a formal complaint with the medical school, arguing that the Program Director was applying a double standard given that Jordan denies citizenship and equal rights as citizens to its majority Palestinian population yet her Co-Chief Resident's research project in Jordan had been approved [27]. Therefore, the Program Director's decision—according to the US State Department's definition of anti-Semitism, "Applying double standards by requiring of it (Israel) a behavior not expected or demanded of any other democratic nation"—qualified as anti-Semitism [28]. Following a lengthy appeal, Dr. Simcha was able to eventually gain her Program Director's approval to participate in her chosen program. However, by the time she went, the research program had already begun. She had endured unnecessary hardship and had been unable to fully benefit from her grant.

BDS advocates who seek to limit the collaboration between Israeli academics in all fields of medicine, with psychiatry being no different, would be loath to learn that many important academic and clinical breakthroughs in medicine occur in the Jewish state. Legendary PTSD researcher, Dr. Arieh Shalev, who is currently Psychiatry Professor at NYU, also served as the Chair of Psychiatry at Hadassah Medical Center and Hebrew University Medical School from 1997 to 2011 [29]. Additionally, Harvard-trained bipolar disorder expert, Dr. Robert H. Belmaker, has been a Professor of Psychiatry at Ben-Gurion University of the Negev for over 30 years [30].

Israel is legendary for developing innovative treatment modalities such as Brainsway, a deep transcranial magnetic stimulation (TMS) methodology. This was invented by Israeli researchers, Zangen and Yiftach Roth, while they were working at the National Institutes of Health (NIH) [31]. Brainsway has been shown to effectively treat severe brain disorders and has been FDA-approved to treat forms of depression that are refractory to other treatment methodologies [32].

Not only is Israel a leading source of academic expertise and methodology but also of psychopharmacology. Teva—one of the world's leading psychopharmacology manufacturers and one of the largest producers of clozapine tablets—is headquartered in Tel Aviv [33]. These examples serve to point out the irresponsibility of BDS advocates who would seek to destroy the critical academic and industrial productivity of the Jewish state even within the apolitical field of psychiatric medicine.

Case 3

The same discrimination faced by American physicians like Dr. Simcha who want to spend time in Israel is also experienced by Israeli-trained physicians who want to practice in America. One such example is that of Dr. McAlister who completed medical school in Israel and elected to do his residency training in America. After graduation and passing his board exams, Dr. McAlister joined a well-known local practice in Boston. Upon his arrival, Dr. McAlister proudly hung his medical school diploma, residency diploma, and board certification on the wall. Dr. McAlister was taken aback when his first patient—an attorney originally from Pakistan with a history of an anxiety disorder—walked into the office and began questioning the doctor's credentials. In an example of demonization of Israel, the patient then said, "I understand that you are Board Certified, but I am not working with an Israeli thug." When Dr. McAlister responded by pointing out that he was neither Israeli nor Jewish, the patient answered, "Then why would you go to work in a country with International War Criminals?" Dr. McAlister answered that his training at Ben-Gurion University was unaffiliated with any political entity. The patient continued, "You cannot be complicit in Israeli war crimes and also be my doctor," before storming out of the office, still cursing Dr. McAlister. The patient then reentered the room, "That's right, I'm BDS-ing your sorry behind back to Tel Aviv!" before he slammed the door a second time.

Examples such as these may potentially be transference reactions stemming from the patient's own experiences. They may also be learned reactions based on personal exposure, culture, or propaganda. What is certain is that patients can miss out on high-quality treatment because of such unfounded prejudice. Moreover, psychiatrists who are perceived to have any association with Israel can be vulnerable to anti-Semitic and anti-Israeli abuse.

Conclusion

Anti-Semitism and anti-Zionism are seemingly irrevocably intertwined in academia. In the field of psychiatry, it is particularly important to be aware of anti-Zionistic sentiment as it can be explored within the therapeutic relationship and lead to deepened understanding on both sides. Barriers of communication, whether they arise from transference and countertransference reactions or from brainwashing, are difficult to surmount. Politics doesn't belong in psychiatry—what does belong is understanding of where the other person is coming from and engaging in a dialogue that allows both parties to see each other as human beings and not as representatives of "the enemy."

Unfortunately, BDS's efforts to delegitimize the Jewish state serve as a powerful tool that anti-Semites use to legitimize their beliefs. They take advantage of a platform that is protected by the First Amendment for scurrilous purposes. As psychiatrists, it is our duty to break down barriers and ensure that patients can receive the treatment they require. One of the ways that this can be achieved is by promoting academic freedom through the recognition that anti-Israel sentiment is a blatant form of anti-Semitism.

Furthermore, supporting Israel as a lone democracy in a sea of dictatorships within the Middle East should be a priority for the field of psychiatry, which has historically set as its goal the championing of the right of every individual to live a peaceful and healthy life on his or her own terms, free of religious or military oppression. Rev. Dr. Martin Luther King Jr. famously recognized Israel "as one of the great outposts of democracy in the world, and a marvelous example of what can be done, how desert land can be transformed into an oasis of brotherhood and democracy" [34].

Acknowledgments The authors would like to thank Dr. Steve Moffic as well as the other editors for their help with this chapter. They further recognize the contributions of Dr. Ronald Pies in coordinating this important effort.

References

1. Anonymous. Challenge anti-Semitism. Nature.Com. 2019. https://www.nature.com/articles/d41586-018-04926-3.
2. Anti-Defamation League. What is … anti-Israel, anti-Semitic, anti-Zionist? 2019. https://www.adl.org/resources/tools-and-strategies/what-is-anti-israel-anti-semitic-anti-zionist.
3. Sharansky N. 3D test of anti-Semitism: demonization, double standards, delegitimization. Jew Polit Stud Rev. 2004;16:3–4.
4. Rosenthal H. Remarks at the 2011 B'nai B'rith international policy conference. U.S. Department of State. 2011. https://2009-2017.state.gov/j/drl/rls/rm/2011/178448.htm.
5. Barnavi E. A historical atlas of the Jewish people: from the time of the patriarchs to the present. New York: Schocken Books; 2003.
6. Kaplan EH, Small CA. Anti-Israel sentiment predicts anti-Semitism in Europe. SAGE J. 2006;50:548–61. https://www.journals.sagepub.com/doi/pdf/10.1177/0022002706289184.
7. O'Donnell G. BDS movement causes backlash against Jewish college students and employees I INSIGHT into diversity. Insightintodiversity.Com. 2018. https://www.insightintodiversity.com/bds-movement-causes-backlash-against-jewish-college-students-and-employees/.
8. Dershowitz A. The case for peace. Hoboken: Wiley; 2011.
9. Kogan I. Anti-semitism and Xenophobia. Am J Psychoanal. 2017;77(4):378–91. https://doi.org/10.1057/s11231-017-9113-6.
10. Encyclopedia Britannica. Anti-Semitism in medieval Europe. Anti-Semitism. 2019. https://www.britannica.com/topic/anti-Semitism/Anti-Semitism-in-medieval-Europe.
11. Plaut WG. The rise of reform Judaism: a sourcebook of its European origins. World Union for Progressive Judaism. OCLC 39869725, and YIVO I Orthodoxy. Yivoencyclopedia.org. 1963. Retrieved 15 Aug 2012.
12. Hoge W. Group spotlights Jews who left Arab lands. NY Times. 2017. https://www.nytimes.com/2007/11/05/world/middleeast/05nations.html.
13. Kantor Center. Antisemitism worldwide – 2018 – general analysis. http://www.kantorcenter.tau.ac.il/sites/default/files/Antisemitism%20Worldwide%202018.pdf.

14. Glasberg R. The treachery trope: anti-Semitism as indicative of a psycho-spiritual disease associated with the Betrayal of cultural ideals and of the self. J Relig Health. 2018;57(1):311–27. https://doi.org/10.1007/s10943-017-0533-7.
15. Jewish Telegraphic Agency. Swedish doctor bullies Jewish staff, colleagues charge. 2018. https://www.jta.org/2018/11/15/global/department-head-swedish-hospital-quits-following-alleged-anti-semitic-bullying.
16. The JC. Swedish hospital's chief surgeon on gardening leave over "Jewish ghetto" remark. 2018. https://www.thejc.com/news/world/swedish-karolinska-university-hospital-chief-surgeon-on-gardening-leave-over-jewish-ghetto-remark-1.472451.
17. Karolinska University Hospital. Investigation started on reported discrimination at Karolinska University Hospital. Karolinska.Se. 2019. https://www.karolinska.se/en/karolinska-university-hospital/news/2018/11/investigation-started-on-reported-discrimination/.
18. Ama-Assn. AMA code of medical ethics. 2016. https://www.ama-assn.org/sites/ama-assn.org/files/corp/media-browser/principles-of-medical-ethics.pdf.
19. Fox News. Cleveland clinic resident fired over threat to give Jews "wrong meds" went to Jewish Medical College. 2019. https://www.foxnews.com/us/cleveland-clinic-resident-fired-over-threat-to-give-jews-wrong-meds-went-jewish-medical-college.
20. Touro College. Jewish heritage. Touro.Edu. 2019. https://www.touro.edu/about/jewish-heritage/.
21. The Jerusalem Post. Belgian doctor refuses treatment to Jewish patient. 2014. https://www.jpost.com/Jewish-World/Jewish-Features/Belgian-doctor-refuses-treatment-to-Jewish-patient-369591.
22. BDS Movement. BDS means freedom, justice and self-determination. 2011. https://bdsmovement.net/news/bds-means-freedom-justice-and-self-determination.
23. English (English) | European Forum On Antisemitism. European-Forum-On-Antisemitism. Org. 2019. https://european-forum-on-antisemitism.org/definition-of-antisemitism/english-english.
24. Washington Examiner. Hold BDS accountable for anti-Semitism on campus. 2019. https://www.washingtonexaminer.com/opinion/op-eds/hold-bds-accountable-for-anti-semitism-on-campus.
25. Algemeiner. When BDS comes to campus, antisemitism follows. 2018. https://www.algemeiner.com/2018/12/21/when-bds-comes-to-campus-antisemitism-follows.
26. Ynetnews. We cannot ignore link between BDS and anti-Semitism. 2019. https://www.ynetnews.com/articles/0,7340,L-5446395,00.html.
27. Gabbay SM. The status of Palestinians in Jordan and the anomaly of holding a Jordanian passport. OMICS International. 5 Feb 2014. www.omicsonline.org/open-access/the-status-of-palestinians-in-jordan-and-the-anomaly-of-holding-a-jordanian-passport23320761.1000113.php?aid=23346.
28. U.S. Department of State. Defining anti-Semitism. 2016. https://www.state.gov/s/rga/resources/267538.htm.
29. ISTSS. Dr. Arieh Shalev Honored with the lifetime achievement award. Istss.Org. 2008. http://www.istss.org/education-research/traumatic-stresspoints/2008-may/dr-arieh-shalev-honored-with-the-lifetime-achievem.aspx.
30. Robert H. Belmaker. Research Gate. 2019. https://www.researchgate.net/profile/Robert_Belmaker. Accessed 12 Mar 2019.
31. Blackburn N. Israel's Brainsway stimulates a magnetic remedy for depression | Weizmann USA. American Committee for the Weizmann Institute of Science. 2019. https://www.weizmann-usa.org/news-media/in-the-news/israels-brainsway-stimulates-a-magnetic-remedy-for-depression.
32. Brainsway. Brainsway's noninvasive treatment for MDD & OCD – how does it work? 2019. https://www.brainsway.com/how-does-it-work/.
33. Israel. Tevapharm.Com. 2019. https://www.tevapharm.com/teva_worldwide/international_markets/teva_in_israel/.
34. Rabbinical Assembly. Conversation with Martin Luther King. 1968. http://www.rabbinicalassembly.org/sites/default/files/public/resources-ideas/cj/classics/1-4-12-civil-rights/conversation-with-martin-luther-king.pdf.

Understanding the Current Resurgence of Anti-Semitism: The Situation in France

Jean-Claude Stoloff

We discover with astonishment that progress has allied itself with savagery. (Sigmund Freud, Moses and Monotheism, p. 131).

In 1945, after the trauma of the Shoah, it seemed possible to believe that the world would henceforth be free of anti-Semitism. But, very quickly, it became obvious that the opposite was, in fact, true. In the Soviet Bloc, the end of the Stalin era was marked by court trials of Jewish leaders such as Rudolf Slansky, hero of the struggle against Nazism and Fascism. These men became the target of public wrath, falsely accused of membership in an international Zionist conspiracy. What stands out particularly in this era is the *complot des blouses blanches* or the "doctors' plot" during which Stalin's Jewish physicians were accused of conspiring to poison him. In Poland, immediately after the end of the war, there were new pogroms, notably the one in Kielce.

Later on, the geographic nucleus of anti-Semitism shifted to the Middle East. During the Israeli-Arab conflict, newspapers in the region were filled with anti-Jew cartoons, similar to those seen in pre-war France in *Gringoire* or *Je suis partout*, two far-right political weeklies. The anti-Semitic tidal wave grew to engulf non-Arab nations such as Iran, Pakistan, and Indonesia, countries with very few Jewish inhabitants. This manifestation of anti-Semitism (or anti-Judaism) in Muslim lands brought attention to several anti-Jewish aspects of Islam, already noticeable, according to Ben-Asher [1] in reading the Koran. The constant reoccurrence of this phenomenon, which has now once again invaded Western countries like France,

Translated from the French by Mary V. Seeman

J. -C. Stoloff (✉)
Société Psychanalytique de Recherche et de Formation (SPRF France), International Psychoanalytical Association (IPA), Paris, France
e-mail: jc.stol@wanadoo.fr

© Springer Nature Switzerland AG 2020
H. S. Moffic et al. (eds.), *Anti-Semitism and Psychiatry*,
https://doi.org/10.1007/978-3-030-37745-8_21

inevitably leads to questions, and these are the very questions that have fueled my own research. It is evident that anti-Semitism or antagonism against Jews has no one simple determinant. The causes are multiple and diverse, and a comprehensive approach to understanding this phenomenon would need to reach far beyond psychiatry and psychoanalysis. The psychoanalytic perspective that I bring needs to be linked to historic, sociologic, theologic, and phenomenologic viewpoints. But, in exploring the unconscious sources of hatred toward Jews, I think that psychoanalysis highlights links that are significant and not otherwise evident in the many diverse writings on this topic. The validity of the psychoanalytic approach lies in its ability to demonstrate the various ways that hostility toward Jews and toward Judaism can be psychologically explained. It is not meant to be a stand-alone, comprehensive explanation.

To be convinced of the utility of the psychoanalytic approach, it is important to read Freud's last great work on questions pertaining to religion, *Moses and Monotheism*. Toward the end of this book, this is how Freud sums up the problem of anti-Semitism: "The deep motives behind anti-Semitism stem from ages long past; they are rooted in the human unconscious and I expect that they will at first seem unbelievable" [2, p., 184].

Freud and Anti-Semitism

Let us consider the term "unbelievable." It must have seemed unbelievable to Freud that he had to leave Vienna and the country of his birth to live in exile in London. It must have been unbelievable to him to witness so massive a resurgence of anti-Semitism in one of the most culturally advanced of European nations, a country to which he was deeply attached intellectually, emotionally, and morally. But perhaps most strikingly unbelievable to him was the fact that the events to which he was a witness actually confirmed his theories; they were in vivo evidence of the powerful rootedness of religion in the unconscious mind.

Freud began his journey into the exploration of religion as early as 1912 with *Totem and Taboo*, but, prior to his attempt to analyze anti-Semitism at the end of his life, his focus had substantially narrowed. After 1930, in the face of the rising anti-Semitism in Europe and the urgency he felt to understand its origins, he began to direct specific attention to monotheistic religions and to Judaism in particular.

Freud had earlier, before arriving at his final views, written:

> A thousand and a half years later, the triumph of Christianity scored a new victory for the priests of Ammon over the God of Akhenaton and this triumph is now being played out on an ever larger stage. Nevertheless, Christianity can be seen as a progressive step in the history of religion in the sense that it represents the return of the repressed. As of that moment, the Jewish religion became, so to speak, a fossil [2]

The priests of Ammon, as readers no doubt know, had brought Egypt back to polytheism after pharaoh Akhenaton's death. It was Akhenaton who had first introduced monotheism to the world, the worship of a single almighty God. Incidentally, by "return of the repressed," Freud meant the return to consciousness of something long forgotten.

But what progressive step was Freud alluding to? Freud was interested in anthropology and in what has been called "the family romance" – fathers and sons vying for the affection of the mother. He believed that in mankind's early years, humans lived in more-or-less wild hordes that consisted of a powerful adult male, his harem of wives, and his children. The sons, as they matured, aroused jealousy in the father who punished them in a variety of ways and even castrated them, circumcision representing a memory remnant of that castration. Ultimately, Freud believed, the sons banded together and killed the father so that they could live and reproduce. Their guilt at having murdered the father, however, survived, and the all-powerful father became the origin of the concept of a God. Freud believed that the guilt arising from the murder of the primal father never died away, but remained engraved in our collective memory. Furthermore, Freud believed that Moses was a disciple of Akhenaton and that he led the Jews in a mission to disseminate the word of monotheism. According to Freud, the Jewish followers of Moses killed him, once again murdering the primal father, but repressing the memory of the crime. Christianity, however, recalled and acknowledged the primal crime and atoned for it symbolically by reenacting it in the crucifixion and resurrection of Jesus.

It is this aspect of Judaism that Freud first held principally responsible for anti-Semitism. Unconsciously, Jews were being blamed for not recognizing and admitting the murder of the father and, as a result, denying the redemptive potential of the Savior, Jesus Christ, and His ability to lead the human race to salvation. According to Christians, "the reproach (against the Jews) goes like this: they don't want to recognize that they killed God whereas we own up to it and have thus cleansed ourselves of this sin. One can plainly see the truth of this reproach." And Freud adds that, because of the unconscious memory of this crime, Jews "have taken on a tragic responsibility which they have to mightily expiate" [2].

Even more startling than the proposition that Moses was not born a Jew, but an Egyptian, is Freud calling the Jewish religion a fossil. Few previous authors have undertaken to analyze this astonishing pronouncement. Everyone agrees that the victory of the priests of Ammon in Egypt was a step backward in the history of religion, a misguided reaction to Akhenaton's monotheistic revolution in Amarna. Precisely on the page in *Moses and Monotheism* that precedes the one where Freud calls Judaism a fossil, he returns to the story of Akhenaton. But now, instead of Judaism, it is Christianity that he terms regressive. "In many ways, the new religion constituted a cultural regression when compared to the older one as is, in fact, a frequent occurrence when significant numbers of human beings, relatively less civilized than a prior group, arrive at a site and take it over. The Christian religion did not maintain the level of spirituality that Judaism had attained" [2].

Continuing along the same line of thought, Freud writes:

> ... one must never forget that all those who today are the very incarnation of anti-Semitism have only lately adopted Christianity; in the relatively recent past, they were forced at knife-point into converting. One could call them badly baptized; beneath a thin layer of

Christianity these peoples have remained what their ancestors were, primitive polytheists. They have not overcome their aversion for their new religion, a religion that was imposed on them against their will, but they have displaced this aversion onto the representatives of the source of Christianity [2].

Let us try to follow Freud's new thinking step by step. In this latter period of his thought, Christianity constitutes a descent from the cultural height attained by the ancient religion of the Hebrews. This is because Christianity brought back certain forms of idolatry and, through the cult of the Virgin Mary, reintroduced the ancient worship of fertility goddesses. Please note that this view is historically correct. When Freud says that the Christian religion has not maintained the high ground reached by Judaism, he is not referring to early Christianity, since he emphasizes that "the Gospels tell a story that takes place among Jews and, in fact, they discuss only Jews...." But later Freud also says, and one needs to read this as something more than just a diplomatic concession to the Church, that anti-Semitism is, fundamentally, merely anti-Christianity, "...and it is not surprising that, in the National Socialist revolution in Germany, the intimate relationship between these two monotheistic religions is evident by the hostile treatment they both receive" [2].

It is patently clear that when Freud, oblivious to the facts, puts Nazi hostility toward Christianity on a par with its treatment of Jews, he is contradicting his original explanation of anti-Semitism. At one point he had attributed Jew hatred to Jewish refusal to convert to the new religion, a religion that had cleansed humanity of patricide through atonement. At another point, and this time much more precisely, he attributes anti-Semitism to the polytheistic bent that Christianity had to adopt in order to prosper in a pagan world. In this new formulation, Christianity no longer comes across as a forward step in the history of religion but, rather, as a step backward from the pure monotheism represented by Judaism.

Freud now asserts that Christianity was a religion that claimed to be monotheistic but which, from the beginning, had to shed itself of certain essentials of monotheism. The consequence of this for him was the fact that two monotheistic religions, based on different forms of faith, continued, each on its own, to evolve in a parallel fashion. This point of view is in radical opposition to the thesis, for a long time asserted by the Church (though recently abandoned), which held Christianity to be *Verus Israel*, the true descendant of Israel. This new view of Freud's contradicts his description of Judaism as a fossilized religion bypassed by history.

Is Judaism a Fossilized Religion?

The designation of Judaism as a fossilized religion seemed unacceptable to me, which was one reason behind my research into the unconscious origins of anti-Semitism. What, in fact, is a fossil if not an organism that has been conserved intact for thousands of years after it has stopped evolving and thus bears direct and trusted witness to life in earlier times? Can one accept this characterization of Judaism without raising one's eyebrows, especially since Judaism has stayed very much alive for 2000 years since the destruction of the Temple? It has constantly renewed itself (*chidush*) through successive reinterpretations of Talmudic texts, producing great thinkers such as Maimonides and Rashi and numerous sages and philosophers, some of whom were Freud's contemporaries.

When we see the current resurgence of anti-Semitism, we are struck by the fact that it has developed most readily in geographic areas where monotheism reigns and rarely goes beyond those areas. As an aside, as Freud himself acknowledged, his explanation of anti-Jewish sentiment leaves out the role played by Islam. I will return to this later.

Monotheistic Kinship and the Question of Paternity

The quote at the beginning of this chapter suggests that it was the rise of anti-Semitism in all its savagery that motivated Freud to more fully examine and identify the origin of monotheism. One can even ask whether all his writings, culminating in *Moses and Monotheism,* were not triggered by what was happening around him. If *Moses and Monotheism* ends on the question of anti-Semitism, it is because this concern is a fundamental issue in the history of monotheism and in the several types of faiths included under this designation. It is also because, and perhaps above all, the three great monotheistic religions are linked by ties of kinship. Within the framework of these familial ties, one can see violence arising from a kernel of hatred at its center, as being at the very heart of the phenomenon of religion. In focusing at the very end of his life on the study of monotheistic religions, Freud was able to validate his past efforts to understand religion as a whole. Why? Because he saw monotheism as doing away with the maternal and feminine deities that are part of other religions and centering itself primarily on the figure of the father. In fact, the essential characteristic of monotheism, according to Freud, is that it is wholly organized around a father (God)-child (man) relationship that, according to him, lends itself inevitably to ambivalence.

Only a few lines before the ones where he calls Judaism a fossilized religion, Freud notes that Judaism is a religion built around a father and Christianity is a religion built around a son. This leads Freud to suggest that the inevitable love/hate relationship between fathers and sons transfers over to a conflicted relationship between these two forms of monotheism. As to Islam, according to Freud, this religion asserts that both Jews and Christians have falsified their religious texts in order to sidestep the only legitimate origin of monotheism – that contained in God's revelation to Mohammed.

Periodic Resurgences of Anti-Semitism

Immediately post war, the trauma of the genocide and the *aggiornamento* (modernization) of the Church with respect to its own attitude toward Jews, especially after Vatican II, made it possible for the world to think that anti-Semitism would soon be extinct. Recent events seem to indicate that the opposite is true. This may well explain part of what Freud referred to as "unbelievable." Beneath the cover of Holocaust denial orchestrated by the great nations of the East led by Iran, and also beneath so-called anti-Zionism, the old anti-Semitism is back, and the traditional themes of Jew hatred are back. They have surfaced in unexpected geographic areas on the outskirts of Asia and in Asia itself, wherever Islam has taken root. This has happened even in regions that are *Judenrein* or, at least, where very few Jews live – a confirmation of the fact that, without, of course, excluding other causes, anti-Semitism is fundamentally linked to monotheistic or Abrahamic religions. It does not exist in China or India where Jews are made to feel even more welcome than Europeans. The violent wars and terrorist acts that we are witnessing today come from an increasingly prevalent form of Islam, which uses identity politics to inspire hundreds of millions of Muslim followers to hate any type of modernity, all Western democracies, and, most of all, the State of Israel. This opposition to democracy has resuscitated old widespread nineteenth- and twentieth-century canards, e.g., about Jews underhandedly dominating the West through control of finance or through various vague occult "lobbies." This may explain how the old Tsarist pamphlet enti-tled *The Protocols of the Elders of Zion* became a best seller in many Arab capitals and beyond.

Monotheistic Religions and Judaism

The decision to narrow his focus to monotheism allowed Freud to introduce into the study of religion the history of kinship among its three different representatives, the transmissions that occurred from one to another, and the associated conflicts.

From this perspective, the term "fossil" can be better understood. To appreciate it, one has to understand Freud's penchant for archaeological metaphors. He had already used this term when referring to circumcision, which he called a *Leitfossil* or "key fossil" (2, pp.109–110), a trace reminder of the compromises that were originally made among a variety of different ethnic groups and streams of thought, which then allowed a merger of somewhat varying beliefs into one encompassing form of worship. A fossil's origin is prehistoric, but it is preserved intact over time, fostering the study of what happens to a once living organism over the course of evolution. By analogy, Judaism is a fossil in that, through the medium of its multiple written texts, it has kept the memory, altered and reinterpreted but very much alive, of its first origins. For Freud, the Jewish religion constitutes a prototypic religion, a means of reconstructing how the larger phenomenon of religion came to be, how the idea of religion was transmitted through space and time, and how it was able to perpetuate itself. This is the task he first set out to accomplish in *Totem and Taboo*, and he did not stray far from his original hypotheses.

Religion: Illusion or Mark of Civilization's Progress?

Freud's thinking about religion is complex and often contradictory. He understands history as a progression toward Enlightenment such that illusory religious beliefs are gradually displaced by reason. It was this understanding that led him to describe

Christianity as having surpassed Judaism, a thesis that recalls similar thinking on the part of Hegel, Kant, Feuerbach, and even Marx.

But if one follows the other direction of Freud's thinking, the one where he refers to monotheism, the purest form of which, according to him, is found in the Judaism of the period of exile after the destruction of the second temple by Titus (70 CE), as "the most elevated form of spirituality," then one reaches an exactly opposite conclusion to the one above. From a cultural and spiritual point of view, both Christianity and Islam would then be seen as false forms of progress – Christianity because of its regression to various forms of idolatrous worship and its acceptance of graven images of the divine, even going as far as believing that a man of flesh and blood could be the incarnation of God and Islam because it places the pursuit of political victory and territorial conquest above all other obligations of the faithful.

This orientation of Freud's thinking highlights a specific characteristic of the essence of monotheism [2]. On that score, Freud's thinking, without his realizing it, approaches that of his contemporary, Hermann Cohen, who saw Judaism as a rational religion, as a religion of exile that does not seek to proselytize but firmly adheres to fundamental ethical principles. On the other hand, one has to recognize, as did Franz Rosenzweig and Walter Benjamin [3], that the so-called progress that came with the Enlightenment and its "Christian spirit" was unable to prevent the eruption of sadistic tendencies in the hearts of "enlightened" human beings. The scandal that was Nazism was not so much its brutality, since that was already foreshadowed in *Mein Kampf* and the speeches of the Führer. The real scandal was the absence of a corrective measure capable of stopping it. Two thousand years of a monotheistic faith that preached love of one's neighbor and equality of all before God were swept aside in a few years like wisps of straw. This was particularly scandalous in deeply Christian nations such as Germany and Poland [4]. These facts appear to confirm Freud's thesis that the conversion to monotheism of the pagan European masses served only as a thin veneer of Christian values that could not resist the surge of barbarian aggression.

Over time Freud underwent a shift in his thinking that ultimately allowed him to take better measure of the importance of pure monotheism and the significance of the father figure in the "progress of the life of the spirit." Writing *Civilization and Its Discontents* played a major role in this shift. This work highlights man's natural inclination toward evil, an inclination that can never be eradicated. Judaic texts constantly refer to this evil (*Yetser hara*), and Jews believe that Torah constitutes its antidote.

As Freud weaves through these problematic issues of progression and regression in the history of religion, he asks a much more fundamental question: should religion be considered an illusion, or, on the contrary, does it serve to advance human civilization, as defined by Freud, by its ability to arouse strong emotional links among individuals? The etymology of religion (*religare*) does, in fact, suggest the idea of linkage. By the 1930s, Freud had recognized, in a total turn around to what he maintained in *The Future of an Illusion,* that no strict demarcation exists between religion, which he had once considered an illusion that alienates and divides, and rational atheism that, he had thought, held monopoly over truth and reason. The idea of progress, which he had already questioned in *Civilization and Its Discontents,* and regression in the history of religions around which the ending of *Moses and Monotheism* is built, brings Freud to the conclusion that non-illusory phenomena are also part of religion. At the end of his life, he is much more inclined to recognize the nugget of truth in religion just as he later accepts that truth can be found at the core of all delusional ideas.

From this new Freudian perspective, religion is no longer an ideology of illusion but, rather, a symbol of what's to come, a collective transitional object, a way by which humans attempt to understand the cosmos – a cosmos which remains, by definition, fundamentally mysterious and unknowable, impossible to reduce to merely reason and science. This was later Winnicott's position and also that of several of Freud's famous opponents: Lou Andréas-Salomé, Pastor Pfister, and Romain Rolland.

There is another reason why we cannot characterize Freud's idea of religion as an example of routine, ordinary atheism [5], the classic kind of atheism that relegates spirituality to the "wastebaskets of history." To the contrary, on many occasions Freud deliberately differentiates himself from philosophers who think that God is only essential for the ignorant masses and not for people of superior intelligence. One example of this latter thinking is Spinoza, with his famous claim of three degrees of knowledge. Neither does Freud believe, as do Descartes or Leibnitz, for instance, that the existence of God is self-evident. Freud sees "theological philosophy" as simply another illusion on a par with other anti-religion ideologies that were gaining ascendance at the beginning of the twentieth century. He clearly affirms the need for religion in *Civilization and Its Discontents* when he underscores the fact of man's basic aggressive instincts, which, had they not been tamed by religion, would have prevented human beings from living together in ever larger communities.

Religion, Psychoanalysis, and the "Taming" of Basic Instincts

After his pivotal moment of change, which I would say occurred sometime in the 1930s, Freud was no longer able to ignore the important function served by religion in "taming" (Freud used this term in *Analysis Terminable and Interminable,* an important text written during this same period – 1937) man's basic instincts. Already in 1908, Freud had established (in *"Civilized" Sexual Morality and Modern Nervous Illness*) that "sexual drives are irrepressible." From that moment on, the question for Freud became: if one admits that instincts cannot be curbed by drill or instruction then what, other than religion, could allow humans to live communally? Hardly had he finished writing his plea that religious illusions be replaced by science (in response to Pastor Pfister's arguments) than Freud begins expressing doubts about the validity of this position [6]. At this juncture, it is to psychoanalysis, and especially to psychoanalytic therapy, that he accords the starring role of instinct tamer. The aim of analytic therapy, he writes, is to bring sexual and aggressive instincts into the open. "Where id once was, there shall ego be. Psychoanalysis is a civilizing task comparable to draining the Zuider Zee" [7]. Civilizing certainly, but does it ipso facto facilitate communal living? After 1915, when he wrote about the ravages of the Great War, Freud never ceased to reiterate that civilization was incapable of transforming man's evil, murderous innate nature. But, by the same token, was psychoanalysis capable of effecting such a transformation? Was faith in psychoanalysis anything more than another illusion? In *Warum Krieg* (*Why War*) [8], Freud writes that the reign of reason [9] might ultimately permit mankind to do without religion. But such a regime must not be "a reign of virtue," an external imposition along the lines of Robespierre. The taming must come from the inside, from within the human spirit; it must, in effect, constitute a victory over oneself. What interests Freud is to understand how self-mastery is able to transform human nature, how innate biology can be controlled, and how a human being can become peaceable and civilized. This question began to haunt him after the disaster of 1914–1918; his conclusion was that a very few people can, in fact, succeed at self-mastery. Why is that? His answer is, "Because they are unable to do otherwise." There are people, he thinks, like himself and Einstein, who could not ever become violent, as if this way of being were etched into their organic, biologic, and genetic heritage.

Let us admit that Freud's answer is not very convincing and leaves us facing a real difficulty. Is spirituality so fundamentally linked in our unconscious with instinctive violence that separating the two is impossible, if not potentially explosive? Is religious belief ingrained in us? In the same way as man is a social and political animal, is he also, for all time to come, a religious animal?

These questions, which Freud did not further develop – do they impact our understanding of the modern world?

The Perennial Endurance of Religion

What we can definitely say about religion other than that all attempts to remove it by terror have failed, whether we look at national socialism or the Russian revolution or the other totalitarian regimes that followed. On the contrary, the perennial nature of religious feelings, and the need to believe in the sacred, have led, in the wake of attempts to undermine monotheistic beliefs based on the transcendence of God, to fanatical regressions. For instance, at the time of the pharaohs, such attempts led to mummification, to revolutionary leaders, and to all kinds of new forms of idolatry. When compared to the abstract nature of pure monotheism, these phenomena are evidence of a cultural regression. The disenchantment with the world shown by the retreat of established religions has not prevented the resurgence of novel, unusual forms of spirituality in the form of sects or diverse ideologies, such as those termed "New Age." The diminution of the delicate sounds of liturgical chants sung a cappella has given way to loud exhortations that transport massive crowds into hypnotic ecstasies, like those in Nuremberg, on Red Square, or on Tiananmen Square during the Chinese cultural revolution.

Finally, with respect to anti-Semitism, we see it returning in unexpected places. This refers to Muslim lands, which confirms its link to Abrahamic religions since it does not occur in non-monotheistic regions such as China or the main parts of India.

The French Situation

With this in mind, let me stop for a minute to consider the case of France. One again hears in the streets of Paris shouts such as "Death to Jews." This is coming from demonstrations attended not only by fanatic Muslims or so-called anti-Zionists but also by a large wing of the extreme left. At the same time, movements identified as belonging to the extreme right continue to profess a generalized xenophobia aimed at Arabs, Blacks, and Jews – demonstrating a traditional anti-Semitism that often draws on Catholic sources. These resurgences of anti-Semitism lean on works published by so-called researchers who question the reality of the Shoah. They call themselves revisionists. In France, there has been an explosion of anti-Semitic acts aimed at religious buildings and cemeteries, but also individuals. There have been murders; certain suburbs of big cities have become essentially uninhabitable for Jews or for Jewish institutions.

Since the time of the French revolution and the first Napoleonic era that granted status to Jews, a latent anti-Semitism has always existed in France. Besides the anti-Judaism of the Church, there was a tendency toward anti-Semitism among significant sections of the labor movement. The famous socialist theoretician, Proudhon, directly attacked Jews, whom he considered to be the personification of capitalism. The Dreyfus case flared up at the beginning of the twentieth century – a Jewish officer falsely accused of being a German collaborator by a coalition of the army and the Church. Finally, thanks to the works of Robert Paxton, we all remember the anti-Semitic complexion of Pétain's collaborationist government and the ideology of the *révolution nationale* that supported him. The case of contemporary France is interesting because it exemplifies the different forms of Jew hatred – Islamic, anti-Israeli of the extreme left, old-school anti-Semitic of the extreme right – and coalesces them into an explosive cocktail that has led many French Jews to want to emigrate, mainly to Israel, the USA, or Canada. One has to ask the question: is there not an essentially unconscious commonality among all these forms of hatred against Jews?

Religious Violence and Anti-Semitism

One of the main objectives of this chapter is to show that anti-Semitism, including its current resurgence, convincingly demonstrates, as Freud suggests at the end of *Moses and Monotheism*, a core of violence within the phenomenon of religion. Each religion believes that its truth is the one and only truth so that, as in families, as in sacred texts, and as in what we understand to have taken place in ancient societies, sibling rivalries explode into acts of aggression. According to Freud, anti-Semitism almost unbelievably (to use his very term) illustrates the ambivalence (awe/fear/jealousy/hatred) that sons naturally feel toward their fathers and that the two other monotheistic religions feel toward their progenitor – i.e., Judaism.

Viewed from this angle, but only from this one angle, Judaism is, indeed, a fossil, a reminder that the primeval father was vindictive and all-powerful but was put to death, making way for a father (the God of monotheism), who was both merciful and just. Judaism is a living fossil, which retains the indelible and unforgettable trace of the original ambivalence toward mankind's primitive conception of God. By refusing all idolatry, Judaism continues to symbolically murder primitive Gods, while the two other great monotheistic religions have symbolically exonerated themselves from the crime, Christianity by the crucifixion of God's son, Jesus, and Islam by its total submission to Allah. Muslim means "one who has submitted to God." Thus, Muslims believe that the commentaries in the Hebrew Talmud are heresies because man must not question the meaning of the word of God.

In summary, Freud's view was that an unconscious kernel of anti-Semitism exists in everyone. This is clear in France, a former colonial power with a large immigrant population from North and sub-Saharan Africa. The immigrants come from countries where the Jewish population used to be second-class citizens only to see Jews flourishing, relative to the Muslim population, in today's France. In addition to unconscious reasons, French Muslims have conscious economic reasons for hating Jews, on top of which, to them, Israel represents a modern colonial aggressor vis-à-vis Palestine.

It is impossible to understand the Shoah without taking into account the centuries of anti-Jewish hatred that preceded it [10]. The constancy of this hatred, which seems to be ever present and to erupt periodically in different parts of the world, cannot be denied even though the word, "anti-Semitism," was not in use until the end of the nineteenth century. Different words can be used – Judeophobia, anti-Judaism, racial anti-Semitism, and anti-Zionism – but the basic antagonism cannot be disguised by changing the word. A clear-cut distinction between religious anti-Judaism and racial anti-Semitism appears to me to be specious, since hostility to the religion of the Jews has always been accompanied, at least since the Gospel of John, by a hatred directed not only against individual Jews but against the Jewish people in their entirety. Therefore, the different terms used are only variations on the same theme of hostility toward Jews as individuals and as a people. Although we need to be careful to not overstate the case for the unconscious, it is hoped that this essay contributes to an appreciation that anti-Semitism, no matter the precise term used to describe all the related phenomena, refers to an interconnected web of emotions, an "organized body of images partially or wholly unconscious" [11].

Since unconscious prejudices are, to a large extent, transmitted from generation to generation, what, then, is the remedy for anti-Semitism? Since it is during early childhood that biases, such as antagonism toward Jews, are formed, it seems likely that social and community psychiatry, combined with early childhood education, can help to dispel them. Institutions dedicated to the mental health of children (and their parents) can, I believe, serve as powerful antidotes to the spread of this venomous undercurrent in our society.

References

1. Bar-Asher MM. Les juifs dans le Coran [Jews in the Koran]. Paris: Albin Michel; 2018.
2. Freud S. L'homme Moïse et la religion monothéiste [Moses and Monotheism]. Paris: Gallimard; 1986.
3. Mosès S. L'ange de l'histoire [The Angel of History]. Paris: Gallimard; 2006.

4. Favret-Saada J, Contreras J. Le christianisme et ses juifs, 1800–2000 [Christianity and its Jews, 1800–2000]. Paris: Seuil; 2004.

5. Hirt J-M. Vestiges de Dieu, Athéisme et religiosité [Vestiges of god, atheism, and spirituality]. Paris: Grasset; 1998.

6. Freud S. Le malaise dans la culture [Civilizations and its Discontents] OCF XVIII PUF; 1994.

7. Freud S. La décomposition de l'appareil psychique, Nouvelles conférences d'introduction à la psychanalyse [The decomposition of the Psychic Apparatus, in New introductory lectures on psychoanalysis]. Paris: Gallimard; 1984.

8. Freud S. Pourquoi la guerre, Nouvelles conferences d'introduction à la psychanalyse [Why War? In New introductory lectures on psychoanalysis]. Paris: Gallimard; 1984.

9. Major R. Cruelle démocratie [Cruel Democracy]. Galilée; 2003.

10. Gribinski M. En relisant Eric Michaud, Penser/rêver, La maladie chrétienne [Upon re-reading Eric Michaud in To Think/to Dream, the Christian Malady] Edition de l'Olivier, #11, 2007, p.161–79.

11. Laplanche J, Pontalis J-B. Vocabulaire de la psychanalyse [The vocabulary of psychoanalysis], 1967. https://www.amazon.fr/Vocabulaire-psychanalyse-Jean-Laplanche/dp/2130560504.

Childhood Experiences of Anti-Semitism in Argentina (1976–1983): Stories of Trauma, Resilience, and Long-Term Outcome

22

Sigalit Gal

Since I remember myself, I knew that I am Jewish, and that someone can tell me something about it, but I did not realize that something bad can happen to us because of this.
– Tomas

Introduction

This chapter explores the long-term mental health impact of childhood experiences of anti-Semitism during the military dictatorship in Argentina (1976–1983), among adult Jewish Argentinian immigrants to Israel. Despite the successful integration of Jews who immigrated as early as the end of the eighteenth century, Jews in Argentina have always been subject to anti-Semitism and xenophobia [1, 2]. The literature shows that the severity of the manifestation of anti-Semitism escalated according to each period's political circumstances and reached its peak during the sixth military dictatorship [3].

Substantial literature has researched the effects of exposure to identity-focused discrimination such as anti-Semitism, from interpersonal microaggressions to structural-level political agendas of state-sponsored persecution and genocide, most notably the Holocaust which took the lives of over six million Jews and directly affected millions more. Researchers have explored many domains of the long-term effects of the experiences of anti-Semitism on mental health, including psychopathology [4], resiliency [5], and the co-existence of both negative and positive outcomes [6]. This narrative study, which is focused on the experience of an understudied population of adult Argentinian immigrants to Israel, illuminates the possible connection between the experience of anti-Semitism during childhood and mental health consequences of adult Jewish Argentinian immigrants to Israel. As such, it

S. Gal (✉)
Faculty of Arts, Social Sciences, McGill University, Montreal, Canada
e-mail: Sigalit.gal@mail.mcgill.ca

© Springer Nature Switzerland AG 2020
H. S. Moffic et al. (eds.), *Anti-Semitism and Psychiatry*,
https://doi.org/10.1007/978-3-030-37745-8_22

can provide mental health practitioners with a greater understanding of the mechanisms involved, which ultimately could impact the development and the improvement of existing services and interventions.

There were several reasons for my investigation into this topic. Apart from addressing the gap in the existing knowledge about the long-term impact of childhood political trauma experienced in one's country of origin on adult immigrants' mental health, my curiosity about this subject emerged from my own personal experience as a cultural minority in Canada, which includes a complex psychological realm that is based on a continuing and evolving dialogue between my emotional history in my country of origin, Israel, and my partial adaptation to the Canadian culture. Furthermore, I can see how choosing to focus on the experience of Jewish immigrants to Israel in general, and in particular on the experience of Jewish Argentinian immigrants to Israel, is strongly related to my identity as a Jewish person and as an Israeli native. It is also associated with my exposure to anti-Semitism during my work as a Foreign correspondent in France (2001–2002) who investigated, researched, and wrote articles, particularly on anti-Semitism.

In addition, during my doctoral fieldwork as a clinical counsellor, I met with emotionally distressed adult Jewish immigrants in Montreal, and I listened to their life stories that often shifted between childhood experience in immigrants' countries of origin and their immigration experiences as adults. This experience has given me the opportunity to hypothesize that, in some cases, childhood adversity and emotional history may reflect in different ways on current experiences, perceptions, and interpretations of the internal and external reality as adult immigrants, as well as on the strategies that are chosen by these individuals to deal with various immigration stressors.

When searching for a more specific population to serve as a case study for my research, I was reflecting on one of my visits in Israel. During this visit, I had an opportunity to talk with some Jewish adults who immigrated to Israel from Argentina after escaping the sixth military dictatorship. My exploration of the existing knowledge suggested minimal research on the long-term impact that their childhood experience of anti-Semitism and human rights abuse may have on their mental health.

Long-Standing History of State-Sponsored Anti-Semitism in Argentina

Understanding the long-standing history of state-sponsored anti-Semitism in Argentina can provide the context of its escalation 30 years after the end of the Second World War, during the sixth military dictatorship. This is pertinent to the Argentinian government's unofficial support of Nazi Germany, prior, during, and following the war [3, 7]. Apart from the adoption of German military ideology during and after the Second World War [8, 9], Argentina opened its doors to thousands of Nazi war criminals at war's end [10]. Some of these men rose to powerful positions in government, allowing them to transmit to others the principles of the Third

Reich's methods of persecution and to contribute to the escalation of existing anti-Semitic attitudes [3]. All of these methods found a place in government policy, decades later [11, 12].

Shortly before the military dictatorship replaced the democratic government led by Isabel Peron, there were already key figures in Peron's government who expressed Nazi ideology in the public sphere (e.g.: Alberto Ottalagano, the administrative head for universities) [13, 14].

Other factors that contributed to the escalation of anti-Semitic attitudes and to the demonization of the Jew [15] were the Catholic Church [16, 17] and the capture of Nazi Adolf Eichmann in Argentina by the Israeli secret service in 1960s [18–20]. From then on, anti-Semitism in Argentina manifested itself in anti-Zionist attacks by the political left and by defenders of the Arab cause – an attitude that was adopted by the political right and added to their existing "old" anti-Semitism [3, 18, 19].

Escalation During the Sixth Dictatorship

Few studies on the implementation of anti-Semitism in the policy of the military dictatorship exist. For this reason, I use Kaufman's [30] mixed methods, based on an archive of reports, interviews, and testimonies of former Jewish prisoners. Reports by the Amnesty International, the Inter-American Commission on Human Rights, and the US State Department provide additional evidence that, during the 1970s, Argentina had the highest prevalence of anti-Semitism of any South American country, even when compared to countries with similar military regimes [3].

Despite the immense efforts of the post-dictatorship regime to eliminate all documentation of its actions [21], archive information collected from 27 detention centers in Argentina and testimonies of former Jewish prisoners show strong evidence that Jews were particularly and intentionally selected for abuse. They were jailed in separate facilities and suffered more extensive physical punishment, both in quantity and in quality, than the general population at that time [3]. In addition to physical abuse, there was also verbal anti-Semitic abuse, which included accusations of a Jewish international conspiracy to establish a second Jewish state in southern Argentina, a general perception of Jews as the embodiment of the anti-Christ and the use of Nazi terminology during interrogations [3]. Third Reich persecution strategies were used, as well as the practice of forcing Jews to change their Hebrew names and convert to Catholicism [3].

Anti-Semitism was also practiced in the public sphere through the distribution of Nazi and other anti-Semitic literature, accusations of Jewish disloyalty, and public physical and verbal attacks [11].

To this day, we can only estimate the total number of victims (Jews and non-Jews) murdered during the military regime, as military officials made sure to destroy any evidence well before their regime came to its end [21]. The current estimate is 30,000 "disappeared" [22, 23]. This number includes 3000 Jews, a number that is disproportionately high given that, at that time, Jews made up approximately 1% (0.8–1.2%) of a population of about 26 million [11, 24, 25].

Current-Day Anti-Semitism in Argentina

The anti-Semitism in Argentina did not end with the restoration of democracy in 1983. During the 1990s, there was again a significant increase in anti-Semitism, illustrated by two disastrous attacks against Jews during that period: on March 17, 1992, there was a terror attack on the Israeli embassy in Buenos Aires, and on July 18, 1994, there was the "AMIA bombing," an attack on the *Asociación Mutual Israelita Argentina* building in Buenos Aires, during which 85 people were killed and hundreds were injured [10].

About 300,000 Jews live in Argentina, which is the largest Jewish community in South America and the seventh largest Jewish community in the world [26]. Although the anti-Semitism in Argentina currently does not result from government policy, it still shows itself through multiple incidents in the public sphere. For example, during 2019, the following anti-Semitic incidents occurred: anti-Semitic posts on social media, Swastika graffiti sprayed on the walls in Jewish neighborhoods, physical and verbal attacks on rabbis, vandalization of Jewish gravestones, and a series of threats made against the Delegation of Argentine Jewish Associations (DAIA) over social networks [26, 27]. In addition, in recent years, anti-Semitism seems to have made its way from the public sphere to the Argentinian political arena [26–28].

Anti-Semitism has been one of the main reasons for Argentinian Jews to immigrate to Israel. Yet, despite having been a part of Israeli society for many decades, and although the Argentinian community consists of more than 100,000 people [29], the voice of this community has been relatively silent both in public discourse and in academic research [30]. There is a significant gap in the literature focusing specifically on those who escaped to Israel following the military dictatorship in Argentina. The limited scholarship available is focused on their rescue from Argentina [31, 32], their lack of adjustment into Israeli society, their invisibility within it [10, 33, 34], and their concern over the years in relation to the fate of their disappeared family members [35].

Anti-Semitism and Mental Health Consequences

In the same way that all Adverse Childhood Experiences (ACE) have long-term negative consequences [36], scholars argue that political trauma may impact the child long into his or her adult life taking the shape of various psychiatric disorders such as depression, suicide attempts, mistrust in people, anxiety disorders, oppositional defiant disorders, complex PTSD, aggression, lack of impulse control, attention problems, and problems with adult relationships [37–40]. Among the variety of negative mental health outcomes, it is argued that PTSD is the most common diagnosis [41].

In contrast to the definition of trauma as "an event from which you never fully recover" [42, p. 253], some scholars are of the opinion that no event can be considered inherently traumatic, meaning that each individual may react in a different way to the same event depending on many variables, both internal (e.g.: age when experiencing the trauma) and external (e.g.: social support) [43–46]. The variety of long-term reactions that survivors of childhood political trauma experience is well illustrated in the wealth of literature focused on child Holocaust survivors.

Mental Health Associated with Child Holocaust Survivors

The experience of child Holocaust survivors offers a well-documented example of the long-term psychological reactions of victims of an oppressive political regime, an example that may provide guidance in the analysis of the cases in this study.

The first body of research is comprised of studies that show the way that prolonged exposure to conditions during the Holocaust correlated with a long-term negative impact on child survivors' mental health [4] and specifically with the manifestation of PTSD [47]. Nevertheless, there are also research findings of positive long-term outcomes, such as successful functioning during adulthood in various life domains, namely, career, relationships, and family [48].

A third body of research argues for the *co-existence* of negative and positive outcomes: good adaptation to life and resilience, as well as the manifestation of high level of post-traumatic symptomatology [6, 49].

Apart from the three main bodies of research, there is also a fourth growing body of research on Holocaust survivors that looks for the possibilities of *positive* transformations from this trauma, which may go beyond resilience: Post-Traumatic Growth (PTG) [48]. In the same way that pathology and resilience can co-exist, so can PTSD and PTG [50]. This duality has been called operating on "parallel tracks" [48].

Based on this understanding, I developed a conceptual framework for the current study that includes Beiser and Simich's [51] interactive paradigm of "resettlement and mental health," which demonstrates the interplay of risk and protective factors in the context of immigration and mental health. Another element in my framework is Kirmayer's [37] definition of political trauma, which includes four main components: a) wounding violence; b) violence that has lasting effects on physical and mental health, which is emblematic of PTSD; c) states of extremity that break all bounds of reason, containment, and control and violently disrupt and destroy the social order; and d) an open-ended set of diverse and shifting sorts of events that are linked metaphorically to one of the first three meanings [37, p.389]. Other components in my framework include concepts such as resilience [52], Post-Traumatic Growth [53], and complex PTSD [38]. This model (Fig. 22.1) represents a presumed reciprocal and ongoing interchange between the past (individuals' experience of anti-Semitism during childhood in their country of origin) and present events (immigration, post-migration adjustment) and the assumed link of these elements to a range of possible long-term negative and/or positive outcomes for mental health in adulthood.

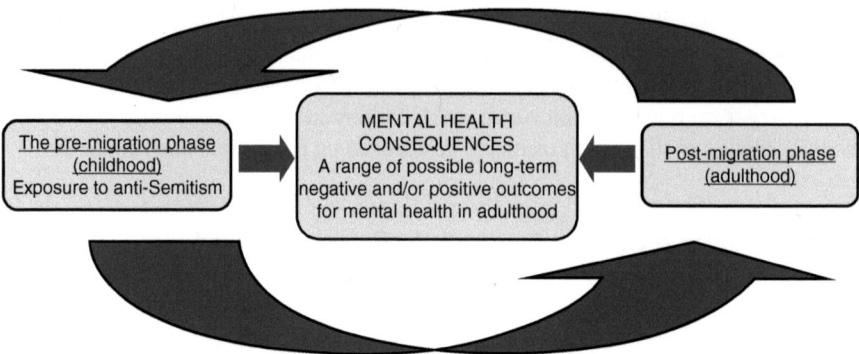

Fig. 22.1 Childhood experiences of anti-Semitism and adult immigrants' mental health

Research Design and Method

The findings presented in this chapter are part of my doctoral dissertation research. The purpose was to identify the risk and protective factors underlying the mental health consequences of childhood political trauma (Argentina 1976–1983) among adult Jewish Argentinian immigrants to Israel.

The following strategies were used to recruit the participant population for this study: (1) snowball sampling, starting with my personal acquaintances (Argentinian immigrant Jews) who forwarded the study invitation to their social networks and encouraged eligible individuals to contact the researcher; (2) advertising about the study on social media; (3) promotional scripts and letters which included an easy-to-read text in Hebrew about the study, its purpose and objectives, and ways to contact the researcher directly while retaining confidentiality; and (4) I expanding my sources by contacting "Argentinian Kibbutzim" and asking the Kibbutzim's administration office to connect me with some of the residents.

The final participants were 15 adult immigrant Jews, 9 males and 6 females between the ages of 48 and 53 years, who had immigrated from Argentina to Israel and who were children at the time of the military dictatorship in Argentina (1976–1983). The mean age of this sample was six at the beginning of the dictatorship. They all had sufficient Hebrew proficiency to take part in the interviews; the duration of their residency in Israel ranged from three to four decades. By means of a distress screening script [54], I excluded those who were struggling with extensive emotional distress and had no access to coping resources.

Following the formal approval for the study from the Research Ethics Board of McGill University, I met in person with each of the participants in different geographic locations in Israel for an average time of 2 hours. All the interviews were audio-recorded and transcribed. Given that it was an exploratory retrospective study, the narrative method [55] was utilized and included a two-phased narrative interview [56]. The first phase was an open life story, the main narrative. This was followed by semi-structured questions (when necessary). Demographic information was collected at the end.

Aligned with the purpose of the study, an exploration of the participants' emotional and behavioral reactions in the present day, observations before, during, and after the interviews were also considered part of the study method [57].

I used a holistic approach to data analysis, so as to include both form and content analysis of the narrative [58], an approach similar to an intuitive reading of clinical sessions. The thematic textual analysis of these interviews was focused on the emotional and behavioral manifestations of these immigrants' past experiences in their present lives. Finally, I triangulated reported and observed data and drew my conclusions.

Since I conducted the interviews in Hebrew, in order to establish the accuracy of the translation (from Hebrew to English), the interviews were independently translated by an additional bilingual person, and the two versions were compared. In addition, back translation has been used by both me and the bilingual person in order to establish accuracy.

As a qualitative researcher, I continuously engaged with self-reflection and reassessed my positioning throughout the different stages of my study. This self-reflection helped me to identify how my positionality was impacting my attitude, my responses, and my interpretations in relation to my research subjects. A special attention was given to my theoretical and professional clinical bias as doctoral student (my doctoral work was a result of a collaboration between the division of Social and Transcultural Psychiatry and the Department of Social Work at McGill University), being a cultural minority in Canada, having an emotional and nostalgic attachment to Israel as my homeland, and holding stereotypical cultural beliefs in relation to the Argentinian culture, which I knew very little about at the time of my study.

Findings

The content of the interviews was focused on two periods of the participants' lives: childhood experience in Argentina and adult immigration experiences in Israel. These were categorized into two main themes: a) retrospective descriptions of the manifestation of anti-Semitism during the dictatorship and b) ways participants believed that these childhood experiences had impacted their mental well-being as adults.

Childhood Experiences of Anti-Semitism

During the interviews, participants described how, in addition to the suffering caused by the dictatorship's human rights abuses, their families and themselves were subject, as Jews, to "special treatment" from both their peers and the Junta. Participants described how the fear of being harmed or murdered at any time was very tangible. One example was the possibility of being kidnapped in route to school. Fernando (this is a pseudonym, as are all participants' names in this chapter) remembers his parents' concern each time he had to pass by two military camps on his way to school: "The possibility of being kidnapped by these soldiers was always in the back of my mind" (Fernando).

While arbitrary arrests were experienced by many civilians, in the case of Jews, there was additional vulnerability and risk. This is how Fabian described an incident when he and his friends were arrested while innocently walking in the street:

> At the police station, they asked us: 'Are you Jewish?' and suddenly I see that behind the counter, one policeman opens his locker and on the back of the locker's door there is a big sign of a swastika. We were so scared, because they already knew that we were Jewish, and we see that they adore the Nazis! So we were convinced that this is it: the worst is about to come. (Fabian)

Anti-Semitism was manifested also in elementary school. Pablo, Laura, and Mariano described how their school curricula and lectures included anti-Semitic ideas. Complaining about it was useless, as illustrated by Pablo:

> [In my school] I had a teacher who was praising Hitler and the 3rd Reich and who said that the Jews in Argentina will pay the price. I tried to have two of my Jewish teachers to back me up and I went to complain about it, but the school principal said I am rebellious, expelled me, and kept the Nazi teacher at school. (Pablo)

Pablo also described how gradually his school began to resemble a military camp, which included harsh discipline, an increasing atmosphere of fear and terror, and the sudden "disappearance" of some students.

Findings show that anti-Semitism at school was not only expressed by the teachers but also by peers. For example, Laura described how at the school cafeteria she was subjected to daily anti-Semitic bullying: "they kept blaming me for killing Jesus" (Laura), and Fernando remembered daily bullying and harassment from his peers on his way to school: "They were telling all the horrible jokes about Jews, like: 'the Nazis took good care of you, they made soaps from you'. So I grew up with it as a child" (Fernando).

Another experience of anti-Semitism was the psychological and physical abuse endured by older teens during their compulsory service in the Argentinian military. In their interviews, Lorenzo, Fabian, and Fernando described their experiences as Jews in the Argentinian military, which included "special" physical punishments for Jews and humiliations that at times resulted in suicide attempts: "I can't say that how they treated us was a big surprise. We had to endure it in elementary school, on the streets; it was not the first time" (Fabian). However, some participants were shocked by the anti-Semitism. As put by Tomas: "Since I remember myself, I knew that I am Jewish, and that someone can tell me something about it, but I did not realize that something bad can happen to us because of this" (Tomas).

Apart from participants' "first-hand" experience of anti-Semitic abuse, they also mentioned their parents' experiences. For example, Fernando vividly remembers a time when his mother was attacked by neighbors after expressing criticism of

Argentina's participation in the Falklands War: "These neighbors almost killed her, they cursed her saying: 'you dirty Jew' and all those 'nice' things" (Fernando). Victor recalls the day when his mother, who was the only Jewish teacher at a non-Jewish school, came back home in tears after seeing graffiti on the school walls saying: "we don't want Jewish teachers here!" Participants also mentioned the stories they heard as children about the torture inflicted on Jewish political prisoners, the ways the Junta took over Jewish businesses, and about the experiences of discrimination against Jews in places of work.

As for participants' reactions to anti-Semitism during the dictatorship, these included behavioral and emotional protective strategies such as the need to hide their Jewish identities (e.g.: taking off the symbol of the Star of David on the Jewish elementary school uniform; avoiding attending synagogue; celebrating the Jewish holidays in secrecy; and conducting Jewish educational weekend activities in hidden locations). As put by Fernando: "The dominant feeling is that you better not reveal that you are Jewish, and that I needed to protect myself, because in Argentina – Judaism is an ugly thing" (Fernando). Other behavioral defense strategies included not going out at night; never going out alone during daytime; lying when necessary; destroying "incriminating" material such as phonebooks, which contained names and addresses of personal contacts that could have led to the arrest of their family members and friends; keeping one's silence; and keeping "a low profile." In addition, some participants showed their ability to contain and endure daily physical and psychological abuse and humiliation in nonviolent ways, by using rationalization and guided imagery, by adopting extensive methods of self-reliance, and by finding support from Jewish and non-Jewish allies. In contrast, in some cases, suffering extensive and prolonged anti-Semitic abuse had led to suicide attempts.

For participants who did not escape to Israel during or immediately after the dictatorship, the escalation of anti-Semitism during the 1990s was a wake-up call. As put by Valentina: "After the dictatorship we did not believe that it could happen again, but it did" (Valentina).

Long-Term Representations of Childhood Traumatic Memory

Immigration to Israel brought a sense of liberation and relief to many given that there was no longer a need to hide one's Jewish identity, but after several decades, participants who were affected by anti-Semitism and human rights abuses during childhood still exhibit negative behavioral and emotional reactions. For instance, as adults, they use the same defense strategies they used as children during the dictatorship.

One such strategy is an excessive lack of trust. As explained by Fernando: "if I will not protect myself no one else will protect me [...] I really believe in it, that you cannot count on anyone" (Fernando). This lack of trust has been demonstrated also by participants' reported attitudes toward their own family members, other Argentinian immigrants in Israel, and toward governmental institutions in Israel. As put by Pablo: "I am nearly 40 years in Israel, and I still do not trust any government's institutions. I will never ever trust them, not in Argentina and not in Israel, and not anywhere in the world" (Pablo).

In addition, observations of participants' behavior before, during, and after the interviews show that most of them exhibit a high level of suspicion: I was the subject of an "interrogation" regarding my "real" motivation to do this study and my personal connection to Argentina. In addition, some participants used false names until they met with me in person.

Another defensive strategy is keeping one's silence: Most participants admitted that these interviews marked the first time they had revealed the whole story of their experiences under the dictatorship as children. As explained by Tomas: "[during the dictatorship] we were not able to talk freely [...] So I am still trying to keep control. Whoever is over 50 years old feels that fear. You cannot speak. You cannot tell" (Tomas). In addition, in some cases, participants exhibited anxiety after the interview, fearing they may have "talked too much," that they had revealed information they had not planned to expose. Pablo, for example, described his interview as an "interrogation," despite it being a narrative interview, in which there is minimal intervention by the researcher.

Yet another defense strategy was living in survival mode. Most participants expressed the need to be mentally and physically ready to face the worst at any given moment and said that they always carry their identification documents with them "as a habit". Some participants, like Lorenzo, take this a step further and do not leave their homes without carrying a "survival kit", in case they are caught by the security forces and never come back to their homes. This survival mode is also evident in their mental readiness to escape from Israel, an urge triggered by the Middle East conflict and by their fear of a military coup in Israel. As explained by Nadia: "I am connecting what happened there [in Argentina] and what is happening now in Israel [...] I came to Israel carrying all this, and I am scared that it will happen again" (Nadia).

In addition to the above, one of the main themes raised by all participants was their complex attitudes toward the Israeli Defense Forces, which range between two extremes: at one end of the scale extensive fear, while at the other end: unconditional admiration. The fundamental anxiety triggered by the sight of an armed soldier or a police officer in Israel was reported by all participants, although, in some cases, that fear, reportedly, had gradually decreased over time. For example, Mariano reported a decrease of his anxiety when seeing Israeli security forces in the streets, but he still experiences immense stress when arriving at military checkpoints in Israel: "I am still very careful not to look them [the soldiers] in the eyes" (Mariano).

Another form of avoidance is participants' reluctance to return to Argentina even on a visit. Participants described how even family visits in Argentina evoked anxiety and fear for their personal safety and how, for them, it is like coming back to a scene of a crime, even though democracy has been restored in Argentina since 1983. "You need to be on guard all the time" explains Nadia. "A policeman in Argentina could arrest you illegally, and take you in with no reason, so you do not want a policeman to see you" (Nadia). "I suffered every minute of being there" said Lorenzo "All the memories that I had about the military over there haunted me" (Lorenzo).

It is interesting to see that, despite their paradoxical constant urge to flee Israel, most participants admitted that, compared to Argentina, it is in Israel where they feel most safe. As explained by Pablo, "even with all the wars and the Intifada, I feel much safer in Israel then in Argentina" (Pablo). "I finally felt that I am part of something" explained Fernando "that I am not alone, that I do not need to defend myself as a Jew and to hide my heritage" (Fernando).

In addition to the above, participants reported that as adults they have been experiencing flashbacks about physical and emotional abuse by Argentinian security force. They suffer from vivid and detailed memories and strong feelings of shame and guilt for "abandoning" their family and friends in Argentina and for not being able to fully comprehend their situation as children. As explained by Valentina: "it was only years later that I understood what was the meaning of the screams that we heard that night when passing by that military base [...] but what I could have done, go to the police?" (Valentina). Among the emotional reactions were also feelings of personal and collective anger and the belief in the "damaged self." As put by Daniela: "All these anxieties that I have, it is something that is there" (Daniela).

Furthermore, observations of participants' behavior during the interviews showed that most of them exhibited anxiety, hyperarousal, and strong emotional reactions (e.g.: crying, detachment, somatic reactions, temporary amnesia). In addition, some participants used the present tense when describing traumatic events that they experienced as children, indicating that they were reliving their past trauma. In addition, although participants were asked to tell the story of their lives, most of them stopped talking after they finished describing their experience as children during the dictatorship, signaling that this is where their life story ends (as well as their interview). It was only after I asked "and then…?" that they continued to talk about their experience as adults.

Using Childhood "Survival Skills" as Adults

Resilience was also manifested. None of these participants interviewed for this study had ever been hospitalized for mental health problems. Furthermore, according to the interviews, it seems that they all function reasonably well, with everyone having managed to start a family and hold a job. Only one participant had been treated with psychiatric medications. Furthermore, participants' narratives revealed their pro-active behavior, such as resourcefulness, reaching out for and using family and social support (both in Argentina and in Israel), and contributing to the general society by initiating social activity and community involvement (e.g.: volunteering, political activism).

In addition, some participants' childhood "survival skills" were transferred into their adulthood and helped with coping as immigrants in Israel. As put by Daniela: "I have learnt during my childhood in Argentina to get adjusted to whatever reality brings you" (Daniela). Or in Sofia's words: "I think that all the difficult things that I went through [in Argentina] have made me stronger. What happened built my ability to cope" (Sofia).

Did Something Get Lost in Translation?

Given the profound lack of trust in others most participants have harbored since the dictatorship, especially toward people from Argentina, the fact that I am not Argentinian and do not speak Spanish actually greatly contributed to participants' feelings of safety and comfort when revealing their stories. However, this also caused some limitations in relation to data collection and analysis. Although one of the inclusive criteria for participation in this research was proficiency in Hebrew, I noticed that some participants instinctively switched from Hebrew to Spanish, especially when describing emotional events. Although they immediately translated what they said to Hebrew, and although I later verified how to write these expressions in Spanish so as to include them in my data, I was concerned that I might have missed the full subtlety and nuance of their meaning in the translation. At times, some participants expressed their frustration at not finding "the right word" in Hebrew to describe their stories and emotions. On other occasions, I suspected that they used the language barrier to avoid responding to questions they did not want to answer.

Also, given that all interviews were conducted in Hebrew, as none of the participants spoke fluent English, after the data analysis was complete, I had to translate more than 30 hours of interviews into English (my second language). Although I tried to be very meticulous in my translation work and provided some of my work for evaluation and review by an additional person who spoke both Hebrew and English, there were still times when I felt that I was unable to fully transmit the nuances of Hebrew slang into English.

Conclusion

The findings of this study correlate with existing knowledge about severe anti-Semitism during the military dictatorship (1976–1983) in Argentina [3, 11]. Participants described how, as well as suffering like everyone from the dictatorship's human rights abuses, they, as Jews, were the targets of prolonged anti-Semitic psychological and physical abuse and also witnessed the various ways anti-Semitism affected their parents and their peers. Experiencing such a prolonged and severe anti-Semitism had forced them as children to use various emotional and behavioral defense strategies.

Some of these childhood behavioral defense strategies, which may have been useful during the dictatorship, were still in evidence (e.g.: feeling anxious when seeing the security forces in Israel), even in the absence of the original threat. Although the purpose of this study was not to diagnose the participants, nor were any measurements for PTSD or complex PTSD used, participants' persistent use of defensive childhood behavioral strategies as adults suggests symptoms of C-PTSD and PTSD, for instance, feeling constantly threatened and acting or feeling as if traumatic events are recurring or will recur [59–61]. The study also found that negative emotions such as anger, shame, guilt, distrust, and the belief of permanent damage to the self continued to be present in participants' adult lives. In the interview, participants appeared to be reliving their past trauma. This again suggests complex PTSD [59–61].

At the same time, this study found a remarkable adaptability in the face of childhood experiences of severe anti-Semitism. This resilience is even more remarkable given the context of the ongoing political instability in Israel. Furthermore, although the post-traumatic growth inventory was not used in this research, participants also show emotional and behavioral reactions that fit the description of post-traumatic growth (PTG) [53]. Most have managed to turn the emotional strength and survival skills learned as children during the dictatorship into useful coping mechanisms as adult immigrants in Israel.

The co-existence of both negative and positive mental health outcomes, which are manifested simultaneously on "parallel tracks" [48], supports the findings of mental health outcomes of child Holocaust survivors [48].

While this study reflects the long-term impact of anti-Semitism experienced in childhood on a particular group of individuals in a particular time period, it does show that anti-Semitism has a powerful influence on the mental health of those exposed to it. This is a lesson that is generalizable. Mental health practitioners need to recognize both the vulnerability and the resilience of survivors.

References

1. Avni H. The Argentinian Jewish Community: its social status and its organizational structure. Jerusalem: Alfa; 1972.
2. Mirelman VA. Attitudes towards Jews in Argentina. Jew Soc Stud. 1975;37(3):205.
3. Kaufman E. Jewish victims of repression in Argentina under military rule (1976–1983). Holocaust and Genocide Stud. 1989;4(4):479–99. https://doi.org/10.1093/hgs/4.4.479.
4. Kuch K, Cox BJ. Symptoms of PTSD in 124 survivors of the Holocaust. Am J Psychiatry. 1992; https://doi.org/10.1176/ajp.149.3.337.
5. Lomranz J. Endurance and living: long-term effects of the Holocaust. In: Extreme stress and communities: impact and intervention. Dordrecht: Springer; 1995. p. 325–52.
6. Cohen M, Brom D, Dasberg H. Child survivors of the Holocaust: symptoms and coping after fifty years. Isr J Psychiatry Relat Sci. 2001;38(1):3.
7. Leonard TM, Bratzel JF, editors. Latin America during World War II. USA:Rowman & Littlefield; 2007.
8. Martínez TE. Peron and the Nazi war criminals. Latin American Program: USA: The Wilson Center; 1984.
9. Bono A. The troubled Jews of Argentina. Worldview. 1977;20(11):10–3.
10. Rein R. Argentine Jews or Jewish Argentines ?: Essays on ethnicity, identity, and diaspora: Boston: Brill; 2010. p. 67–88.
11. Tarica E. The Holocaust again?: dispatches from the Jewish "internal front" in dictatorship Argentina. J Jew Identities. 2012;5(1):89–110. https://doi.org/10.1353/jji.2012.0001.
12. Timerman J. Prisoner without a name, cell without a number. USA:University of Wisconsin Press; 2002.
13. Finchelstein F. The ideological origins of the dirty war: fascism, populism, and dictatorship in twentieth century Argentina: USA: Oxford University Press; 2017.
14. Ottalagano A. I am fascist. So what? Buenos Aires. Argentina: RO.CA. Publication; 1983.
15. Lerner N. Anti-Semitism and the nationalist ideology in Argentina. Dispersion Unity. 1973;17(/18):131–8.
16. Avni H. Forward, in The Catholic Church and the Jewish, Argentina 1933–1945.2008. ix. Jerusalem: The Hebrew University of Jerusalem, by the University of Nebraska Press.
17. Ben-Dror G. The Turning point: The military Coup and "Catholic Argentina" 1943–1945 in The Catholic Church and the Jews: Argentina, 1933–1945: USA: University of Nebraska Press; 2008. p. 90–110.

18. Rein R. Argentina I. the Jews: Perón, the Eichmann Capture and After. Bethesda: University Press of Maryland; 2003.
19. Rein R. The relationships of Israeli-Argentina, and situation of the Jewish community in Argentina under the shadow of the abduction of Eichmann, in The Zionism; 2001. p. 553–78.
20. Harel I. The house on Garibaldi street. Tel Aviv: Maariv Publication; 1975. p. 158–9.
21. DuBois L. The Politics of the Past in an Argentine Working-Class Neighborhood. J Latin Am Caribbean Anthropol. 2005;10(2):460–2. https://doi.org/10.1525/jlca.2005.10.2.460.
22. Cardenas S. Conflict and compliance: state responses to international human rights pressure. Pennsylvania: University of Pennsylvania Press; 2007. p. 52.
23. Nunca Más – Informe de la Conadep – Septiembre de 1984. http://www.desaparecidos.org/nuncamas/web/investig/articulo/nuncamas/nmas2_01.htm. Accessed: August 21 2018.
24. DAIA Buenos Aires. Informe sobre la situación de los detenidos-desaparecidos judíos durante el genocidio perpetrado en Argentina 1976–1983. 2007. http://www.daia.org.ar/2013/uploads/documentos/15/Desaparecidos.pdf. Accessed: November 14 2017.
25. COSOFAM. La violación de los derechos humanos de argentinos judíos bajo el regimen militar (1976–1983), Comisión de Solidaridad con Familiares de Presos y Detenidos en la Argentina (Commission in Solidarity with the Families of Prisoners and Detainees in Argentina, (pp. 69–78), Buenos Aires, Argentina: Milá; 2006. p. 69–78.
26. The Coordination Forum for Countering Antisemitism (CFCA). 2019. From: https://antisemitism.org.il/en/advanced-search/.Accessed: July 28 2019.
27. Times of Israel. Anti-Semitism in Argentina. 2019. https://www.timesofisrael.com/topic/anti-semitism-in-argentina/. Accessed: July 28 2019.
28. Times of Israel. Anti-Semitic Argentine politician kicks off campaign, vows to expel Israel envoy. May 28 2019a. https://www.timesofisrael.com/anti-semitic-argentine-politician-kicks-off-campaign-vows-to-expel-israel-envoy/. Accessed: July 28 2019.
29. Ministry of Aliah and Integration. The Israeli immigration ministry research department, Statistic about the immigration from Argentina to Israel 1972–2016. 2017.
30. Roniger L, Babis D. Latin American Israelis: the collective identity of an invisible community, Section 3: Latin -American Jewish culture in identities. In: Bokser De Liwerant J, Ben-Rafael E, Gorny Y, Rein R, editors. An era of globalization and multiculturalism, Latin America in the Jewish World. Leiden/Boston: Brill; 2008. p. 297–320.
31. Brown J. From Auschwitz to the May square: the story of a freedom fighter, Mekomit. https://mekomit.co.il/. April 28, 2014. Accessed: July 21 2018.
32. Zohar M. Let my people go to hell: blue and white treason. Tel Aviv: Tzitrin Publication; 1990.
33. Sznajder M, Roniger L. From Argentina to Israel: escape, evacuation and exile. J Lat Am Stud. 2005;37(2):351–77. https://doi.org/10.1017/S0022216X05009041.
34. Yazarsky R. Present-day Aliya from Latin America to Israel: ideology, ethnicity and religion, Hed. Haulpan Hachadash. 2015;103:23–31.
35. Rein R, Davidi E. Sport, politics and exile: protests in Israel during the world cup (Argentina, 1978). Int J Hist Sport. 2009;26(5):673–92. https://doi.org/10.1080/09523360902722666.
36. Felitti VJ, Anda RF, Nordenberg D, Williamson DF, Spitz AM, Edwards V, Koss MP, Marks JS. Relationship of childhood abuse and household dysfunction to many of the leading causes of death in adults: the Adverse Childhood Experiences (ACE) study. Am J Prev Med. 2019;56(6):774–86. https://doi.org/10.1016/S0749-3797(98)00017-8.
37. Kirmayer LJ. Wrestling with the angels of history: memory, symptom, and intervention. In: Hinton A, Hinton D, editors. Genocide and mass violence: memory, symptom, and recovery. New York: Cambridge University Press; 2014. p. 388–420.
38. Van der Kolk BA. Developmental trauma disorder: toward a rational diagnosis for children with complex trauma histories. Psychiatr Ann. 2017;35(5):401–8. https://doi.org/10.3928/00485713-20050501-06.
39. Fazel M, Reed RV, Panter-Brick C, Stein A. Mental health of displaced and refugee children resettled in high-income countries: risk and protective factors. Lancet. 2012;379(9812):266–82. https://doi.org/10.1016/S0140-6736(11)60051-2.
40. UNICEF. Children in War. 2015. http://www.unicef.org/sowc96/1cinwar.htm. Accessed: July 21 2018.

41. Kinzie JD. Guidelines for psychiatric care of torture survivors. Torture. 2011;21(1):18–26.
42. Garbarino J, Bruyere E. Resilience in the lives of children of war. In: Fernando C, Ferrari M, editors. Handbook of resilience in children of war. New York: Springer; 2013. p. 253–66.
43. Fazel M, Wheeler J, Danesh J. Prevalence of serious mental disorder in 7000 refugees resettled in western countries: a systematic review. Lancet. 2005;365(9467):1309–14. https://doi.org/10.1016/S0140-6736(05)61027-6.
44. Steel Z, Chey T, Silove D, Marnane C, Bryant RA, Van Ommeren M. Association of torture and other potentially traumatic events with mental health outcomes among populations exposed to mass conflict and displacement: a systematic review and meta-analysis. JAMA. 2009;302(5):537–49.
45. Kinzie JD. Refugees: stress in trauma. In: Fink G, editor. Stress: concepts, cognition, Emotion, and behavior: handbook of stress series: USA:Academic Press; 2016. p. 377–83.
46. Galatzer-Levy RM. Psychoanalysis, memory, and trauma. In: Appelbaum PS, Uyehara LA, Elin MR, editors. Trauma and memory: clinical and legal controversies. Oxford: Oxford University Press; 1997. p. 138–57.
47. Fridman A, Bakermans-Kranenburg MJ, Sagi-Schwartz A, Van IJzendoorn MH. Coping in old age with extreme childhood trauma: aging Holocaust survivors and their offspring facing new challenges. Aging Ment Health. 2011;15(2):232–42. https://doi.org/10.1080/13607863.2010.5 05232.
48. Lev-Wiesel R, Amir M. Growing out of ashes: posttraumatic growth among Holocaust child survivors–is it possible. In: Calhoun LG, Tedeschi RG, editors. Handbook of posttraumatic growth: research and practice. New York/London: Psychology press; 2006. p. 248–63.
49. Barel E, Van IJzendoorn MH, Sagi-Schwartz A, Bakermans-Kranenburg MJ. Surviving the Holocaust: a meta-analysis of the long-term sequelae of a genocide. Psychol Bull. 2010;136(5):677. http://doi.org.proxy3.library.mcgill.ca/10.1037/a0020339
50. Lev-Wiesel R, Amir M. Posttraumatic growth among Holocaust child survivors. J Loss Trauma. 2003;8(4):229–37. https://doi.org/10.1080/15325020305884.
51. Simich L, Beiser M. Immigrants and refugee mental health in Canada: lessons and prospects. In: Bhugra D, Susham G, editors. Migration and mental health. Cambridge, UK: Cambridge University Press; 2011. p. 323–36.
52. Agaibi CE, Wilson JP. Trauma, PTSD, and resilience: a review of the literature. Trauma Violence Abuse. 2005;6(3):195–216.
53. Berger R, Weiss T. The posttraumatic growth model: an expansion to the family system. Traumatology. 2009;15(1):63–74.
54. Alessi EJ, Kahn S, Chatterji S. 'The darkest times of my life': recollections of child abuse among forced migrants persecuted because of their sexual orientation and gender identity. Child Abuse Negl. 2016;51:93–105. https://doi.org/10.1016/j.chiabu.2015.10.030.
55. Denzin NK, Lincoln YS. Methods of collecting and analyzing empirical materials, narrative inquiry. In: Denzin NK, Lincoln YS, editors. The sage qualitative research. Thousand Oaks: Sage; 2005. p. 641–52.
56. Rosenthal G. Reconstruction of life stories: principles of selection in generating stories for narrative biographical interviews. Narrative Study Lives. 1993;1(1):59–91.
57. Merriam SB, Tisdell EJ. Qualitative research: a guide to design and implementation: Sun Francisco, CA: Wiley; 2015.
58. Lieblich A, Tuval-Mashiach R, Zilber T. Narrative research: reading, analysis, and interpretation: USA:Sage; 1998.
59. Resick PA, et al. A critical evaluation of the complex PTSD literature: implications for DSM-5. J Traumatic Stress. 2012;25(3):241–51.
60. Courtois CA. Complex trauma, complex reactions: assessment and treatment. J Psychother Theor Res Pract Train. 2008;41(4):412–25.
61. Cloitre M, Courtois CA, Ford JD, Green BL, Alexander P, Briere J, Van der Hart O. The ISTSS expert consensus treatment guidelines for complex PTSD in adults. Retrived from: https://istss.org/education-research/istss-research-guidelines; 2012.

Anti-Semitism in Cults and Hate Groups

23

Steven Hassan and Jon Caven-Atack

> *I know but one freedom, and that is freedom of the mind.*
> *—Antoine de Saint-Exupéry*

Anti-Semitism

Before anti-Semitism can be defined, readers must understand that the definition of who is a Jew is in itself complicated [1]. Judaism is a religion, but Jewish identity is not necessarily defined by religious belief [2]. According to a 2012 Gallup poll, "Only 38 percent of the Jewish population worldwide considers itself religious, while 54 [percent] sees itself as non-religious and 2 percent categorizes itself as atheist."[1] While Jews, as a group, consider themselves as descendants of the twelve tribes of Israel, there have, of course, been many marriages and conversions along the course of history. Jews share many cultural traditions and foods and rituals, but these vary according to geography and religious practice. Elias Canneti put it this way: "No people is more difficult to understand than the Jews … Jews are different from other people, but, in reality, they are most different from each other" [3]. Since the creation of Israel, in 1948, many Jews around the world – though far from all – identify with a political belief in its continued existence as a Jewish state. This is

---

[1] New Poll Suggests Atheism on Rise With Jews Found to be Least Religious. Haaretz, August 20, 2012.

S. Hassan (✉)
The Program in Psychiatry and the Law. Massachusetts Mental Health Center, a teaching hospital of Harvard Medical School, Boston, MA, USA
e-mail: hassan@freedomofmind.com

J. Caven-Atack
Independent Scholar, Nottingham, UK
e-mail: joncatack@gmail.com

© Springer Nature Switzerland AG 2020
H. S. Moffic et al. (eds.), *Anti-Semitism and Psychiatry*,
https://doi.org/10.1007/978-3-030-37745-8_23

generally known as Zionism. Many Jews and non-Jews are Zionists.[2] Essentially, Jews are people who privately or publicly identify themselves as Jews or who are so-labelled by others. To hate Jews is to hate people who are perceived as somehow "other" than oneself, who are not to be trusted, and who deserve to be shunned, mocked, and disgraced [4].

The persecution of the Jews has a long history. Probably the most influential propaganda text in modern anti-Semitism is *The Protocols of the Elders of Zion*.[3] Historian Norman Cohn shows that the *Protocols* is a revision of a critique of Napoleon III, *The Dialogue in Hell Between Machiavelli and Montesquieu* [5], of 1864 – more than 25 years before Nathan Birnbaum first used the term Zionism ("the return to Jerusalem") [2]. The revision was made by the Russian secret police (the Okhrana), to undermine anti-Tsarist groups and to justify pogroms. As Cohn remarks, "there is a cruel irony in the fact that a brilliant but long-forgotten defense of liberalism should have provided the basis for an atrociously written piece of reactionary balderdash which has swept the world."

The spurious *Protocols* was adopted by the Nazis to justify the systematic extermination of the Jews in the Shoah or Holocaust. Credulous people the world over have used this crass forgery to justify hatred of all who identify themselves as Jews. As Hitler said, "The very enormity of a lie contributes to its success ... The masses of the people easily succumb to it, as they cannot believe it possible that anyone should have the shameless audacity to invent such things ... Even if the clearest proof of its falsehood is forthcoming, something of the lie will nevertheless stick."[4]

At the extreme, contemporary anti-Semites believe in a grand conspiracy which unites all those who identify as Jews as part of the Zionist Occupation Government or ZOG.[5] These ideas were spread in the novel *The Turner Diaries*, written by neo-Nazi William Luther Pierce [7]. The novel was a key inspiration for Timothy McVeigh who, along with Terry Nichols, murdered 168 people in the bomb attack in Oklahoma City in 1995.[6] As Voltaire said, "Those who can make you believe absurdities, can make you commit atrocities."[7]

A plethora of anti-Semitic and white supremacist groups continues to spread. The United States has witnessed the rise of not only the KKK [8] but also the Aryan Nations, Identity Christians, Stormfront, Hammerskin Nation, White Aryan Resistance, the Freemen, and the Council of Conservative Citizens [9]. The Identity Evropa group has been rebranded as the American Identity Movement.[8]

---

[2] Herzl, *Judenstaat*, 1894, cited in Tuchman.

[3] https://www.britannica.com/topic/Protocols-of-the-Elders-of-Zion

[4] Hitler, A. *Mein Kampf*, cited by Louis Golding [6].

[5] ZOG https://www.adl.org/education/references/hate-symbols/zog

[6] Oklahoma City Bombing Fast Facts April 8, 2019 CNN Library. https://www.cnn.com/2013/09/18/us/oklahoma-city-bombing-fast-facts/index.html

[7] Voltaire, *Questions sur les miracles*.

[8] https://www.splcenter.org/fighting-hate/extremist-files/group/identity-evropa

These groups have created an Internet presence that has spread division and hatred. Their disinformation campaigns have been instrumental in instigating terrorist attacks upon Jews. The situation has been made far more dangerous through the concept of "leaderless resistance," first introduced, as a proposed guerilla response to a Communist takeover of the United States, by Colonel Ulius Louis Amoss shortly before his death in 1961.[9] The idea was promoted by former Klansman Louis Beam in a 1983 essay.[10] Leaderless resistance urges the formation of "phantom cells" as small as a single person that commit terrorist acts.

In 2015, Dylann Storm Roof was convicted of the murder of nine African-Americans during a service at the Emanuel African Methodist Episcopal Church in Charleston. He was hoping to ignite a race war that would overthrow the Jewish domination of American society (through "the Jewish agitation of the black race").[11] In his manifesto, *The Last Rhodesian*, Roof insisted that it was necessary to "destroy the jewish [sic] identity." He says, "If we could somehow turn every jew [sic] blue for 24 hours, I think there would be a mass awakening because people would be able to see plainly what is going on." Roof was greatly influenced by the website of the Council of Conservative Citizens, an openly anti-Semitic forum, where we are told, for instance, "Martin Luther King was personally directed and controlled by a Jewish U.S. Communist Party leader" [11].

Among the worst of many anti-Semitic attacks in the United States were the synagogue murders at Chabad of Poway, in San Diego in April 2019 [12], and the Tree of Life, in Pittsburgh in October 2018 [13]. There have been many other attacks on Jews in the United States [14]. The echo chamber of the World Wide Web has seen an increase in racist, Islamophobic, and anti-Semitic attacks, based upon disinformation and incitement to violence. In May 2019, Nolan Brewer was sentenced to 3 years in prison for defacing the Congregation Shaarey Tefilla in Carmel, Indiana, with swastikas. His lawyer claimed that he was influenced by Stormfront, a neo-Nazi website [15]. Brewer does not appear to have had any contact with other neo-Nazis except online.

The echo chamber of the web can influence individuals to become thoroughly indoctrinated by spending countless hours exposed online. These fringe actors seem to adopt for themselves the characteristics of the BITE model spending long hours sleep deprived, isolated in their rooms, watching radicalization videos, and interacting in secretive chat rooms.

The BITE Model

To explain mind control and destructive cult behavior in general, Hassan [16] has added to Festinger's tripartite theory of cognitive dissonance [17] the element of control of information. Hassan argues that if you regulate the supply of information,

---

[9] Kaplan [10]. Louis Beam published in the Seditionist #February 12, 1992, written in 1983.

[10] Beam, Louis. The Seditionist, issue 12, February 1992.

[11] Roof, *The Last Rhodesian*, published online.

you manipulate a person's experience and restrict the ability for self-determination. Four components of mind control – behavior, information, thought, and emotion – form the BITE model of mind control that all destructive cults use to control their members (see Fig. 23.1).

Cult organizations distinguish themselves from normal, healthy social groups by subjecting members to systematic control of behavior, information, thought, and emotion to keep them dependent and obedient. The BITE model of mind control describes an extensive list of strategies included in the four components. These include deceptive recruitment, control of sleep, control of time, loaded language, thought-stopping techniques, and many other variables to induce phobia indoctrination. More recently, Daesh has been reported to use drugs like Captagon in their control of its members.[12]

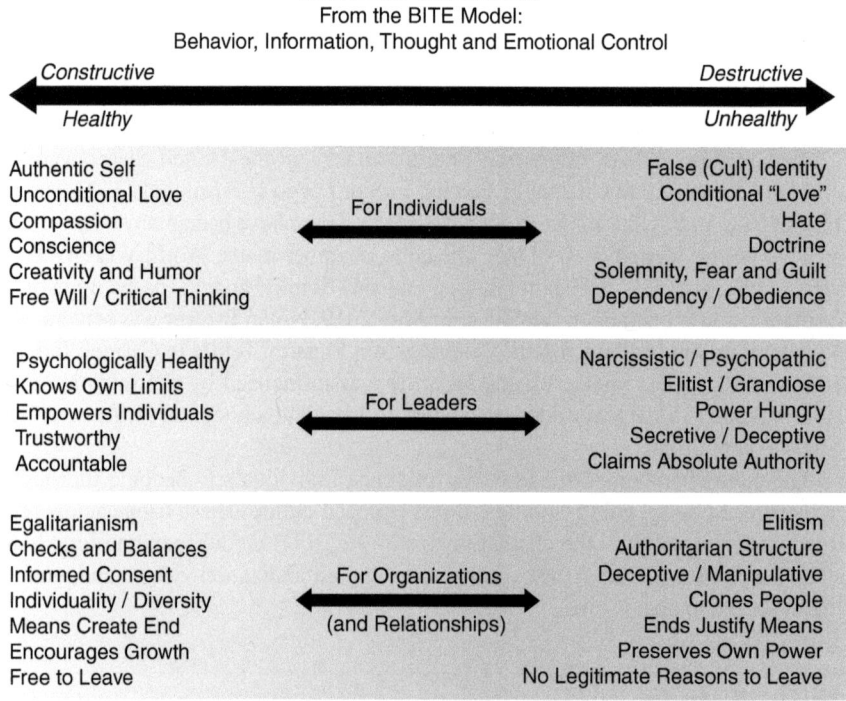

Fig. 23.1 The BITE model influence continuum. (Used with permission from Hassan [16])

---

[12]$1.4 M ISIS cache of "jihadists drug" seized, U.S. says June 18, 2018 CBS News.

Mind Control and the Mental Health Profession

The fifth edition of the *Diagnostic and Statistical Manual of Mental Disorders* (DSM-5), a classification of mental disorders compiled and published under the auspices of the American Psychiatric Association, defines Other Specified Dissociative Disorder 300.15 as an: *Identity disturbance due to prolonged and intense coercive persuasion: Individuals who have been subjected to intense coercive persuasion (i.e. brainwashing, thought reform, indoctrination while captive, torture, long-term political imprisonment, recruitment by sects/cults or by terror organizations) may present with prolonged changes in, or conscious questioning of, their identity.*[13]

Mental health practitioners and therapists, however, are largely unaware that mind control meets the diagnostic criteria of a psychiatric disorder and are not familiar with the specialized approaches that have been pioneered and developed to treat it. The dual identity model of mind control offers an important conceptual tool which is significant when interacting with cult members[14] (see Fig. 23.2).

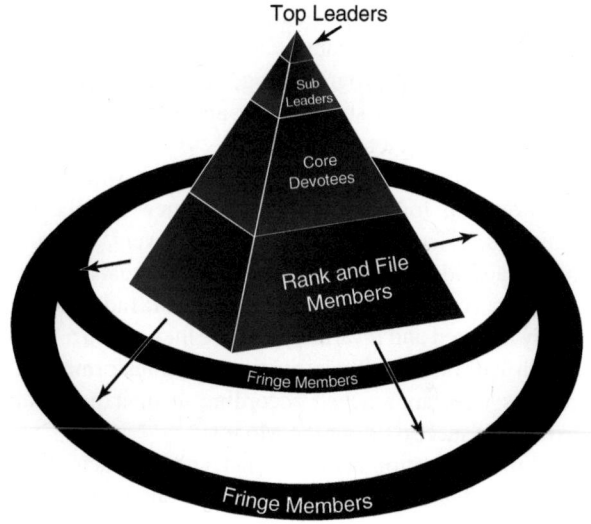

Fig. 23.2 Destructive cult structure. (Used with permission from Hassan, S. Combating Cult Mind Control)

---

[13] https://dsm.psychiatryonline.org/doi/book/10.1176/appi.books.9781585629992

[14] Erich Fromm coined the term "pseudo-self" in Escape from Freedom, 1941, reprinted by Ishi Press, NY, and Tokyo, 2011. The term "pseudo-identity" was used by Louis Jolyon West and Paul Martin [18].

Recruitment into Anti-Semitism

There are many ways that people can be recruited to join a group. All cults prefer recruits who are intelligent, talented, and successful. As a result, members are often powerfully persuasive and seductive to newcomers. The convinced and steadfast members whom a newcomer meets may be as convincing as the actual doctrine or ideology of the cult itself.[15]

One of the authors of this chapter (SH) was recruited into Sun Myung Moon's Unification Church (the "Moonies") at the age of 19, while a student at Queens College. He spent the next 27 months recruiting and indoctrinating new members, fundraising, and organizing political campaigns. He ultimately rose to the rank of Assistant Director of the Unification Church at its U.S. headquarters. Following a serious automobile accident, he was deprogrammed by former Moonies. He did not understand that the group was anti-Semitic until after he exited and reflected on Rabbi James Rudin's critique on what he was actually taught to believe [19].

In 1999, Steven Hassan started the Freedom of Mind Resource Center, Inc. – freedomofmind.com – a consulting, counseling, and publishing organization dedicated to upholding human rights, promoting consumer awareness, and exposing the abuses of undue influence, mind control, and destructive cults. He pioneered an approach called the Strategic Interactive Approach (SIA) to help victims of mind control. Unlike "deprogramming," this is a noncoercive approach that shows family and friends how to strategically and ethically influence someone who has been influenced to join a hate group.

As a recruiter for the Moonies, Hassan was taught to use a personality model comprised of four "gates" to recruit new members. People were categorized as "thinkers," "feelers," "doers," or "believers." Thinkers approach life with their minds and identify themselves as intellectuals, feelers are led by their emotions, doers are action-oriented and fixed on "bravado and brawn," and believers are spiritually oriented and invariably believe they are on a "holy mission" for a noble cause, which will often be social justice and transformation. Once categorized, potential recruits were approached according to their personality, and this method proved extremely successful for the Moonies.

With the creation of the Internet, and the reach of social media, online destructive cult recruitment has largely replaced one-on-one recruitment. Hundreds of front groups can be created such as matchmaking websites or blogs that attract lonely, dissatisfied individuals. Potential recruits can be "love-bombed" – or flattered – online and then contacted by members of the cult. Potential recruits are told to be careful not to tell anyone about secret insider activities. Movies, video games, books, and Hollywood-style videos are used to attract and indoctrinate. Personal information about recruits is often easily accessible on the dark web to help

---

[15] Cults use celebrity members in their promotion – Madonna for Kabbalah Centre, Tina Turner for Nichiren Shoshu, and a raft of celebrities including Tom Cruise and John Travolta for Scientology.

manipulate and blackmail specific targets. Members can be kept awake all night watching their computer screens (thus rendering them more vulnerable to mind control) via discussion boards and endless videos.

It is interesting to note that it appears there is a greater percentage of Jews involved in cults compared with their representation in society [20]. Groups that include ideologies that are anti-Semitic in that they either propose that Jews killed Christ or that they are not fully legitimate and theologically intact have successfully recruited Jewish people. Some cults go so far as to justify the Holocaust, as the Moon cult did. Recruitment is done deceptively, and members who are Jewish usually do not learn of the anti-Semitic beliefs until they are deeply embedded in the cult. Contrary to a popular assumption, Jews in anti-Semitic cults are not self-hating, nor are they angry at their religion of birth. What makes Jews more susceptible to the appeals of these groups? One theory that makes sense is being raised in the belief of "Tikkun Olam," or the "repair of the world," that Jews are obligated to make the world better than it was before they entered into it. Jews are also raised to be life learners and be open to new ideas and perspectives. This makes them more vulnerable to cult recruiters.

Differences Between Ethical and Unethical Social Influence

Constructive, healthy influence empowers a person to maintain an internal "locus of control" concerning their personal, authentic identity, which includes their conscience, creativity, volition, and ability to make independent decisions. Access to a wide range of information and the freedom to critically evaluate it is fundamental.

Destructive, unhealthy influence involves engendering an external "locus of control" and a cult pseudo-identity which makes a person dependent and obedient to the leader or the cause. Undue influence is used in many ways to program and control the person to become a "clone" of all other members and to succumb to group think. Both authors have written significant volumes that describe the social influence phenomenon [16, 21].

Lifton and Festinger

Robert Jay Lifton is regarded by many as the foremost authority on mind control and thought reform. As a psychiatrist with the US Air Force during the early 1950s, he interviewed American servicemen who were prisoners of war (POWs) during the Korean War, as well as priests, students, and teachers who had been held captive in "reeducation" camps in China. Lifton also interviewed Chinese students who had been subjected to indoctrination in Chinese universities. He published his findings in the 1961 book *Thought Reform and the Psychology of Totalism: A Study of "Brainwashing" in China* [22], where he described his Eight Criteria of Thought Reform and the coercive techniques used in the People's Republic of China's "reeducation" program that he labelled "thought reform" (*szu-hsiang kai-tsao*) or, acknowledging the popular media term, "brainwashing" [22]. In 1999, Lifton applied his model of thought reform to the Aum Shinrikyo cult in *Destroying the World to Save It* [23]. Contemporary China has reeducation camps influencing over one million people.[16]

Lifton's Eight Criteria are milieu control, mystical manipulation, demand for purity, the cult of confession, sacred science, loading the language, ideology over experience, and dispensing of existence. Through the demand for purity, believers become "isolated and engulfed" [24] by the dogma. They adopt the loaded language of the group – so, Jews have been dismissed as "subhuman" or "vermin" – and conform their behavior, their thoughts, and their emotions to the mores of the group they have joined. Even when it is an online or virtual group, it will also limit their information. Anything that disagrees with the dogma will be dismissed through natural confirmation bias to avoid the cognitive dissonance of disagreement with strongly held beliefs.

Hassan's Strategic Interactive Approach relies on these as well as Festinger's theory of cognitive dissonance. Festinger argued that the three principal components of cognitive dissonance are *control of behavior, control of thoughts*, and *control of emotions*. In 1950, Festinger summarized his basic principle as follows: *If you change a person's behavior, his thoughts and feelings will change to minimize the dissonance*. In other words, if any one of the three components change, the other two will shift to reduce dissonance [17].

Cognitive dissonance theory helps to explain heightened commitment to a cause. According to Festinger, people need to maintain order and meaning in their life. We have to believe we are acting according to our self-image and following our own values. If our behavior changes for any reason, our self-image and values realign to reduce dissonance. It is crucial to recognize that authoritarian cult groups deliberately create dissonance and exploit it to control their followers. Government agencies and the mental health community have generally underestimated how psychologically astute destructive cult organizations can be.

The Experience of Ex-Anti-Semites

The experience of ex-anti-Semites is informative. Derek Black grew up in the Ku Klux Klan. His father was a Grand Wizard in the Klan. As a child, Derek created the website Kids' Stormfront. As Derek Black has said, "The fundamental belief that drove … my family, over decades, was that race was the defining feature of humanity … and that people were only happy if they could live in a society that was only this one biologically defined group" [25]. Derek was isolated from the wider community through home-schooling but later enrolled at New College of Florida where

---

[16]Farooq, Umar. China Has Detained a Million Muslims in Reeducation Camps. The repression picked up dramatically in 2016, after a top party official who had put down unrest in Tibet was sent to Xinjiang. The Nation November 27, 2018.

he first met Jewish students. These new friends invited him to a Shabbat dinner and, after a few visits, his childhood conditioning broke down. At the age of 22, he renounced white nationalism [26]. His story was reported by Eli Saslow in the book *Rising Out of Hatred* [27].

Arno Michaelis was the lead singer with the "hate-metal" band Centurion and led an international skinhead, racist organization. A chance encounter with a server at a McDonald's changed his perception of the world. As he says:

> I had managed to convince myself that white people were superior to everyone else and that there was a worldwide Jewish conspiracy to wipe us out. I was terrified of the world around me and confused enough to call that feeling of terror 'courage' … The many people who crossed the street rather than pass me on the sidewalk were wise to do so. But that first time I walked into the McDonald's where you worked, I was met with your smile, as warm and unconditional as the sun.

At his third visit, the server asked him about the swastika tattooed on his finger. She said, "You're a better person than that. I know that's not who you are." He ran from her and got drunk listening to blaring white power music with his white power friends. It took another 7 years for the seed of that conversation to grow. Along with Pardeep Singh Kaleka, Arno now runs Serve2Unite[17] and has published an autobiography, *My Life After Hate* [28]. The two of them later published a book together, *The Gift of Our Wounds* [29].

Recommendations

Combating destructive mind control requires a holistic, complex systems approach involving policymakers, health and social care providers, faith leaders, and educational providers.[18] "Inoculation" programs (facilitated by former members of destructive cults) in workshops and online can protect people from being infected by mind control by teaching them about the techniques that destructive cult organizations use. Such programs apply to all hate groups.

Former members of destructive cults and hate groups who have received specialized counseling and training are uniquely suited to share their stories of indoctrination with others and should feature prominently in inoculation programs.

An educational program that trains mental health practitioners, religious leaders, and educational providers to identify what makes people vulnerable to undue influence should be implemented.

The media have an important role to play in combating mind control. They should not only report the sensational aspects of the former members' experiences but must also show how cult mind control is perpetrated.

---

[17] https://www.giftofourwounds.com/serve2unite

[18] The Ninth International Conference on Complex Systems 2018 Sponsored by NECSI. https://freedomofmind.com/the-ninth-international-conference-on-complex-systems-2018-sponsored-by-necsi/. July 16, 2018.

Online activism must be put in place to counter the cult recruitment process by engaging recruiters and exposing the flaws and weaknesses of their beliefs and actions.

Many former members of destructive cults are misdiagnosed by mental health professionals who prescribe psychotropic medications that fail to address the underlying difficulties. Mental health professionals need specialized training so that they can formulate approaches that take into consideration not only the upbringing of their patients but also the psychosocial and political influences exerted on them.

Conclusion

Well-funded anti-Semitic groups are aggressively looking for ways to ensnare and indoctrinate new believers. Disaffected youth, some traumatized veterans, and people who have been subjected to unfair treatment are especially vulnerable to recruitment into hate groups. The political actions of both the American and Israeli governments since the Trump presidency have generated a great deal of anger and resentment toward Jews worldwide. The Internet has become a breeding ground for extremist hatred, and it encourages "leaderless resistance," a form of lone terrorism that is almost impossible for law enforcement to detect. As citizens, we all need to be more aware of the signs of developing extremism.

Mental health professionals need to understand the social influences and psychological determinants of violent extremism and the unethical techniques that cult and terrorist organizations use to recruit people to join their ranks.

If we are to truly counter violent extremism, politicians, faith leaders, educational providers, and mental health practitioners must make a sustained and concerted effort to raise awareness of the powerful effects of undue influence and mind control and organize and commission events and workshops in schools, mosques, churches, synagogues, and at primary and secondary health and social care settings, as well as online programs. Short accessible videos showing the basic methods of recruitment and the characteristics of predatory people and their agents are needed. Both authors have produced books, articles, as well as videos and placed them online to help explain the psychology of due and undue influence [21, 30]. As the methods of mind control are better understood, we will see a decline in extremist violence [31]. As separate ethnic groups share their beliefs and customs with others, we will see a diminution in hatred of outsiders and, eventually, a healthier and more cooperative society.

References

1. Kertzer MN. What is a Jew? New York, NY: Touchstone; 1953, 1960, 1996.
2. Sand S. The invention of the Jewish people, London/New York: Verso; 2009.
3. Canetti E. Crowds and power. New York: Gollancz; 1962.
4. Tuchman B. The bible and the sword. NY: Ballantine; 1956, 1984.
5. Joly M. Dialogue Aux Enfers Montesquieu et Machiavelli. Bruxelles: Tous les libraires; 1864.

6. Golding L. The Jewish problem. Harmondsworth: Penguin; 1938.
7. Berger JM. Alt history: how a self-published, racist novel changed white nationalism and inspired decades of violence. The Atlantic; September 16, 2016. https://www.theatlantic.com/politics/archive/2016/09/how-the-turner-diaries-changed-white-nationalism/500039/.
8. Clark A. How "Birth of a Nation". Revived the Ku Klux Klan. https://www.history.com/news/kkk-birth-of-a-nation-film.
9. Serwer A. White nationalism's deep American roots. April 2019. https://www.theatlantic.com/magazine/archive/2019/04/adam-serwer-madison-grant-white-nationalism/583258/.
10. Kaplan J. Leaderless resistance. Terror Polit Violence. 1997;9(3):80–95. https://doi.org/10.1080/09546559708427417.
11. Council of Conservative Citizens. Martin Luther King: FBI Reveals Jewish Communist Controller, Sex Scandals, November 2017. http://cofcc.us/.
12. Miller S. When Houses of Worship Become Targets of Hate. USA Today, April 28, 2019.
13. Londberg M. Pittsburgh Synagogue Attack Worst in US History. USA Today, October 27, 2018.
14. Fattal I. A Brief History of Anti-Semitic Violence in America. The Atlantic, October 28, 2018.
15. Mettler K. A Nazi sympathizer pleaded guilty to defacing a synagogue. His lawyer says conservatives helped radicalize him. Washington Post, May 28, 2019.
16. Hassan S. Combating cult mind control: the #1 bests-selling guide to protection, rescue and recovery from destructive cults. Newton, MA: Freedom of Mind Press; 2015. (first edition 1988).
17. Festinger L, Riecken HW, Schacter S. When prophecy fails: University of Minnesota Press; 1956.
18. West LJ, Martin P. Pseudo-identity and the treatment of personality change in victims of captivity and cults. In: Lynn SJ, Rhue JW, editors. Dissociation: clinical and theoretical perspectives. New York\London: Guilford Press; 1994.
19. Rudin AJ. Jews and Judaism in Rev. Moon's Divine Principle: A Report. http://www.ajcarchives.org/AJC_DATA/Files/7A35.PDF.
20. Clendinen D. Jews Act to Stop Young from Defecting to Cults. November 22, 1981 NY Times. https://www.nytimes.com/1981/11/22/us/jews-act-to-stop-young-from-defecting-to-cults.html.
21. Atack J. Opening minds: the secret world of manipulation, undue influence and brainwashing. Colchester: Trentvalley Ltd.; 2015. 2018
22. Lifton RJ. Thought reform and the psychology of totalism. New York: Norton; 1961.
23. Lifton RJ. Destroying the world to save it: Aum Shinrikyo, apocalyptic violence, and the new global terrorism. New York: Henry Holt; 2000.
24. Stein A. Terror, love and brainwashing: attachment in cults and totalist systems. London: Routledge; 2017.
25. Fresh Air, NPR. How a rising star of the white nationalism broke free from the movement, September 24, 2018.
26. Enzinna W. Renouncing hate: what happens when a white nationalist repents. September 10, 2018. https://www.nytimes.com/2018/09/10/books/review/eli-saslow-rising-out-of-hatred.html.
27. Saslow E. Rising out of hatred: the awakening of a former white nationalist. New York: Doubleday; 2018.
28. Michaelis A. My life after hate. Milwaukee, WI: Authentic Presence Publications; 2012.
29. Kaleka P, Michaelis A, Fisher RG. The gift of our wounds: a sikh and a former white supremacist find forgiveness after hate. Milwaukee, WI: Authentic Presence Publications; 2012.
30. Hassan S. Freedom of mind: helping loved ones leave controlling people, cults and beliefs. MA: Freedom of Mind Press Newton; 2012.
31. Hassan S. The cult of Trump: a leading cult expert explains how the president uses mind control. New York: Simon and Schuster; 2019.

Harnessing the Power of Film and Storytelling to Challenge Anti-Semitism

24

Ahmed Hankir

Introduction

> Life is indeed darkness save when there is urge, and all urge is blind save when there is knowledge, and all knowledge is vain save when there is work, and all work is empty save when there is love. (Khalil Gibran)

I vividly remember reciting the above lines from the twentieth-century Lebanese mystic Khalil Gibran's poignant poem at the inaugural World Psychiatry Association – Transcultural Psychiatry in Mediterranean Countries Conference in Tel Aviv in 2012. I continue to think that this was an extraordinary feat; a Lebanese man reciting Lebanese poetry to a largely Israeli audience in the capital of a country that was and remains officially at war with Lebanon. Perhaps that in and of itself is a remarkable achievement that indicates at least some progress, no matter how seemingly small or trivial, had been made in promoting peaceful co-existence between the two warring nations? This chapter will provide background information about how I got to that junction in my life and where I went from there. It will also discuss and describe how we can harness the power of film both as a therapeutic instrument to heal psychological wounds and as a tool to challenge anti-Semitism.

Operation Peace for Galilee

Identity can be a difficult issue to describe. "Where are you from?" is a question that I am often asked. It is a question that evokes a degree of consternation in fact for it isn't really so straightforward to answer. Does where I'm from mean where I was born? Or does it mean what passport I bear? Or is the interrogator alluding to my

A. Hankir (✉)
South London and Maudsley NHS Foundation Trust, London, UK
e-mail: ahmed.hankir@slam.nhs.uk

© Springer Nature Switzerland AG 2020
H. S. Moffic et al. (eds.), *Anti-Semitism and Psychiatry*,
https://doi.org/10.1007/978-3-030-37745-8_24

307

ethnicity (which invariably tends to be the case)? To try to appease all those concerned, my spiel is something along the lines of, "I was born in Ireland, lived most of my life in England and I am of Lebanese descent". But the concept of identity is seldom that simple. What role does religion play in all of this? And how about the language that one speaks? The platforms are indeed many and the layers multiple.

After qualifying from Cairo medical school in the early 1980s, my father decided to migrate to Belfast where I was born. A major factor that contributed to his decision was the 1982 Lebanon War also known as, "Operation Peace for Galilee". This was a brutal and bloody war that involved the Multinational Forces (MNF) which included American troops. It was in Operation Peace for Galilee that more than 200 US Marines were killed from a suicide bomber, viewed at the time as one of America's largest losses outside of the Vietnam War.

The infamous Sabra and Shatila massacre also took place during the 1982 Lebanon War. Up to 3500 people perished during the massacre, mostly Palestinian and Lebanese Shiites. Memories of those dark days have not faded and indeed continue to influence the collective consciousness of all those who were involved: the Palestinians, Lebanese and Israelis (this will be discussed later in this book chapter). I do not want to delve too deeply into the 1982 Lebanon War. Suffice to say that the point I wanted to illustrate was how war can profoundly shape a person's life and trajectory even before he or she is born.

Before leaving Lebanon, my parents witnessed the destruction and collapse of their country and the devastating loss of human life. Although as a child I myself was not physically in Lebanon during the war in the 1980s, I still "felt" the effects. Karam et al. published a paper entitled, "Major depression and external stressors: the Lebanon Wars" in the European Archives of Psychiatry and Clinical Neuroscience. They examined the effect of war events and pre-war depression on the prevalence of major depression during war in Lebanon and revealed that individual levels of exposure to this type of conflict and a history of pre-war depression predict the development of depression during war [1]. Many of my mother's family and friends were killed in the 1982 Lebanon War, and this was deeply distressing and depressing for her. My mother's depression influenced my upbringing and cast a melancholic hue on my childhood memories. It is important for psychiatrists to be mindful of this when assessing and treating patients whose parents migrated from conflict zones and the manner in which the trauma of war can be transmitted from one generation to the next.

There Is No Place Like Home

We moved to England from Ireland in 1990 where my father started work as an obstetrician. Although we had a good quality of life in England and there was stability and security, my parents were starting to miss home. So, in 1995, we relocated to Lebanon. This was a huge turning point in my life; psychosocial stressors such as the language barrier (I was unable to converse in Arabic at the time) and adjusting to a culture that was seemingly alien to the one that I was raised in placed a tremendous amount of strain and stress on my mental health. Indeed, Potochnick and colleagues revealed how migration was associated with an increased risk of developing common mental disorders among migrant youth aged between 12 and 19 years. Using logistic regression, they evaluated how migration stressors (i.e., traumatic events, choice of migration, discrimination) and migration supports (i.e. family and teacher support, acculturation and personal motivation) were associated with depressive symptoms and anxiety [2]. Migration aside, it seemed that the odds of developing mental health difficulties were already stacked against me; according to the World Health Organization, half of all mental illnesses begin by the age of 14, and neuropsychiatric conditions are the leading cause of disability in young people in all regions [3].

Returning to Greener Pastures

Living in Lebanon in the 1990s during the aftermath of the civil war was not easy; there were many households that did not have 24-hour electricity, and there was only one road connecting Beirut to the South of Lebanon which is where we were residing. Since prospects were not looking favourable, my parents felt that it would be best for me to return to the UK after I finished high school. So, on the tenth of July 2000 at 17 years of age, I bade farewell to my family in Rafic Hariri Beirut International Airport and boarded a plane to England. Upon arriving on British shores, I had to find work fast since I had very few resources at my disposal. The first job I could secure was working in a van in Malvern Hills selling burgers and kebabs for a living. I remember customers asking me if I could speak English, and my dream of qualifying as a doctor seemed very distant if not far-fetched. However, I was determined to enter medical school no matter how hard I had to try and no matter how long it would take me. I worked 70 hours per week stacking shelves as a stock advisor in a supermarket by day and cleaning floors as a janitor at night. Indeed, the callouses on my hands were testaments of my toil. I did this for a year and saved up enough money to enroll into a school that would enable me to take the exams to enter medical school. I continued to work full-time whilst preparing for the pre-med exams, and this was a constant threat to obtaining the necessary grades, but thankfully, by the grace of God, after 2 years of hard work and sacrifice, I secured a place in Manchester medical school. My dream of qualifying as a doctor was starting to become true.

Medical School and the 2006 Lebanon War

I matriculated into Manchester medical school in 2003. When I was a third-year medical student in 2006, I woke up one morning to discover that my hometown in Lebanon had been bombed by Israeli warplanes and that hundreds of people were killed overnight, many of whom were civilian. I feared that my family were among the dead and I reacted to the onslaught; I developed a debilitating episode of psychological distress, which derailed me completely [4]. I was forced to interrupt my studies, and, with my student loan severed, I was rendered impoverished and homeless. In my despair, I contemplated suicide; however, I resisted the urge to act upon these thoughts since suicide is forbidden in Islam [5].

During medical school I forged a very close friendship with a Jewish student. This student welcomed me to his home; he and his family provided me with care and comfort when I was at my most vulnerable. I look back at those days and I am utterly astonished by how compassionate and altruistic this family was towards me. Indeed, if it were not for this Jewish family, I would never have resumed my medical training and I wouldn't be composing this chapter as a doctor. I will forever remember the kindness that this Jewish family showed me. I can only pray that one day I will be as generous and compassionate to those who are less fortunate as this Jewish family were to me. God bless them always.

As a medical student with mental illness, I did not find the thought of taking psychiatric drugs (or "chemical cosh" as it is referred to by members of the anti-psychiatry community) too appealing. What I did gravitate towards, however, was the power of film, literature and poetry [6]. I remember how deeply therapeutic and profoundly cathartic it was for me to watch movies at the cinema (I was utterly captivated and blown away, for example, by the 2005 dystopian political thriller film V for Vendetta as I felt I could identify with the protagonist's determination to achieve his goal), read novels (mostly fiction of the magical realism variety from Gabriel Garcia Marquez) and recite verses conceived by Dylan Thomas and Rudyard Kipling (who, interestingly, both allegedly suffered from a major mood disorder as I did). Moreover, there were no "adverse effects" associated with these activities. I therefore developed an intense interest in how we can leverage the power of film to heal psychological wounds, but I did not want to limit film's potential there. Perhaps, I would muse to myself, we could also harness film's power to address societal ills?

The Colossal Power of Film

> If you really want to understand a man you have to slip into his shoes and walk around in them…. (Atticus Finch, *To Kill a Mockingbird*)

Each of us has our own favourite line or scene from a film that has deeply moved us in one way or another. Indeed, cinema possesses extraordinary power. Through the journey of a single film, we can take a roller coaster ride across the spectrum of human emotion. Film can enthral an entire auditorium heaving with people, or it can silence and even reduce them to tears. Movies can also provide viewers with a precious qualitative insight into the minds of people with mental illness so that we may, *Slip into their shoes and walk around in them.* By virtue of cinema, we can learn more about what mental illness is like from the inside and this, in turn, can help us to have a better understanding of what it is like to have a psychiatric disorder, be that the narrowing of repertoire in autism as poignantly depicted by Oscar winning actor Dustin Hoffman in Peter Guber's production *Rain Man* [7] or the insidious and devastating fragmentation of memory caused by dementia as masterfully portrayed by Oscar winning actress Meryl Streep in *The Iron Lady* [8].

Films are extremely popular across the different cultures. India is the country that produces the largest number of films every year. In 2009 alone the Hindi film industry Bollywood produced a staggering 1288 Indian feature films [9]. The USA, Hong Kong and Nigeria are examples of other regions where film industries are booming.

One could argue that as long as human beings continue to seek entertainment and escapism for, as the twentieth-century Noble Laureate T.S. Elliot said, *mankind cannot bear very much reality* – cinema will remain deeply embedded in our societies. The storylines of films are influenced by the societies we live in. Given that one in four of us has a mental illness at some point in our lives [10], mental illness and the psychiatrists who treat these illnesses play huge roles in our societies and on our screens.

In view of the above, the former president of the World Psychiatric Association, Professor Dinesh Bhugra, examined Bollywood films produced since the early 1960s as a means to analyse the changes in Indian society's attitudes towards mental health issues [11]. Bhugra's analyses revealed how in post-colonial India in the 1950s and 1960s there were many films featuring people with mental illness who were subjected to ridicule, but there were also some films with sympathetic portrayals of sufferers of mental illness. In the 1970s and 1980s when the country was going through major economic, social and political upheavals, there were films that portrayed psychopaths who couldn't rely on the system to provide for the vulnerable so they became vigilantes who took the law into their own hands. The image of those suffering from mental illness transformed in the 1990s when there were many motion pictures that portrayed the theme of morbid jealousy. These films typically involved men who were trying to control women and who viewed them as a kind of commodity. This period overlapped with the economic liberalization taking place in India at the time, which gave people the power and freedom to own property and other objects. Many men extended this to include women (i.e. they viewed the socio-political changes in India at the time as a means to justify the "objectification" of women) and viewed them as property that they could (and should) rightfully own [11].

The Royal College of Psychiatrist's Initiatives to Use Film to Improve Public Understanding of Psychiatry and Drive Recruitment into the Profession

The Royal College of Psychiatrists created a section on its website on psychiatry and film entitled, "Minds on Film". According to the website, "'Minds on Film'" is a monthly blog that explores psychiatric conditions and mental health issues as portrayed in a selection of readily available films" [12]. The founder of "Minds on Film," Dr. Joyce Almeida, a consultant psychiatrist, reviews movies with a psychiatric theme. She has reviewed the motion picture, Aviator, a biographical film about the American billionaire, Howard Hughes, that presents a thoroughly well-researched and accurate portrait of the development of his obsessive compulsive disorder (OCD) – the director Martin Scorsese actually consulted an OCD specialist in order to ensure the veracity of the portrayal of the protagonist's psychopathology and make certain that the representation of this psychiatric condition was as realistic and accurate as possible [13]. She also reviewed The Diving Bell and the Butterfly, which narrates the true life story of *Elle* magazine editor in chief, Jean-Dominique Bauby, who suffered a brain stem cerebrovascular accident and consequently developed locked-in syndrome. Each review consists of an introduction, a brief description of the film, and discusses the relevance that the film has to the field of mental health [14].

The Royal College of Psychiatrists also helped to found the UK's first ever medical film festival, "MedFest". The purpose of MedFest is to explore the relationship between medicine and cinema and, in doing so, to challenge preconceptions people hold about psychiatry and psychiatrists. The aim of the 2012 festival was, "To stimulate debate of the social, political and ethical implications of portrayals of health and illness on our screens" [15].

Film as a Therapeutic Tool

Film had been increasingly recognized as a therapeutic tool to treat mental illness, and the term "cinematherapy" had been coined to reflect this. Cinematherapy was defined as:

> A form of therapy or self-help that uses movies, particularly videos, as therapeutic tools. Cinematherapy can be a catalyst for healing and growth for those who are open to learning how movies affect people and to watching certain films with conscious awareness. Cinema therapy allows one to use the effect of imagery, plot, music etc in films on the psyche for insight, inspiration, emotional release or relief and natural change. Used as part of psychotherapy, cinema therapy is an innovative method based on traditional therapeutic principles [16].

Over the last few years, the UK has used film as a "therapeutic tool" for service receivers. For example, a recent paper on marital disharmony reports that there are some relationship therapists who recommend couples who engage with their services to watch a film that specifically revolves around the theme of discord amongst partners. The couple is then invited to return for a further session for a detailed discussion about the film in a facilitated environment, all of which may yield new insights and consequently ameliorate discord [17].

Films have also been used for character building and as a means to make apparent the benefits of virtuous character traits. Niemiec et al. have used positive psychology models portrayed in film to illustrate a number of character strengths, notably wisdom, knowledge, courage, humanity and justice. Such an approach also looks at matters such as love, kindness, citizenship, hope, humour and spirituality, sentiments one can develop using models from films. Although the films that use some of these models may be fictional, they can nonetheless be understood and applied in a real-world setting [18].

World Psychiatry Association – Transcultural Psychiatry Conference in Mediterranean Countries

In 2012, in my second year as a doctor working for the National Health Service, I responded to an invitation to submit an abstract for the World Psychiatry Association – Transcultural Psychiatry Conference in Mediterranean Countries in Tel Aviv.

The abstract was about the portrayal of post-traumatic stress disorder (PTSD) in the 2008 Israeli animated war film, "Waltz with Bashir" written and directed by Ari Folman. Waltz with Bashir depicts Folman in search of his lost memories of his experience as a soldier in the 1982 Lebanon War [19]. The Scientific Committee clearly liked the abstract. They not only accepted it but also invited me to deliver a Keynote Address entitled, "Waltz with Bashir Two Views: Lebanon and Israel" following the screening of the film. I had informed my friends about this, many of whom strongly encouraged me to decline the invitation to give a Keynote Address in Israel since I would be "shaking hands with the enemy". I refused to subscribe to such an absurd notion, and I was determined to deliver the message of peaceful co-existence and to challenge anti-Semitism in any of its many forms. Moreover, since 2012 was the 30th year commemoration of the Sabra and Shatila massacres, I thought, "what better time to attempt to promote peaceful co-existence?" On reflection, the main driving force behind my determination to present in Tel Aviv was the Jewish family who had taken care of me when I was a medical student during the 2006 Lebanon War. I will never, ever forget how kind and compassionate they were towards me, and this particular life experience continues to shape my values and worldview. So, I boarded the plane from Manchester Airport to Ben-Gurion International Airport in Tel Aviv.

"I'm an alien, I'm an illegal alien, I'm a Lebanese man in Israel…"

Upon my arrival in Israel, I felt incredibly apprehensive. I had heard stories about how Muslims were detained and interrogated in Tel Aviv. Many of these Muslims were hoping to travel to Jerusalem to pray in Al-Aqsa Mosque and to visit holy Islamic sights such as the Dome of the Rock, and they were invariably refused entry. The memories of what ensued after disembarking from the aircraft and arriving in Ben-Gurion International Airport will remain indelibly etched in my mind for the rest of my life.

As I was approaching passport control, I noticed a man holding a placard with my name on it. Contrary to what I had been told (i.e. that I would be treated with suspicion and hostility), the man welcomed me and shook my hand. Without laying a single finger on me or asking me a single question, he opened the gates of Tel Aviv, gently ushered me in and then vanished. I was completely taken by surprise by what had occurred. I had expected hours of interrogation and harassment; however, I was granted entry into Israel with a minimum of fuss. The first and most overwhelming feeling that I experienced was that of fear, not of Israel, but rather the fear of betraying the trust that had been placed in me. What had just occurred was a very "human" act (i.e. rendering oneself vulnerable and placing trust in another) despite what many in the Arab community believed that Israelis and Jews were "inhumane".

During the conference itself, I opened my Keynote Address with the first two lines of the Lebanese mystic Khalil Gibran's poem. I then discussed and described how "humanizing" Folman's portrayal of PTSD in Waltz with Bashir was and how I, as a survivor of psychological distress, sensed a kindred spirit with him and was able to derive solace from the shared experience. The entire audience collectively and categorically condemned the Sabra and Shatila massacres (I had heard that many Israelis and Jews celebrated the death of Palestinians during the massacres; this was clearly not the reality), and I received a standing ovation.

Closing Remarks

In this chapter, I have provided an insight into how migration and trauma can precipitate mental health difficulties in adolescents and how this can be transmitted from one generation to the next and how we, as mental health professionals, should be mindful of this. I have also illustrated how we can use the power of film to challenge anti-Semitism. I hold no illusions. It will take many films to challenge the deeply entrenched views that many Arabs have about Jews and many Jews have about Arabs, but my personal experiences give me hope that one day Arabs and Jews will be able to live in peaceful co-existence.

I believe that film and storytelling wield a colossal amount of power and that psychiatry must take full advantage of this. The message to those who do provide mental health services is that the portrayal of psychopathology in film can help us to better understand our patients and the harrowing effects that mental illness can have on them. The animated documentary film Waltz with Bashir provides us with a unique insight into what it is like to suffer from PTSD, and this has allowed many to empathize with veterans and civilians affected by war.

On a personal note, both the 2006 Lebanon War and mental illness humiliated me and made me feel powerless. However, by watching films I felt "alive again". The film Waltz with Bashir was particularly poignant because it reconciled both the "cause" and "cure" of my mental illness; it was a film (the "cure," i.e. cinematherapy) about a Lebanon War ("the cause"). I felt that I could reach the "hearts and minds" of Israeli people through the message Waltz with Bashir contained: That we are all human, that our suffering is one and, in the words of Queen Rania of Jordan, the voice of the human heart needs no translation. I was determined to share that message of unity in the heart of Israel itself. By presenting a Keynote Lecture in Tel Aviv, I had taken a leap of faith by defying apprehension and social outcry, and, in return, the people of Israel had taken a huge leap of faith in me. The outcome? A memory that I shall cherish forever and a story of hope that I will share with the world.

Take-Home Messages for Mental Health Professionals

1. Film possesses an extraordinary power and offers an unrivalled medium for entertainment and escapism. Films are extremely popular across different cultures, and there are many films that have a mental illness theme.

2. Films can provide a precious qualitative insight into minds afflicted with mental illness for the families of people who have a psychiatric disorder, for mental healthcare providers and for members of the general public, thus allowing them to develop a better understanding of the subjective experience of what it is like to suffer from psychopathology.
3. Films have the power to *heal* and the term *cinematherapy has been coined* to reflect this. Cinematherapy must, however, be facilitated by a mental healthcare professional in an appropriate setting.
4. Film has the power and potential to promote peaceful co-existence and can be used as a tool to challenge anti-Semitism and discrimination in all its forms.

References

1. Karam EG, Howard DB, Karam N. Major depression and external stressors: the Lebanon wars. Eur Arch Psychiatry Clin Neurosci. 1998;248(5):225–30.
2. Potochnick SR, Perreira KMJ. Depression and anxiety among first-generation immigrant Latino youth: key correlates and implications for future research. J Nerv Ment Dis. 2010;198(7):470–7.
3. https://www.who.int/mental_health/maternal-child/child_adolescent/en/
4. Hankir A, Zaman R. Jung's archetype, 'The Wounded Healer', mental illness in the medical profession and the role of the health humanities in psychiatry. BMJ Case Rep. 2013;2013:bcr2013009990. Published 2013 Jul 12. https://doi.org/10.1136/bcr-2013-009990.
5. Hankir A, Carrick FR, Zaman R. Islam, mental health and being a Muslim in the West. Psychiatr Danub. 2015;27 Suppl 1:S53–9.
6. Hankir A, Kirkcaldy B, Carrick FR, Sadiq A, Zaman R. The performing arts and psychological well-being. Psychiatr Danub. 2017;29(Suppl 3):196–202.
7. Guber P. The four truths of the storyteller. Harv Bus Rev. 2007;85:52–9142.
8. Wessely S. Dementia and Mrs Thatcher. Lancet. 2012;379:210–21.
9. Annual report 2009 (PDF). Central Board of Film Certification, Ministry of Information and Broadcasting, Government of India. Retrieved 10 September 2010.
10. The world health report 2001 – Mental Health: New Understanding, New Hope. The World Health Organization website. Published 2001. Updated 2001. Cited 2019. http://www.who.int/whr/2001/en/.
11. Deakin N, Bhugra D. Families in Bollywood cinema: changes and context. Int Rev Psychiatry. 2012;24:166–72. https://doi.org/10.3109/09540261.2012.656307.
12. https://www.rcpsych.ac.uk/news-and-features/blogs/cultural-blogs/minds-on-film-blog.
13. http://www.rcpsych.ac.uk/mentalhealthinfo/mindsonfilmblog/theaviator.aspx.
14. http://www.rcpsych.ac.uk/mentalhealthinfo/mindsonfilmblog/thedivingbellandbutterfly.aspx.
15. Aref-Adib G, Kowalski C, Conn R. Dr Kamran Ahmed. Psychiatr Bull. 2012;36:ibc. https://doi.org/10.1192/pb.bp.112.038588.
16. Cinema Therapy. (n.d.) Segen's Medical Dictionary. (2011). Retrieved June 21 2015 from http://medical-dictionary.thefreedictionary.com/Cinema+Therapy.
17. Bhugra D, Gupta S. Editorial. Int Rev Psychiatry. 2009;21:181–2.
18. Niemiec RM, Wedding D. Positive psychology at the movies: using films to build virtues and character strengths. Gottingen, Hogrefe & Huber; 2008. p. 2.
19. Hankir A, Agius M. An exploration of how film portrays psychopathology: the animated documentary film Waltz with Bashir, the depiction of PTSD and cultural perceptions. Psychiatr Danub. 2012;24(Suppl 1):S70–6.

Consensus, Coalitions, and Division: Today's Jewish Community Counters Antisemitism

25

Elana Kahn

On Saturday morning, Oct. 27, a white supremacist walked into a Pittsburgh synagogue and murdered 11 people. For most Americans, it was a wake-up call, with the resounding message that antisemitism is alive, well, and again murderous in the country that, for generations, has been the Golden Land for Jews. For the organized Jewish community, however, the attack was not a complete surprise; like Jewish institutions across the country, the leaders of that three synagogue complex in Pittsburgh had prepared for the many threats facing Jews and Jewish institutions. Staff and volunteers had participated in trainings that included ways to respond to active shooter situations.

For American Jewish institutions, threat of violent antisemitism is always in the backdrop. Before the Pittsburgh attacks, most Jewish communities already employed full-time security professionals, who focused not only on facility security but also on maintaining ongoing relationships with local law enforcement officials. Even in the good years—with waning antisemitism and Pew [1] confirming that Americans feel more warmly toward Jews than any other religious group—calm was punctuated with multiple deadly shooting incidents, including the 1999 shooting at the Los Angeles Jewish Community Center, the 2006 shooting at the Jewish Federation of Greater Seattle, the 2009 shooting at the U.S. Holocaust Memorial Museum, the 2014 killings at the Overland Park Jewish Community Center, and the 2018 phoned-in threats to Jewish community centers across the country.

These attacks and threats elevate the level of insecurity within the Jewish community, punctuating a sense that racial- or ethnicity-driven acts of hate are always somewhat about the Jews. Even when other communities and institutions are attacked, as with the 2012 shootings at the Oak Creek Sikh Temple near Milwaukee and Sandy Hook Elementary School in Newtown, Connecticut, American Jews feel an increasing sense of vulnerability. After such attacks, the Jewish community raises its alert level and often implements additional security measures.

E. Kahn (✉)
Jewish Community Relations Council, Milwaukee Jewish Federation, Milwaukee, WI, USA
e-mail: elanako1001@gmail.com

© Springer Nature Switzerland AG 2020
H. S. Moffic et al. (eds.), *Anti-Semitism and Psychiatry*,
https://doi.org/10.1007/978-3-030-37745-8_25

Still, after the brutal Pittsburgh attack, which is considered the largest attack on the Jewish community in American history, the Jewish community stepped up security. Within a year, Jewish institutions across the country looked very different, with many of them installing bulletproof glass, employing armed security, requiring sign-in sheets, and employing other security measures. While most synagogues increased training for staff and increased vigilance during events, one synagogue in Milwaukee went so far as to hire its own full-time security guard.

Responsive and Proactive Measures

However, direct security measures are only one way that the Jewish community counters antisemitism. The community also defends itself through a variety of longer-term responsive and proactive measures that include responding directly to incidents, working to implement proactive programs to increase tolerance of and respect for Jews and other minority groups, educating people in positions of power to know and feel positively toward Jews and the Jewish community, influencing public policy in a way that ensures safety for Jews and the Jewish community, and ongoing strategic relationship building.

When hate incidents occur, Jewish Community Relations Councils, defense agencies such as the Anti-Defamation League, and other Jewish professionals and volunteers step in to work with schools and other agencies to implement measures that will keep Jews and other minorities safe. In these cases, the incidents are often an opportunity to hold the hosting institutions accountable and then work with them to implement positive changes. One recent example of such engagement followed the 2018 online publication of a photo of students from a central Wisconsin high school's prom, posing with their arms raised in a Nazi salute. The Jewish Community Relations Council of the Milwaukee Jewish Federation (JCRC) rallied organizations, faith communities, and leaders from across the state to co-sign a statement of condemnation. It also worked with the school district to implement a series of educational programs designed to increase knowledge of, comfort with, and respect for Jews and other minority groups.

Similarly, in a 2019 incident, a University of Wisconsin-Milwaukee student protested beside a Jewish student gathering with a placard of a swastika and other hateful symbols. Campus organizations, Jewish faculty, and the JCRC represented the community by speaking with the student, communicating with university administration, and then serving on a task force formed to address hate and bias incidents on campus. Though the university task force addressed bias incidents and culture for all vulnerable populations, the JCRC was the only non-campus group represented on the task force, reflecting the Jewish community's commitment to participating in broad efforts to protect all minorities. That philosophy is fundamental in American Jewish life; Jewish security is inextricably tied to that of other faith, ethnic, and racial communities.

Such an approach is not only philosophical but also pragmatic. There is abundant evidence that white supremacists and those who target Jews are also hateful toward people of color, immigrants, Muslims, and other minorities. A community that allows expressions of bigotry toward one vulnerable population will also tolerate such expressions toward others. Knowing that, it is important to quantify and qualify the amount and level of antisemitism in our communities. In Milwaukee, the JCRC continually monitors and responds to antisemitic incidents, compiling incidents into an annual audit that it shares with national and local organizations. Nationally, the Anti-Defamation League and the Southern Poverty Law Center, among others, conduct similar audits. Consistently, when incidents against Jews increase, so do they rise against other minority populations, including immigrants and LGBTQ people.

When possible, the Jewish community seeks to work in coalition with others. That approach took hold after the August 2018 Unite the Right rally in Charlottesville, Virginia, which gathered members of the far-right and included self-identified members of the alt-right, neo-Confederates, neo-fascists, white nationalists, neo-Nazis, Klansmen, and various right-wing militias. In Milwaukee, the Jewish community worked with the YWCA to declare a weekend dedicated to countering hatred, inviting people and institutions from the local community to hold programs dedicated to fighting hatred and increasing understanding. The effort garnered a mayoral proclamation.

Defense Through Relationships

In many ways, the organized Jewish community was shaped by the need to respond to and protect itself from acts of antisemitism. In the 1930s, it founded a series of defense agencies, such as the ADL, American Jewish Committee, and local community relations councils. In founding those organizations, it understood that protecting the community required a multipronged approach; not only must the community directly call out antisemitism, but it must also develop ongoing relationships with elected officials, civic leaders, and influential individuals. Community security depends on building networks of allies, among neighbors and people in power, so that the Jewish community would never again be alone. The Jewish community stands alone in the American social landscape for investing in a field—community relations—that has as its goal security through ongoing relationships.

The community relations field is built on the understanding that everything—every policy and law, every action that contributes to workplace or school culture—is based on relationships. Even governmental policy is determined through relationships elected officials determine how to vote on legislation because of whom they know. So the Jewish community works to ensure that when a member of Congress votes on something with bearing on the Jewish community, he or she will consider how it will affect people who matter to him or her.

That approach can be seen in Jewish community programming too. Community relations councils actively pursue interfaith and intergroup efforts of many varieties. Over the years, the Milwaukee JCRC has founded and run intentional alliances with Catholic, Latino, Muslim, African American, and Presbyterian communities.

JCRC is among the founders of the Interfaith Conference of Greater Milwaukee and maintains leadership roles in the organization. Other Jewish organizations also pursue robust and positive relations outside the Jewish community: Jewish museums regularly hold programs that draw on themes that are common with other minority communities; social justice and social action problems regularly partner with churches and other community groups; community-wide commemorations of Kristallnacht and Holocaust Remembrance Day always include leaders from other faith communities.

Openness is not incidental but essential to organizations and agencies throughout the community. Jewish community centers, which include athletic facilities, childcare, camps, and cultural programs, are used as neighborhood gathering places and boast a high percentage of non-Jewish membership. Jewish Family Services, which began by serving the Jewish community, now serves a clientele that is primarily not Jewish. Milwaukee's Jewish Food Pantry, staffed mostly by volunteers from the Jewish community, is located in a non-Jewish neighborhood with economic need and serves mostly non-Jews. Jewish museums and Holocaust education programs reach well beyond the Jewish community and focus on issues of shared concern, such as civil rights and bullying.

The Jewish community advocates issues of concern to other targeted communities, often leading or standing with those communities. When the Native American community in Wisconsin advocated prohibiting schools from using Native American symbols or language in schools or team mascots, the Jewish community stood with them. The JCRC was among the lead organizations in the Community Coalition for Quality Policing, a criminal justice effort in Milwaukee. Jewish organizations, synagogues, and individuals have taken a lead in advocating immigration reform. Such advocacy reflects the deep understanding that we cannot afford to be alone; we need such alliances to defend ourselves. The post-Holocaust moniker "never again" refers not only to genocide but also to the belief that Jews should never again be without allies and friends who are willing to risk themselves for the safety of Jews.

Those connections are not merely strategic. Jews often naturally feel an affinity for other communities that have experienced multigenerational trauma. The emerging study of epigenetics, the understanding that trauma at critical time periods can leave a chemical mark that affects the expression of a person's genes and that this effect can then be passed down to subsequent generations, can shift how Jews understand themselves and can motivate them to feel allied with other communities that still struggle with the effects of their ancestors' trauma. While some interpretations of studies in epigenetics remain controversial and disputed [2], they shape how affected groups (such as Jews and African Americans) understand themselves and form alliances in contemporary America. Even without the science, it is clear that targeted groups often internalize the oppression that they experience, resulting in a set of distinct behaviors. It is not a stretch to say that American Jews embrace a collective self-description of resilience and toughness, of doing whatever is necessary to survive and thrive, as a direct response to years of persecution. Other communities have similarly internalized and responded to their collective experiences.

As such, understanding and sharing collective trauma can be an effective way to increase empathy between communities. In my interfaith and intergroup relations, it has become clear that people are more inclined to empathy when sharing personal stories of hardship and trauma, even if those experiences are from generations past. African Americans and American Jews, for example, are more inclined to see each other as allies when they share stories of lived experience with oppression and suffering. Understanding that, I make personal sharing, particularly about families and their journeys, memories and values, hurts and memories, a central part of our dialogue.

Division on Community Approaches

Not everyone in the Jewish community embraces the Jewish communal responses to antisemitism, broadly defined as proactive relationship building and increased security. To the first, some in the Jewish community criticize this friend-building approach, preferring more direct and aggressive defense (which features publishing public statements, heavy handed media ads, etc.) Indeed, it is difficult to measure the efficacy of alliance building because so much of the work is preventative and behind the scenes. The Pittsburgh attacks gave the Jewish community the opportunity to measure the quality of its alliances as many communities gathered for services and vigils. In Milwaukee, as in many communities, hundreds of faith leaders, elected officials, civic leaders, and other non-Jewish allies showed up to demonstrate solidarity with the Jewish community. People throughout the country wore and posted stickers expressing that solidarity and shared the conviction that such acts of hate directed at Jews were anathema to their understanding of America.

Still, some in the Jewish community posit that we cannot afford to seem vulnerable or acquiescent to communities that have had some role in harming Jews. To them, interfaith relations are not to be trusted. Those who hold these views can understand activities such as a Muslim–Jewish dialogue or interfaith programs in churches as a betrayal to the charge of Jewish self-defense; they can be interpreted as feckless acts of overlooking how these communities have been complicit or overt actors in antisemitism. After the JCRC participated in a vigil against violence in a local cathedral, I received a note from an Orthodox Jewish leader asking if the church would ring its bell once for each Jew who died as a result of their complicity during the Holocaust. According to that perspective, which is widespread in the American Jewish Orthodox community, Jews should never enter churches, partially because of the memory of Christian oppression. I have also been criticized for Muslim-Jewish programs with a litmus test approach; Muslim participants should be required to condemn Muslim antisemitism and Hamas violence toward Israel. Such an all-or-nothing approach remains a minority view, but it is a continual point of tension within the Jewish community.

Once an issue on which the Jewish community enjoyed broad consensus, security—how the community protects its members—is increasingly becoming a fault line in American Jewish life. Though the presence of police cars or armed guards in front of synagogues on Shabbat (Sabbath) leads some to feel safer, for others that presence is a reminder that they are not safe. triggering feelings of insecurity and anxiety. That experience is heightened for Jews of color, who comprise an estimated 10–20% of the American Jewish population.

Such an experience is understandable, considering the well-publicized killings of unarmed African Americans and Latinos. The direct result of the September 11 terror attacks, America's War on Terror, has led to the militarization of law enforcement—including not only arming local police S.W.A.T. teams with military grade weapons, body armor, a fierce warrior approach to policing, but also increased militarization of border patrol and immigration enforcement agents [3, 4]. Many law enforcement officials view these militarized units as necessary for public safety, but there is strong evidence that such tactics leave many feeling insecure, targeted by the very professionals who are tasked with protecting them. A 2018 study of 9,000 law enforcement agencies found that police militarization not only did not reduce violent crime, but it also eroded public confidence in police departments [5]. A 2018 article by Vesla Weaver, "More Security May Actually Make Us Feel Less Secure," points to the negative effects of police interactions, including an increase in post-traumatic stress disorder; declining grades and test scores among youth; legal estrangement; strategic avoidance of people, places, and institutions; isolation from peer networks; and aggravated perceptions of racial discrimination [6].

As antisemitic incidents increase and become more deadly, with the Pittsburgh synagogue attack as a turning point, American Jewish organizations and synagogues have become resigned to the need for higher-grade security systems, armed guards, and even armed congregants. But some American Jews are speaking up, asking about the psychological effects of arming Jewish institutions. They are as follows: are we raising children to be part of "the lockdown generation," who expect attack and carry with them an elevated level of anxiety about the inevitability of violence and hate? How do we ensure that Jewish spaces are not only secure but also welcoming to Jews of color and members of other communities, including people of color? Do weapons in Jewish spaces make us feel safer or more vulnerable, a physical reminder of trauma? Our communities will need to grapple with these questions in a thoughtful and inclusive way, including Jews of color, as well as Jews with European heritage and Jews from across the political and religious spectrum.

Israel and Partisan Politics

Another complicating factor of the American Jewish response to antisemitism involves polarized discourse about the modern state of Israel. Like with security, American Jews once overwhelmingly agreed in their strong support for Israel, but such consensus has been lost to political and ideological tensions. It has become commonplace for progressive Protestant church associations and academic associations to call for supports of the Boycott, Divestment, and Sanctions movement against Israel. For the first time, in 2018, two people who openly support the BDS movement were elected to Congress. Most American Jews view the BDS movement as unfairly targeting Israel; by ignoring countries with horrific human rights records and holding Israel to a unique standard, the movement itself seems driven by anti-semitism. Some Jewish communities have responded by drawing red lines for the allocation of funds and co-sponsorship, refusing to support or work with organizations that support the BDS movement. Consequently, members of the Jewish community who define themselves as non- or anti-Zionist, or even robustly critical of Israel's policies, say that they feel unwelcome in the Jewish community.

Cynically, some of that genuine tension has been exploited by political and civic leaders, who use antisemitism and criticism of, or support for, Israel to score partisan political points. As Jeremy Burton, executive director of Boston's JCRC, said during a session at the 2019 Jewish Council for Public Affairs conference, "People are moving towards more extreme, more fractured, more oppositional spaces, and it's creating a really complicated place for ... organizations like JCRCs." [7]

In 2019, antisemitism became a cudgel in partisan politics like never before in the American Jewish community. American Jews have disagreed over Israel and over antisemitism in the past, but this is different. Now, political actors, including members of Congress, on the right claim that the left is antisemitic and anti-Israel, and those on the left claim that they are being unfairly accused of antisemitism when they actually just mean to criticize Israeli policy. Each claims that the other side is weaponizing antisemitism in its political game.

For example, in January 2019, after it had been revealed that leaders of the national Women's March had supported antisemitism, tacitly or actively, many Jews backed away from the march. Some, however, insisted on engagement and defended the march leaders. (This raises interesting questions about allegiance and tribe: which element of our identity supersedes others when we are pressed to choose?) Notably, a group of Jewish women of color rallied to participate in the controversial national event. Women who participated talked about the powerful experience of not walking away but, instead, staying engaged in the march in spite of the leaders' antisemitic statements and actions. It was not a one-time event. In February 2019, when freshman Congresswoman Ilhan Omar (D-Minn) tweeted that support for Israel in Congress was "all about the Benjamins," she was roundly condemned for trading in old antisemitic tropes about Jewish financiers buying and controlling American politicians. It was one of many statements that attributed malicious power to Israel and to Jews, such as a previous statement about Israel hypnotizing the world to force them to overlook the state's evil acts. Support for her was divided along political lines.

While some parts of the political left are claiming their stake in criticism of Israel and the minimization of the deleterious effects of antisemitism, the political right is firmly narrating itself as supportive of Israel, although this support sometimes neglects the interests of actual American Jews. In August 2019, President Donald Trump tweeted and then said that American Jews who voted for Democrats were being disloyal "to Jewish people and very disloyal to Israel," tapping into classic antisemitic canards of dual loyalty. Amid widespread outrage, some Jews rushed to his defense, turning their ire on Jews with other political persuasions. What is common in these stories is a culture of partisan antipathy.

These rifts along political lines threaten to dismantle the consensus-building approach that has allowed Jews to come together not only for prayer but also to solve communal problems, safeguard rights, and advocate as a community, in spite of political differences. Such new conditions challenge the organized Jewish community in new ways as it works to prevent and counter antisemitism without the almost universal support it previously enjoyed. Community leaders will need to consider how to navigate multiple interests—building coalitions while supporting segments of the community that do not participate in interfaith and intergroup relations, increasing security measures while attending to the anxiety and inherent complications, ensuring that the community is welcoming to people who hold a variety of political opinions while not submitting to polarized rhetoric of politics. It is clear that this age—simultaneously considered an era of increased security and a time of deep insecurity—will require new kinds of leadership.

References

1. Pew Forum. Americans express increasingly warm feelings toward religious groups. 2017 Feb. https://www.pewforum.org/2017/02/15/americans-express-increasingly-warm-feelings-toward-religious-groups/.
2. Khazan O. Can trauma be inherited between generations? 2018 Oct. https://www.theatlantic.com/health/archive/2018/10/trauma-inherited-generations/573055/.
3. Kain E. Police militarization in the decade following 9/11. 2011 Sept. https://www.forbes.com/sites/erikkain/2011/09/12/police-militarization-in-the-decade-following-911/#2d130f6e5d7e.
4. Rizer A, Hartman J. How the war on terror has militarized the police. 2011 Nov. https://www.theatlantic.com/national/archive/2011/11/how-the-war-on-terror-has-militarized-the-police/248047/.
5. Mummolo J. Militarization fails to enhance police safety or reduce crime but may harm police reputation. Proc Natl Acad Sci U S A. 2018. https://www.ncbi.nlm.nih.gov/pmc/articles/PMC6140536/.
6. Weaver V. More security may actually make us feel less secure. Proc Natl Acad Sci U S A. 2018. https://www.ncbi.nlm.nih.gov/pmc/articles/PMC6166813/.
7. Hanau S. JCPA makes expansion push amid increasingly treacherous politics. 2019 Feb. https://jewishweek.timesofisrael.com/jcpa-makes-expansion-push-amid-increasingly-treacherous-politics/.

Stemming the Tide of Anti-Semitism: The Roles of Psychiatrists and Psychiatry

James L. Fleming

Introduction

As reports emerge of increased levels of anti-Semitism in the U.S., Europe, and elsewhere in the world [1], the question of whether and how both individual psychiatrists and organized psychiatry should respond grows in importance. This chapter will focus primarily on the situation in the U.S., starting with events leading up to the national elections in November of 2018 and culminating in what has been described as the deadliest attack against the American Jewish community in U.S. history, namely the mass shooting at the Tree of Life Jewish synagogue in Pittsburgh on October 27, 2018 [2]. I will present a case for both individual psychiatrists and the psychiatric profession as a whole to speak out against anti-Semitic words and actions and against the broader phenomenon of hate speech, which all too often leads to hate-based crimes through incitement of a small minority of individuals predisposed to such violence.

At the outset, I would like disclose some of my own background and experience, which may help readers understand both my perspective and the source of my interest in the issues covered in this chapter. I come from Irish roots and a Christian background and was raised in the Midwest United States. I learned to meditate in 1972 while in college and went on to become an instructor of Transcendental Meditation and to study the Vedic tradition of India. Daily meditation since then, along with travel to Central America, Cuba, Brazil, Egypt, Israel, and the Palestinian territories, has helped me foster an appreciation for the wide variety of world cultures and religious traditions. Concerns about the Israeli–Palestinian conflict and tensions in my local community surrounding this and other issues among Jews and Muslims led me to begin engaging in interfaith dialogue in 2009. This dialogue led me in 2011 to help found an "Abrahamic" interfaith group in the Kansas City area called "People of Faith for Peace." The group, which includes local Jews, Christians,

J. L. Fleming (✉)
Psychiatric Medical Care, Kansas City, MO, USA
e-mail: jflemingmd@yahoo.com

© Springer Nature Switzerland AG 2020
H. S. Moffic et al. (eds.), *Anti-Semitism and Psychiatry*,
https://doi.org/10.1007/978-3-030-37745-8_26

and Muslims, engages in shared meals, dialogue, advocacy and community service. I am also a life member of the American Psychiatric Association (APA) and have been a Representative from Missouri to the Assembly, the APA's governance body since 2015; I am currently Chair of the APA Caucus on Climate Change and Mental Health. In 2018, in response to serious concerns about the adverse effects of immigration policies being enacted by the Trump administration, I completed a training course in asylum evaluations through Physicians for Human Rights, began to provide asylum evaluations for immigrants, and organized and presented educational programs for the annual meetings in 2019 of both APA and my district branch of the APA, the Missouri Psychiatric Physicians Association.

Rising Tide of Anti-Semitism

The growth of anti-Semitism internationally is related, at least in part, to the rise of xenophobia, racism, and nationalism, which in turn appear to have been triggered by international mass migration. The extent of this migration has been identified by historians as the most widespread since World War II. In the United States, the arrival of large numbers of migrants at the southern border has been highly politicized, leading to an increase in the public expressions of xenophobic and overtly racist speech. Donald Trump, for example—who had for years promoted the false narrative about America's first African American President, Barack Obama, not being a U.S. citizen by disputing his place of birth—launched his 2016 Presidential campaign with harsh rhetoric about Mexican immigrants, saying that Mexico was sending "criminals, drug dealers, rapists" to the U.S. [3]. Neo-Nazi and white supremacy groups cheered Trump's 2016 election victory, and in the year following the election, according to the Southern Poverty Law Center, which tracks "hate groups," there was a significant increase in the number of such organizations. Neo-Nazi groups showed the greatest growth within the white supremacist movement during this time period (fall 2016 to fall 2017), soaring by 22%, from 99 to 121 [4].

Ethical Basis for Action by Psychiatrists and Psychiatry

While American culture has historically witnessed its share of racist, hate-based dialogue, Americans have never seen the current vitriolic rhetoric being tolerated by, much less generated from, the highest executives in the land. At what point are psychiatrists ethically bound to intervene and how? Possible interventions include speaking out individually, engaging one's professional organization to issue public statements, as well as more "activist" engagement such as protests, political activism, or even civil disobedience. We can also engage professional and nonprofessional activities that aim to address social injustice and/or unjust public policy. In my own case, in addition to providing asylum evaluations on a pro bono basis, the Kansas City interfaith group mentioned above provided several months of after-school tutoring for children of Somali refugees after a Somali teen was murdered in a hate crime outside a local Somali mosque.

Ethical guidance for professional activity by psychiatrists relies on the American Medical Association's Principles of Medical Ethics, and the APA has added "annotations" unique to psychiatry [5]. Both are hereafter referred to as the "Ethics Code" and can be considered to have two aspects: prohibitive ("thou shalt not...") and affirmative (thou shalt..."). Both are relevant to this discussion. A relevant example of a prohibitive guideline is Section 1.2 of the Ethics Code, which states that a psychiatrist *should not be a party to any type of policy that excludes, segregates, or demeans the dignity of any patient because of ethnic origin, race, sex, creed, age, socioeconomic status, or sexual orientation.* The affirmative corollary is found in Section 7, which states: *A physician shall recognize a responsibility to participate in activities contributing to the improvement of the community and the betterment of public health* (note that sections of the Ethics Code with a decimal point refer to the APA's Annotations, whereas those without a decimal point are the AMA's Principles of Medical Ethics from which the Annotations are derived). Section 5 also contains an affirmative responsibility; it urges physicians to *continue to study, apply, and advance scientific knowledge ... [and]... make relevant information available to patients, colleagues, and the public.* All three of the sections of the Ethics Code are expressed in the May 2018 APA Position Statement, entitled "Resolution Against Racism and Racial Discrimination and Their Adverse Impacts on Mental Health" [6]. These aspects of the Ethics Code call for a response to racist, hate-based rhetoric, especially when it originates from public officials.

Responses in the current environment will likely involve public statements and the engagement of government leaders and agencies. However, one could conceive of situations in which engagement in civil disobedience is not only permissible but also necessary to protect patients. Examples may be: 1. refusal to provide information to authorities about the immigration status of patients or families we are treating; 2. for government workers or government contractors, "blowing the whistle" (reporting to other government officials or the media) about unjust policies which an individual psychiatrist believes are harmful to patients, even though this might be in violation of agency rules or protocol.

The Ethics Code does provide some guidance on civil disobedience, though, in my view, is not sufficiently supportive of such activities. Section 3 states: "A physician shall respect the law" but also "recognize a responsibility to seek changes in those requirements which are contrary to the best interests of the patient." Section 3 (an aspect of the psychiatric annotations) notes that physicians "lose no right of citizenship on entry into the profession of medicine" and also recognizes that protesting "social injustices," while possibly being illegal, may not be unethical from a professional standpoint. Many, myself included, would go farther and state that it could actually be unethical to *obey* certain unjust laws.

However, as mental health professionals who serve a diverse spectrum of society, it makes sense, in general, to avoid getting involved in conflicted partisan politics unless doing so is clearly in the interest of our patients, the public, or the profession. A 2015 report from the APA Ethics Committee advises that when making public statements in relation to the policies or behavior (including speech) of government leaders or politicians, whenever possible we should "focus on issues rather individuals" [7], although this is presented as a recommendation rather than an ethical guideline per se. It should also be noted that all aspects of the Ethics Code have been developed as guidelines, not rigid rules or laws, as indicated by this statement from the Forward of the Ethics Code: *The annotations are not designed as absolutes and will be revised from time to time so as to be applicable to current practices and problems.*

One can certainly foresee times when "naming names" is not only unavoidable but also necessary [8, 9], and some have done so, including two psychiatrists/analysts in the wake of the contentious presidential election of 2016 [8] and more prominently in a "best seller" focusing on the issue of "dangerousness" with respect to the winner of that election, Donald Trump [10].

The more prominent and powerful a person is, the more society expects them to uphold standards of decency and respect. That an issue may be politically volatile or might be viewed by someone or some group as "politically partisan" does not exempt one—anyone in my opinion—from a moral or ethical duty. In some ways, the riskier—both personally and professionally—it is to speak out against increasing levels of abuse and oppression, the more necessary it is to do so. Historical records document the hazards of remaining silent in times of growing peril, times when not taking a stand can be deadly, even catastrophic. The late author and Holocaust survivor Elie Wiesel brings these dynamics into sharp focus: "We must take sides. Neutrality helps the oppressor, never the victim. Silence encourages the tormentor, never the tormented. Sometimes we must interfere" [11].

Background of a Modern Anti-Semitic Terror Attack

Before outlining how psychiatrists can appropriately and effectively "take sides" during perilous times, an examination of events surrounding the 2018 midterm elections is in order. The backdrop for this time period involved broad changes in immigration policy by the Trump administration, the most notorious of these being the "zero tolerance" policy, which resulted in the separation of immigrant children from their parents at the U.S. southern border [12]. The APA was the first among several medical organizations to issue a public statement condemning the policy, pointing out the long- adverse effects on child development of such actions [13]. As an APA Assembly Representative, I have continued to engage the APA leadership on this issue.

As the campaign for seats in the U.S. Congress progressed, fear-based rhetoric about immigrants, clearly based on politics rather than available data, started to ramp up as the midterm elections approached. President Trump warned of an "invasion" of criminals and terrorists," repeatedly referring to a "caravan" of Honduran immigrants. He also warned of an "infestation" of our country by diseased immigrants. These warnings of supposed imminent danger ended abruptly after the election, but not before they were echoed on certain cable news outlets and amplified by certain social platforms, some of which made references to the Jewish refugee relief agency HIAS (Hebrew Immigrant Aid Society) and their efforts to assist the migrants. One man, Joseph Bowers, energized by the frenzied anti-immigrant rhetoric and frustrated by the lack of "action," resorted to violence, going into the Tree of Life Jewish synagogue in Pittsburgh with assault weapons and murdering 11 people and wounding six others. Bowers, who had a history of posting anti-Semitic comments on social media, was especially incensed by the work that the HIAS was doing with immigrants and a few hours before entering the synagogue posted this on social media: "HIAS likes to bring invaders in that kill our people. I can't sit by and watch my people get slaughtered. Screw your optics, I'm going in" [2]. This is a clear demonstration of a direct connection between hate-filled, fear-based speech emanating from powerful leaders being repeated, perpetuated, and amplified by like-minded voices in media outlets and then leading to overt violence and mass murder. The community surrounding the Tree of Life synagogue will never be the same again in the wake of this heinous terror attack. And, at the same time, yet another mass shooting burdens the American psyche; Jews around the world have been retraumatized and reminded that just being Jewish and having a place of public worship are potentially life-threatening risks.

A Call to Action in Historical Context: Psychiatric Silence and Complicity

It is important for psychiatrists to help individuals and communities heal in the aftermath of such tragedies, but as health care professionals, I believe that we also have an obligation to go beyond disaster response to identify causative factors. Imagine infectious disease and public health specialists focusing only on the treatment aspects of an epidemic of food poisoning without determining the source of contamination and aggressively addressing it. In my view, there is no justifiable reason to not apply the same approach to incidents leading to violence and the ensuing psychological and emotional trauma it engenders. Then APA President Dr. Altha Stewart agreed with this sentiment in her column in the APA's periodical Psychiatric News, published a few weeks after the Tree of Life massacre: "We members must speak out, use our specialized training and expertise for the public's benefit, and apply it to not only healing, but also preventing psychological trauma and senseless tragedies" [14].

Before discussing further how to heed this clarion call to speak out, we would do well to review—or perhaps learn about for the first time—the role that psychiatrists played during the pinnacle of anti-Semitic hatred, the Nazi Holocaust itself. It would be sad enough if psychiatrists had been simply silent or "neutral" as the malignancy of Nazi agenda became evident. Tragically, not only were physicians overrepresented among German society in the Nazi party, but psychiatrists were actually in charge of the infamous T4 program that sought to purge German society of those deemed as a genetic burden: as many as 100,000 mentally ill and developmentally disabled children and adults were killed (involuntarily euthanized) using execution methods, which became models for the "Final Solution," the extermination of six million Jews [15, 16]. The connection to American psychiatry is indirect but still disturbing: Hitler was said to be inspired by the American eugenics movement, in which psychiatrists played a prominent role by promoting and carrying out sterilization of thousands of mentally ill and developmentally delayed patients [17].

In the effort to avoid repeating errors of silence and complicity, such as those that occurred in Nazi Germany, psychiatrists need to pay close attention not only to "words" but also to the sociopolitical context in which words are spoken, as well as to the power balance between the speaker and the audience, intended or unintended. This context affects our patients, as well as our potential patients, the public at large, especially vulnerable groups who are frequent targets of both verbal and physical attacks. The details become more important when the speaker is in a position of power and prominence; i.e., the "bar" should be raised even higher. Why? It is because speaking out about powerful figures, especially elected officials, carries several types of risks for psychiatrists and for psychiatric organizations:

1. These leaders hold power to seriously harm or even eliminate detractors; world history as well as contemporary, international news reports are full of examples of personal retribution, even in otherwise "free" or democratic societies.
2. Some leaders, despite potentially egregious behaviors and policies, may still be supported by a significant portion of the electorate, and when psychiatrists or psychiatric organizations "call out" these leaders, their supporters may feel personally attacked or criticized. This may adversely affect trust in one's caregiver or may cause mental or emotional distress, though this is likely to be temporary.
3. Elected officials such as the U.S. President could, out of retribution, alter other, related policies (e.g., related to funding of services or programs relevant to psychiatry) in a way that harms the profession and the patients we are charged with serving. As I opined earlier in this chapter, none of these factors have "veto power" over our ethical responsibilities, but we do need to weigh them carefully and be prepared for the consequences of our advocacy, whatever form it takes. In essence, we need to discern, at different times in our history, whether or not we are in the midst of "a Bonhoeffer moment." This was the title of a February 2018 article [9] in the Christian social justice periodical *Sojourners*, which refers to Dietrich Bonhoeffer, a German pastor, theologian, staunch anti-Nazi dissident, who was eventually arrested and executed by hanging for his activism. The authors draw parallels between the current political scene—from the standpoint of government leadership and public support—in the U.S. and that of Nazi Germany, though they are rightly cautious about equating the two. I believe that we should continue to exercise caution in concluding that any modern government is close to replicating the horrors of the Nazi Holocaust, brutal and widespread as it was. But societies would be remiss if they did not at least examine the available "data" to see how close they are to following the trajectory that sets the stage for similar atrocities. The warnings of renowned psychiatrist Robert Jay Lifton, author of a study of "Nazi Doctors," are relevant in this regard [18].

He describes the phenomenon of "malignant normality," present throughout the society of Nazi Germany and also in the Unites States in the "Trump era." Malignant normality involves acceptance as normal, by society at large, of behaviors that at another time would—depending on the circumstances—be viewed on a continuum from mildly abnormal to extreme and, as Lifton put it, "evil." An example of the "malignant normality" at the time of Hitler was the common sight of uniformed German officers sitting in the pews of churches on Sundays, who during the "work week" carried out the horrific policies of the concentration (death) camps [9]. Pastors such as Dietrich Bonhoeffer were very much in the minority.

In this modern era, Lifton asks psychiatrists to be "witnessing professionals" by "bringing our knowledge and experience to bear on what threatens us," as well as on what "might renew us." He believes that malignant normality is manifesting itself in the form of large-scale support for or even mere tolerance of the behavior and policies of the current U.S. President. He suggests that we begin by recognizing "the urgency of the situation in which the most powerful man in the world is also the bearer of profound instability and untruth" [10]. Some may disagree with Lifton on this point, and some readers, who for whatever reason support President Trump, may be offended by such statements. Everyone must ultimately make their own judgments, but psychiatrists should at least consider whether or not their support for any leader is in line with the "prohibitive" guideline from the Ethics Code mentioned above: namely, that a psychiatrist "should not be a party to any type of policy that excludes, segregates, or demeans the dignity of any patient because of ethnic origin, race, sex, creed…"

White Nationalism and Anti-Semitism in the United States

The fear-fueled rhetoric leading up to the 2018 U.S. national election, which many saw as clearly aimed at stirring up hatred and anger at immigrant "invaders," contains some disturbing parallels to that of Nazi Germany, as well as that of other oppressive regimes that single out certain demographic groups as the primary "enemy." Even a superficial review of numerous media reports reveals ties between the rhetoric of President Trump and that of white supremacist, neo-Nazi movements (a Google Scholar search yielded only one article on this connection presumably due to the short amount of time elapsed since Trump was elected). Two examples with extensive media coverage follow. After the Tree of Life terror attack, not surprisingly, President Trump condemned the attack but refused to take any responsibility for the role that his rhetoric regarding immigrants might have played in inflaming fear and hatred. At a campaign rally on October 22, 2018, 5 days before the mass shooting, the President declared: "I'm a nationalist, okay? I'm a nationalist." That he was cognizant of the culturally dangerous implications of this statement made by a white male in the top seat of government is suggested by his introducing the comment by saying: "we're not supposed to use that term" [19].

Consider also the President's repeated refusal to condemn white supremacists and neo-Nazis, including many who gathered for the Unite the Right rally in Charlottesville, NC, in August 2017, when the evening before the main rally approximately 200 people marched with tiki torches chanting (including directly in front of a Jewish synagogue) "Jews will not replace us" and invoking the Nazi chant "blood and soil." In addition to stating that there were "fine people on both sides" (protestors and counterprotesters), Trump focused on the fact that the white nationalist and neo-Nazi protestors "had a permit" as if that justified the hatred that they were promoting. He also referred to the evening rally as "people protesting very quietly" [20], which was clearly not the case as can be seen in videos of event. Many people were reportedly shocked and frightened by the sights and sounds they witnessed, and the next day, a woman was killed when a white nationalist protestor drove a car into a crowd of counterprotesters.

Many Americans, in my experience, including some psychiatrists, do not seem disturbed by these statements from the President, at least not enough to withdraw their support. But we should not miss the significance of the continuous negative references—either overtly offensive statements or more subtle ones—to Jews and Muslims (many of whom are of Semitic ethnicity) and non-white, non-Christians in general. All of these references seem to fuel and empower white nationalist, neo-Nazi groups that have repeatedly celebrated Trump's election victory and continue to voice support for his rhetoric and his administration's policies regarding immigration [21]. The point here is not to try to prove whether or not Donald Trump is trying to emulate or could possibly repeat in any substantive fashion the horrific policies of Adolf Hitler and his cohorts. Rather, the concern is more general and is threefold:

1. Specific connections have been demonstrated between the current presidential administration and rising white nationalist, anti-Semitic activities and sentiments.
2. The white nationalist movement threatens the safety of the American public, as seen in the case of recent domestic terror attacks. Even in the absence of overt violence, hateful rhetoric creates fear, depression, and other forms of emotional distress, particularly in certain minority religious and ethnic demographic groups, including Jews, Muslims, Latinos, and Blacks.
3. Psychiatrists have an ethical obligation to support these (and all) communities and help prevent further trauma and emotional distress.

We also need to be alert to the subtle and not-so-subtle manipulations that escalate during times of increased ideologic polarization, racial tension, and an expanding gap between those with extreme wealth and those of lesser means. It may be the mark of our times that some of those who wield political power in a discriminatory or oppressive fashion try—in a manner that should be recognized as both ironic and sinister— to present themselves to the public as "victims" while simultaneously singling out certain demographic groups as the cause of their alleged victimhood. These manipulations create anguish as well as confusion, add to existing divisions, and in some cases turn deadly.

Just as this chapter was being finalized, a variety of non-Jewish supporters of the President came to his defense after he stirred up another nationwide uproar by tweeting that four Congresswomen of color, all American citizens who had criticized his policies, should "go back" to the countries they came from [22]. The supporters of the President, including political operatives with ties to neo-Nazi groups, conservative politicians, and self-identified Christian supporters of Jews, invoked the charge of "anti-Semitism" against the Congresswomen. The racist trope "go back to where you came from" has been used for many decades in the U.S. against African Americans and for centuries in the U.S. and abroad against Jews. Even though Trump's use of the phrase was condemned in a bipartisan manner and by nonpartisan groups, including the venerable civil rights group the Anti-Defamation League (ADL), one Christian evangelical group (Proclaiming Justice to the Nations) accused the ADL itself of "siding with anti-Semites." *The New York Times* editorialist Michelle Goldberg, who reported on this, wrote that the Christian group "even had the audacity to hurl [the accusation] 'lashon hara' [Hebrew for "evil tongue"] at the Jewish civil rights organization" [22]. Consider the irony and misplaced outrage of the dynamic operating between these two groups: a group of non-Jews, founded in 2005 to "support 'Jews and Israel,'" accusing the ADL of anti-Semitism and another group, formed in 1913, with "a dual mission of securing justice not only for Jews but for all people." This type of dynamic seems like an appropriate opportunity—in the words of Robert Jay Lifton—for "witnessing professionals" to bring "our knowledge and experience to bear on what threatens us," as well as on what "might renew us." Distortion of truth and inappropriate use of the charge of anti-Semitism are just some types of threat that we face, and calling out these distortions and supporting those who do can help renew us. And here, the words of Elie Wiesel also bear repeating: sometimes "we have to take sides … we have to interfere."

A further irony in this dynamic also presents a greater threat: on one hand, there are groups that are so intent on defending a political leader or ideology that they are willing—in the words of Michelle Goldberg—to use Jews as "human shields" and the charge of anti-Semitism as a metaphorical weapon. And, on the other hand, there are true anti-Semites and white nationalists, a small minority of whom get sufficiently agitated by the atmosphere of fear and hate—generated, or at least facilitated, by the former group—that they act out violently using actual weapons, sometimes leading to major tragedies such as the Tree of Life massacre, as well more recent domestic terror attacks.

The backlash over the "go back to where you came from" tweet did bring out some strong responses that can help bring moral clarity to the situation. For example, an open letter from the Montana Association of Rabbis to Montana Senator Steven Daines—in an attempt to defend the President—launched an attack on the Congresswomen on Twitter, calling them "anti-American, anti-Semite, radical Democrats [who] trash our country and our ideals." A portion of the Rabbis' letter is copied here because it illustrates an important "strategic" point for psychiatrists aiming to help stem the tide of anti-Semitism and racism: psychiatrists will only be minimally effective as lone voices trying to speak out against fear and hate-generating speech by leaders, and perhaps more importantly, they will have minimum impact on the large swath of the public that seems to have been empowered or "granted permission" by these leaders to express racist, xenophobic sentiments in a more open and aggressive fashion:

> We refuse to allow the real threat of anti-Semitism to be weaponized and exploited by those who themselves share a large part of the responsibility for the rise of white nationalist and anti-Semitic violence in this country. Accusing these representatives of antisemitism is no justification for telling them 'to go back to where they came from' or inciting violence against them.
>
> At a time when many of the core values and norms of American democracy are under threat, we cannot equivocate or hesitate to challenge the forces of hate, even—and especially—when these forces cloak themselves in the authority of the Senate or the White House. – Montana Association of Rabbis [23]

Making Advocacy Effective

Like other contemporary crises, such as climate change, in which deep ideological rifts get in the way of honest, truth-based (e.g., science-based) dialogue, psychiatrists will be best able to help stem the rising tide of anti-Semitism by learning from and collaborating with nonmedical, nonmental health professionals. This includes groups like the Montana Rabbis and the ADL, as well as other faith leaders, human rights organizations, social scientists, historians, and, in some cases, politicians and current government officials who are brave enough to speak out. Under strain, a culturally diverse, complex, and interconnected society such as the one we live in requires input and collaboration from multiple sources to ensure justice, as well as efficient functioning. Physicians, whose primary role in society is to direct clinical care, a role that requires deep engagement and constant education, may be less inclined to engage in collaboration outside of a purely clinical multidisciplinary approach. But when physicians, including psychiatrists, decide that it is time for action, based on the demands of the times and the responsibilities of their Ethics Code, they will do well to seek out the wisdom of other stakeholders, many of whom have been engaging in exactly the sort of advocacy that is required by the circumstances. In other words, there is no need to reinvent the "rhetorical wheel." In addition, psychiatrists, as well as other physicians with experience in both "crisis management" and long-term caring and healing, could serve as leaders to help educate the public and assist those seeking to unify heretofore "single issue" advocacy groups during times of rising xenophobia, white nationalism, and domestic terrorism [24].

There is another, equally important strategic element to this advocacy, one that tends to come easier to physicians, including psychiatrists: speaking out via one's professional association. This is a force multiplier: news outlets are much more likely to cover press releases from a national organization than from an individual psychiatrist, even a prominent one. An additional force multiplier is engaged when multiple medical organizations work together, as indicated by the lobbying strategy of the called "Group of Six," which includes the APA and five primary care organizations [25]. In general, legislators, agency heads, and other government officials respond better to large organizations, which also tend to have established contacts and lines of communication. Of course, a large organization such as the APA, by necessity, must have procedures in place and a protocol to follow when making public statements. When an official APA policy already exists, such as the Position Statement on racism and racial discrimination mentioned earlier [6], this process tends to be much faster. However, the leadership of the organization still must decide when and how to express its concerns publicly. Individual members can advocate for the leadership to take action, and any individual psychiatrist (or anyone for that matter) can quote the policies of the organization and apply them—one hopes appropriately—to the situation that they believe needs public attention.

Conclusion

Xenophobic, racist, and anti-Semitic rhetoric and violence against "the other" did not begin with Donald Trump, nor will it end after he is out of office. But words matter, and words from powerful leaders matter more. They have the power to do great good but also the power to do great harm. As physicians, healers, and leaders, we have a responsibility to help statesmen "do great good" and to let them and the public know when the opposite is occurring. This means being honest about what we are seeing and hearing and then speaking out and taking other appropriate actions when necessary. Our patients and potential patients, the public, may not always expect this from us, but we do owe it to them.

Acknowledgment The author appreciates comments and information from Mark Komrad, MD, regarding the involvement of psychiatrists in the American eugenics movement, as well as in various aspects of Nazi policies, including the T4 program. Dr. Komrad is on the Faculty of Psychiatry at Johns Hopkins, Tulane, and the University of Maryland.

References

1. Walt V. The hatred stalking Europe. TIME. 2019 July. Online: 2019 June 20. https://time.com/longform/anti-semitism-in-europe/.
2. Robertson C, et al. 11 killed in synagogue massacre; suspect charged with 29 counts. New York Times. 2018 Oct 27. https://www.nytimes.com/2018/10/27/us/active-shooter-pittsburgh-synagogue-shooting.html.
3. Reilly K. Here are all the times Donald Trump insulted Mexico. 2016 Aug. https://www.time.com/4473972/donald-trump-mexico-meeting-insult/.
4. 2017: The year in hate and extremism. Southern Poverty Law Center. 2018 Feb. https://www.splcenter.org/fighting-hate/intelligence-report/2018/2017-year-hate-and-extremism.
5. Principles of medical ethics with annotations especially applicable to psychiatry; Sections 1.2, 3 and 7 of the APA code of ethics. https://www.psychiatry.org/about-apa/read-apa-organization-documents-and-policies/.
6. Resolution against racism and racial discrimination and their adverse impacts on mental health, Approved May 2018. https://www.psychiatry.org/home/policy-finder.

7. APA Commentary on Ethics in Practice. Topic 3.4.7. 2015 Dec. https://www.psychiatry.org/psychiatrists/practice/ethics.
8. Dunlap CE, Ifil-Taylor D. Helping patients heal after a bruising election campaign. Clinical Psychiatry News. 2017 Nov 28. https://www.mdedge.com/clinicalpsychiatrynews/article/118930/anxiety-disorders/helping-patients-heal-after-bruising/page/0/2.
9. Hale LB, Williams RL. Is this a Bonhoeffer moment? Sojourners. 2018 Feb. https://sojo.net/magazine/february-2018/this-bonhoeffer-moment-American-Christians.
10. Lee BX, Lifton RJ, editors. The dangerous case of Donald Trump: 37 psychiatrists and mental health experts assess a president – updated and expanded with new essays. St Martin's Press (originally released in 2017).
11. Wiesel E. Quotation from "Night". 1960. https://www.goodreads.com/quotes/99574-we-must-take-sides-neutrality-helps-the-oppressor-never-the.
12. Smith Trump administration scrambles as outrage grows over border separations. 2018 June. https://www.theguardian.com/us-news/2018/jun/18/us-immigration-border-families-separated-children-kirstjen-nielsen.
13. APA statement opposing separation of children from parents at the border (Public Statement by the American Psychiatric Association). 2018 May. https://www.psychiatry.org/newsroom/news-releases/apa-statement-opposing-separation-of-children-from-parents-at-the-border.
14. Stewart A, Pozios V. Forget about staying in our lane: let's connect the dots. Psychiatr News. 2018 Dec. https://psychnews.psychiatryonline.org/doi/10.1176/appi.pn.2018.12a20.
15. Frielander H. The origins of the Nazi genocide: from euthanasia to the final solution. Chapel Hill: University of North Carolina Press; 1997.
16. Goldhagen D. Hitler's willing executioners: ordinary Germans and the Holocaust. New York: Penguin Random House; 1996.
17. Dowbiggin I. A merciful end: the euthanasia movement in modern America. Oxford: Oxford University Press; 2003.
18. Lifton RJ. The Nazi doctors: medical killing and the psychology of genocide. New York: Basic Books, Inc; 1986.
19. Cummings W. 'I am a nationalist': Trump's embrace of controversial label sparks uproar. USA TODAY. 2018 Oct . https://www.usatoday.com/story/news/politics/2018/10/24/trump-says-hes-nationalist-what-means-why-its-controversial/1748521002/.
20. Coaston J. Trump's new defense of his Charlottesville comments is incredibly false. 2019 Apr. https://www.vox.com/2019/4/26/18517980/trump-unite-the-right-racism-defense-charlottesville.
21. Simon M, Sidner S. Trump says he's not a racist. That's not how white nationalists see it. CNN Politics. 2018 Nov. https://www.cnn.com/2018/11/12/politics/white-supremacists-cheer-midterms-trump/index.html.
22. Goldberg M. Defenders of a racist president use Jews as human shields. 2019 July. https://www.nytimes.com/2019/07/19/opinion/trump-ilhan-omar.html.
23. Franklin RL, et al. Montana Association of Rabbis appalled by Daines' support of president's 'rhetoric of hate'. 2019 July. https://www.missoulacurrent.com/opinion/2019/07/montana-rabbis/.
24. Giroux HA. White nationalism, armed culture and state violence in the age of Donald Trump. Philos Soc Criticism. 2017;43(9):887–910.
25. Richmond LM. APA, coalition lobby lawmakers on MH parity, drug treatment records. Psychiatric News. 2019 July. https://psychnews.psychiatryonline.org/doi/10.1176/appi.pn.2019.7a12.

We Refuse to Hate

27

Omar Reda

Introduction

I had the great pleasure of writing a chapter about the experience of Muslim refugees in the book *Islamophobia and Psychiatry*, and I am extremely delighted and humbled to get invited to contribute to this equally important book, *Anti-Semitism and Psychiatry*.

At critical times in my life, I have received many acts of beauty, kindness, and grace from my Jewish brothers and sisters, and I am grateful for the opportunity to pay them back at their times of distress by raising my voice and declaring loudly that hate is not to be committed in my name or in the name of my religion. Furthermore, as a Muslim psychiatrist, I can add a great deal of healing when it comes to the psychosocial impact of hate on my Jewish clients.

I am doing this not only because of my personal position on justice for all and my strong opposition to the multiple forms and shades of hate and bigotry but also because all Muslims, I believe, hold a special interest in this particular form of malignity and have a moral obligation to bear witness and stand united in solidarity by passionately speaking up against oppression.

Borrowing from the 2017 Runnymede Trust Report [1] about Islamophobia, I would like to define anti-Semitism as "any distinction, exclusion, or restriction toward, or preference against, Jews (or those perceived to be Jews) that has the purpose or effect of nullifying or impairing the recognition, enjoyment or exercise, on an equal footing, of human rights and fundamental freedoms in the political, economic, social, cultural or any other field of public life."

When it comes to the suffering of Jews, many people think only of the Holocaust, but that is a common example of historical ignorance. Different forms of micro- and macroaggression toward Jews existed even before the birth of prophet Moses, as

O. Reda (✉)
Providence Health & Services, Portland, OR, USA
e-mail: omar.reda@providence.org, omar@projectuntangled.org

© Springer Nature Switzerland AG 2020
H. S. Moffic et al. (eds.), *Anti-Semitism and Psychiatry*,
https://doi.org/10.1007/978-3-030-37745-8_27

manifested in the hostility of the Egyptian pharaoh toward the children of Israel. Institutional and systematic discrimination and profiling of Jews is prevalent in many countries, including the United States; it is unfortunate in this time and age to be witnessing the flames of violent anti-Semitic fires ignited by racist media outlets, extremist groups, and deviant politics.

Islam and Anti-Semitism

Going through the painful experience of leaving my home country of Libya and living in exile in different countries and facing multiple forms of racism and profiling from individuals and systems alike, I am a vocal advocate for human dignity for people of all walks of life. It is important to stand by the "coalition of the oppressed" by speaking up against injustice or at least not bearing false witness when people are treated as inferiors or as "others." Beautiful things happen when we start to see everyone as a unique divine gift and when we treat one another as children of God. We are created beautiful in God's image, regardless of our choice of dress before Him, what language our tongues use to supplicate to Him, or what practices and rituals we endorse to kneel before Him. To unconditionally accept, celebrate, and love each other is to praise and glorify Him.

My colleagues, in other chapters, will thoroughly examine the two pure sources of reference in Islam (its holy book, the Quran, and the teachings of its noble prophet Muhammad, the Sunnah) to state the authentic position of Islam on hatred toward Jews. I would argue here that anti-Semitism is an anti-Islamic phenomenon, not only because, as the children of Adam and Eve we are all brothers and sisters, and not only because Arabs, like Jews, are the direct descendants of prophet Noah's son Shem, also not just because prophets Isaac and Ishmael were half-brothers, which makes Jews and Muslims literally cousins, but also because both faiths have had their unfair share of hate and discrimination.

Dallas-based Imam and interfaith champion Omar Suleiman declared that "Anti-Semitism and Islamophobia are probably the two closest forms of bigotry." I can't agree more. The two faiths share many laughs and tears throughout history, through periods of prosperity and hardship. It is very important now more than ever to remain united and not buy into divisive messages.

It is true that language matters. We have seen many labels recently referring to certain religious and ethnic groups, such as calling irregular migrant Latinos "undocumented or illegals." I think the use of the term anti-Semitism to refer to hate toward Jews is accurate. I have always disliked the word Islamophobia. Hostility toward Muslims is not a phobia and has nothing to do with a mental illness or a psychology of fear but has everything to do with an ideology of hate. The term "anti-Muslim sentiment" is also a misnomer; we are talking about not a mere sentiment here but a fatal phenomenon; those who hate are shamelessly walking inside mosques, synagogues, and churches, shooting peaceful worshippers inside their places of safety.

Like Islamophobia, anti-Semitism can literally kill, especially if we continue to be passive bystanders or when some of us end up identifying with the aggressor. Both practices of religion-based hostility represent the dark side of humanity, and our choice of response can prove that humanity has not yet lost its light. We should never remain complacent when others are pushed to the margins. We are at a critical and defining moment in history when it comes to holding true to our core values; to remain silent in the face of oppression is a shameful stain on our collective conscience.

During an Islamophobia conference in Winnipeg, one of the speakers said, "Our collective humanity diminishes with every hate crime we ignore." I would say that it diminishes with every hateful gesture we overlook; microaggressions if not challenged can turn into transgressions. In the same conference, it was stated that "something is seriously wrong with our society when we place the burden of fighting hate on the shoulders of its recipients." We have seen noteworthy examples of solidarity with Muslims, such as people protesting the travel ban or holding hands making human shields to protect mosques or those praying at airports. Muslims also need to do their part and become more vocal in condemning all forms of injustice, not only by simply uttering words but also through action.

It is true that many Muslims confuse Judaism with Zionism. I was in the same boat before moving to the United States. The first is a hatred of a people. The second is the hatred of a political conviction, which can be peaceably discussed and argued.

The US and many European countries support and defend the state of Israel. This political stand has led to a widespread resentment among many Arabs and Muslims toward Jews and a hatred for Zionist ideologies. The politics of the Middle East are beyond the scope of this chapter, but it is unjust to consider that all Muslims, especially those of Arab descent, bear ill will toward Jews. It is a misunderstanding that erases centuries of peaceful coexistence between the two groups. The Israeli–Palestinian conflict should not forever color the Jewish–Islamic relations.

The status quo of violently responding to violence is not working. The world needs to invest in a more compassionate approach. We need to not buy into the current narrative or be part of the problem. To contribute to the solution, we need to start honest conversations and interfaith dialogues that are focused more on humanity and shared values and use religion for bridge building and as a healing, not a hindering, tool. We need to hold sacred spaces in our hearts for each other's narratives and deeply respect diverse convictions and different viewpoints. We need to stand up for one another. As Shahina Siddique of the Canadian chapter of Islamic Social Services Association (ISSA) eloquently stated, "Prayers and thoughts are nice, but they do nothing to dismantle the racist structures." We need to be willing to take a bullet for our neighbors and believe that we are indeed in this dark tunnel together and it is time to light some candles.

One criticism of Judaism has been the foundational belief, held by many tribes, that Jews are God's "Chosen People," a private conviction that has been seen as a source of arrogance and superiority, qualities often attributed to Jews. But the Torah teaches respect and hospitality to strangers. Our children will have a better future if we teach them to love who they are and passionately follow their chosen religion but also to invite "others" into their circles of love.

Throughout my personal and professional career, I have had positive encounters with people of the Jewish faith. Unfortunately, there are representatives of all religions who take texts out of context and misuse religion to promote and advance their own agendas, which can range from exclusion of others to blunt racism to acts of violence. My focus is not on them here but on finding the good in one another. That is not an easy task; it took an honest self-inventory for me to discover and work hard through my explicit and implicit bias.

Due to my low USMLE [2] scores and my immigration status before becoming a US citizen, I struggled to get into a residency program, I received countless rejection letters before the program director at the University of Tennessee in Memphis decided to take a chance on me. His Jewish background did not prevent him from offering a young Muslim dreamer a life-changing opportunity. He went further by supporting my participation in the Harvard Program in Refugee Trauma during my residency and even wrote a letter to the United States Immigration Services to expedite the approval of my green card so that I could travel to Egypt to see my mother after she suffered a heart attack. I am forever grateful for Dr. Allen for all he did and would like to pay tribute to him through this modest effort.

When the F-Word Is the Elephant in the Room

The field of psychiatry had come a long way when it comes to the role of religion in healing. We are now commonly using the bio-psycho-socio-spiritual model to design care plans for our clients.

Many psychiatrists in the United States are Muslims, and with more than four million Jews in the country, chances are that when a Muslim and a Jew come face to face in the inpatient psychiatry unit or the therapy encounter, the F-word (faith) might then become the big invisible elephant in the room.

During my work as a psychiatrist, I have noticed interesting themes when it comes to my Jewish clients and their families. I have had patients who were bluntly open about their Zionist views, about hatred and mistrust of Muslims, and others who felt that they had to apologize for the recent rise of Islamophobia. I think it is healthiest to take a middle stand. As a Muslim, I am not personally responsible for anti-Semitism, and that is exactly what I expect of my Jewish colleagues when it comes to Islamophobia. We need to condemn both, support each other, but not act as victims or feel an obligation to lash out, withdraw, or excessively apologize whenever there is an attack on our common humanity. To treat one another with suspicion is the very goal that these dark ideologies are seeking.

Anti-Semitism is ignorant, cowardly, and deadly. Many people fear and hate what they do not know, and many express their hate through passive aggression, but events like shootings, stabbings, and bombings can be committed by highly educated people and in the brightest light of day. The solution is not education alone. I believe that human connection, especially through children and women activities, has the most potential for healing when it comes to people who fear or hate "others." It becomes hard to hate or fear those with whom you have much in common.

One example is the family of my patient who struggled with psychotic symptoms. The family was very supportive and involved in his treatment plan even though they lived thousands of miles away in Israel. We communicated through telephone and secure emails, and they found my Muslim background comforting for their Jewish son. Somehow, I spoke few words of their cultural language, and my "mere presence" brought safety to their space. Coming from a very traditional close Arab family myself, I appreciated and admired their presence too. Cultural awareness and humility allowed me to get to know their dynamics and open a sacred space in my heart for them. I realized that they were neither "enmeshed" nor "controlling" parents. Psychiatrists can learn many things from people of different faiths and cultural traditions. That is why I love psychiatry and brag about our specialty as the best and most beautiful field of medicine.

Another Jewish client I helped work through an episode of delirium told me, "what you did for me is something divine," but there was nothing magical about our relationship; all I did was offer emotionally available and nonjudgmental listening. It is amazing how easy it can be to comfort people and mend their hearts. We just need to practice more togetherness and being with each other at times of joy and distress. At the end of our time together, my patient and I held hands and prayed for each other in the name of a common God.

Conclusion

Given my own background and my many encounters with the trauma story, I am aware of the deep impact and the risk of transgenerational transmission of trauma, and I am especially sensitive to this possibility in communities of protracted suffering, such as those of Jewish background. Monsters that terrorize someone's sleep might be the actual demons that tormented their parents, and voices that ring in young minds might speak in the exact hateful language heard by their ancestors.

After the New Zealand mosque shooting that left more than 50 people dead, a Jewish neurologist asked to meet with me to offer support and solidarity. He comes from a Holocaust survivor family and experienced his share of hate and discrimination as a young Jewish immigrant, but he wanted to make sure that day that I was taken care of. I reminded him that his story is as important as mine and that tending to my wounds must not allow him to neglect his. We hugged and cried together and renewed our commitment to refuse hate.

I have been more aware of, sensitive to, and involved in the causes of diverse populations and have made meaningful connections and friendships with many Jewish groups and organizations like the Never Again Coalition, and Jewish Voices for Peace, among others.

I am a strong believer in the power of beauty. Either it is in the struggles of someone with mental illness, drug addiction, homelessness or in the stories of those living with dementia, developmental delay, or a physical disability or through visiting the refugees, orphans, and the many more who go unnoticed, are voiceless, and seem invisible and forgotten. I am constantly looking for beauty in everyone I come across, and I am very pleasantly surprised by the potential for good that I find. Kindness and compassion are virtues that are worth sharing, and, when shared, they are often reciprocated many times over. Most people hide unlimited amounts of treasured gold within themselves; what is missing is the digging. We need to invest in and commit to unconditional humility, acceptance, and love and imagine and work toward a world where we celebrate what we truly have in common rather than fight over our perceived differences. We owe it to our children and the future generations to create a world for them that is safer and more beautiful than ours.

Beauty is an essential ingredient for healing, not only in a psychotherapeutic setting or a medical context but in all human interactions. Our interpersonal spaces can, and should, always be places of safety, hope, and beauty.

But when children get shot at or receive bomb threats in the very safety of their schools, when families get separated and people have to make the difficult decision of leaving home to a new land, when believers get targeted by acts of terrorism inside houses of worship, and when, on a daily basis, we have to deal with ugly shades of cruelty and interpersonal violence, one might start to lose faith in humanity, and darkness can then cast its shadow on our world.

Fireflies are not so exotic when flying around in the bright sunlight, and watching fireworks during the day is not that magnificent. But have you ever watched in amazement the face of a full moon? And have your eyes opened in awe and wonder at the sight of the shining stars? The Japanese term *Kintsukuroi* means to use gold to repair what is broken, nicely stating that things can become more beautiful when damaged or tested with trials and tribulations, and people can become stronger and more resilient because of their traumatic experiences. In the wise words of Rumi, "there are beautiful things that you can only see in the dark."

We live in very difficult times, and we have many reasons to hate, but we also have the choice to love. The former brings people down and break hearts; the latter builds bridges and mends broken hearts. Love literally heals. What would you choose? My choice was easy; my choice is to refuse to hate.

References

1. https://www.runnymedetrust.org/uploads/Islamophobia%20Report%202018%20FINAL.pdf.
2. https://www.usmle.org/.

Is There a Cure for Anti-Semitism?

28

H. Steven Moffic

It is the height of chutzpah to think that anyone can find a way to end Anti-Semitism. After all, however it is defined, it seems to have resisted all such attempts for possibly thousands of years. To explain why we should still try requires a lengthy and complex discussion, as well as an appreciation of what our various chapters have already taught us.

If the Passover story has some historical veracity, it can at least be traced back to that time when Jews were depicted in the Jewish Torah as slaves in Egypt and left under duress. What is clearly documented is that negative attitudes toward Jews is found in the writings of an Egyptian priest named Manetho in the third century BCE and that the first-known pogrom in history occurred back then in Alexandria, Egypt. Yet there has been some time since when the Jewish people have thrived in Egypt, and that is one of the many examples of how Anti-Semitism can be overcome and can vary under different circumstances.

The underlying etiology of such a chronic condition as Anti-Semitism is uncertain, but there does seem to be some unique possibilities. Some will say it started with anger about Jewish monotheism at a time of pagan worship. Interestingly enough in regard to Egypt, there was a brief period before Jewish monotheism emerged, when Egyptian pharaoh Akhenaten advocated for a monotheistic sun god. But that was soon opposed, and evidence of it seemed to disappear for centuries. Freud, as he was dying with cancer and on pain medication, later audaciously argued that Moses had been an Egyptian priest and a devoted follower of Akhenaten and was forced to leave Egypt with his followers after Akhenaten died, leading to the reestablishment of monotheism [1]. In this last major work, *Moses and Monotheism*, Freud also pointed out that belief in the invisible god of Judaism, which he himself did not believe in, nevertheless paved the way for developing abstract thinking, as well as the introspection that even led to his own self-analysis and the emergence of modern psychiatry.

H. S. Moffic (✉)
Private Community Psychiatrist, Milwaukee, WI, USA
e-mail: rustevie@mac.com

© Springer Nature Switzerland AG 2020
H. S. Moffic et al. (eds.), *Anti-Semitism and Psychiatry*,
https://doi.org/10.1007/978-3-030-37745-8_28

Over time, a common assumption has been that there is a hidden conspiracy theory that the Jewish people are trying to take over the world. Recent research finds that such conspiracy theories increase when personal alienation or anxiety are combined with feelings that society is unstable [2].

Others will say that it was the ethical part of the ethical monotheistic covenant with the Jewish people that was too uncomfortable for others; changing moral standards is always difficult. Another theory has to do with envy of Jewish social success when given the opportunity, with a resultant sadomasochistic response from the envious. Connected to that envy of success may be the Jewish policy not to proselytize and recruit people to Judaism; that can lead to feelings of rejection and anger toward the Jewish people.

At a more personal level, there can be jealousy at the closeness of Jewish families, especially if one has not had that in their family. That is a setup for the projection of one's sadness and anger onto Jews.

Since religion is involved, it should not be surprising that evil, however that is defined, is associated with Anti-Semitism, but from both sides. Anti-Semitism can be thought of as an evil ideology and Jews themselves as evil.

Perhaps it is something else or a combination of factors that vary with time. Throughout all these centuries, the Jewish population has had a very low percentage in most countries and in the world, leaving the perception that they were a vulnerable people. Thankfully, psychiatry has shown that successful treatment of mental disorders can serendipitously be made without clearly understanding their underlying etiology.

Only 15 years ago in America, Jewish culture could be celebrated in our "15 minutes of fame," ranging from Madonna studying the mysticism of Kabbalah to the television comedy "Seinfeld." This time period in the United States veered toward Philo-Semitism, a love and affinity for the Jewish people. Anti-Semitism was hardly evident, though the rare cultural observer could sense that it lingered in quiet hearts and could return, breaking our hearts. That turned out to be true.

A paradoxical therapeutic view, cynical though it may seem, could look at the "benefits" of Anti-Semitism—that the Jewish people have still survived and thrived in many ways. That response suggests that the Jewish people and their values have often responded with posttraumatic growth and resilience. However, that viewpoint could discount—and never make up for—the losses of all those lives and the unresolved intergenerational transmission of trauma from Anti-Semitism, which probably still haunt almost every Jewish person in some way. This trauma can be passed on by either parental behavior or epigenetic changes in parental DNA before childbearing. The positive point, though, is that all of the repercussions of trauma do not necessarily have to be negative ones.

Even more startling may be the likelihood that a significant degree of Anti-Semitism in a society seems to consolidate Jewish identity and prevent assimilation. In other words, doing away with Anti-Semitism, if that is ever possible, may be Anti-Semitic in the sense that it will lead to lessened Jewish identity.

Given the harm over the years, we still have to try to find a way to end Anti-Semitism, even if that is reminiscent of Don Quixote and "The Impossible Dream" of the popular play *Man of La Mancha*. Don Quixote's quest turned out to be delusional. That the quest is so hard can be explained by human nature. We are hard-wired to be fearful of outsiders who are perceived to be a threat. Nevertheless, there is reason for hope. New findings, though modest, suggest that both explicit and implicit biases can decrease over time, even if how that can be generalized, continued, and maintained is unclear [3].

In addition, there are instances of what might be considered "cures." One is from new relationships forged between the perpetrators and victims of Anti-Semitism or between those at risk for becoming perpetrators and victims. Another kind of "spontaneous" cure sometimes occurs when the hater is moved to reform their ideation. Take this example. One Chicago self-identified "skinhead" said that, like so many others like him, he was searching for identity, community, and purpose: really what everybody searches for sooner or later. What reportedly helped him leave that way of life was

> Ultimately, you know, it was interactions with people of color who, you know, showed me compassion when I least deserved it. And those moments of clarity added up. – Christian Picciolini

This example suggests how ordinary citizens can help reduce Anti-Semitism and the racial targets of White Nationalists. It is the opposite of the passivity of innocent bystanders.

Psychiatrists, however, have had at best a mixed track record of addressing such social concerns as xenophobia, racism, Islamophobia, Anti-Semitism, or, even at times, stigma against the mentally ill. The mentally ill were an early target in Nazi Germany [4]. Psychiatrist Robert Jay Lifton exposed the complicity of German doctors in the Nazi extermination of the severely mentally ill and the Jews [5]. The German Psychiatric Association during the 1930s remained silent as Hitler came to power. Moreover, American organized psychiatry has had periods of not protecting the mentally ill and other groups at risk of discrimination. Back in the 1930s, scores of schizophrenic patients were sterilized, and there was a debate in 1942, right in the middle of World War II, about whether "feebleminded" children and adults should be killed [6]. Later, homosexuality was included as a diagnosable psychiatric disorder until it was removed in 1973. American-organized psychiatry avoided participation in military torture techniques after September 11, 2001, but organized psychology did not [7].

We psychiatrists can do better, though, can we not?

What Is Anti-Semitism?

The reader may be exposed to as many definitions of Anti-Semitism as chapters in this volume. Whole books have focused on the definition [8]. Without an acceptable definition, the prevalence and intervention outcomes are harder to pinpoint. Technically and concretely, the term means being against Semites, including hating them, in this case of the Jewish Semites. In the distant past, Semites also referred to non-Jews in the Middle East. Since 2010, the U.S. Department of State has used this working definition [9]:

> Antisemitism is a certain perception of Jews, which may be expressed as hatred toward Jews. Rhetorical and physical manifestations of antisemitism are directed toward Jewish or non-Jewish individuals and/or their property, toward Jewish community institutions and religious facilities.

Notable in this definition is that Anti-Semitism can be directed to non-Jews, those who support Jews in various ways, as was depicted in the recent movie *The Tobacconist*. Also, this definition includes targeting Israel as a Jewish collectivity but would not include "criticism of Israel similar to that leveled against any other country."

Hatred, as Freud thought, is a normal emotion and therefore not inherently bad [10]. In situations like overthrowing a cruel dictator, it can be put to constructive use as a "noble hatred" [11].

The term did not start coming into popular usage until the nineteenth century in Germany. Interestingly enough, the terms anti-Jews, anti-Jewish, or anti-Judaism have rarely been used, though President Trump began to use anti-Jewish when he affirmed Israel's rights to the Golan Heights, along with his criticism of the Democratic support of the Jewish people [12]. At that time, he also used the term anti-Israel, instead of the more commonly used Anti-Zionism. Anti-Israel technically refers to being against the country of Israel, whereas Anti-Zionism refers to being against the Jewish people having a homeland in Israel. Occasionally, the term Zionophobes is used, which implies (unreasonable) fear of a Jewish homeland in Israel. There is also a related term called secondary Anti-Semitism, wherein one is harshly criticized for protesting Anti-Semitism.

Of course, there may be deeper psychological reasons for such terminology switching. Anti-Jewish is liable to feel much more personal than Anti-Semitism because it strikes at the heart of one's identity with the Jewish people. Zion can refer to a spiritual state, as well as a geographic state. Anti-Israel strikes against the Jews who live there, as well as Jews in the diaspora who view Israel as their ancestral home. To complicate this terminology and identity, even the very definition of Judaism and what it means to be a Jew today is so variable.

Regardless of the precise term used, the problem is a unique hatred. For one thing, it has lasted so much longer than other societal hatreds. For another, it has been cyclical. Perhaps due to the historical ambivalence toward Jews, swinging like a pendulum from hate to admiration, the Jewish people can often be put into an intermediate position between those in power and other oppressed groups. That seems to make the Jewish people a sort of vulnerable buffer group that has some power and privileges until social pressures build up, after which they can be blamed and scapegoated, distracting those groups on the bottom [13]. This being caught in the middle has happened not only internally in a country but between countries, as witness that both Nazi Germany and Communist Russia killed so many Jewish people during World War II. This unstable social position reflects why Jews are sometimes thought to be "white" in America and sometimes not, especially during those past periods where Jews were thought to generally have lighter skin color. This social position may have similarities to the psychology of the middle child in the family.

Unlike Anti-Semitism, racism seems to have been more constant in various societies. If one is both Jewish and Black, the discrimination can be both constant and cyclical. The same may be true of sexism. Indeed, the Jewish community is becoming more diverse due to intermarriage, cross-cultural adoption, and the influx of immigrants from various countries. Philo-Semitism must include this diversity to be truly considered Philo-Semitism.

The study of Anti-Semitism has long been marked by academic debates, starting with the spelling. This, too, is more than an academic exercise as even the spelling can have psychological implications. Is it Anti-Semitism, as in this chapter, which is chosen to emphasize its importance? Or Anti with a small "a," as in anti-Semitism, or just the word antisemitism, capitalized or not? Two very popular recent books on the subject spell it differently, in part due to whether there is actually something called Semitism [14]. Therefore, the name of this condition still needs clarification and consensus.

Another complexity is that Anti-Semitism has morphed over time and in different situations. In current times, sometimes Anti-Semitism can be expressed and disguised as Anti-Zionism, when criticism of Israel is unfounded and used for other purposes. Anti-Semitism can vary in intensity and repercussions. It can even seem contradictory, that is, Jews are all-powerful but also subhuman. Or take assimilation. If Jewish people do not want to assimilate, there are suspicions of why not, but if they do assimilate, what are they up to? It exists even where Jews are absent or have died (in cemeteries). Jews seem to be an all-purpose scapegoat. The irony is that the term "scapegoat" originated in the Jewish Bible (Leviticus 16), where on the Day of Atonement, the priest placed all the sins of the community from the previous year onto a goat, which was then beaten and driven into the desert. Perhaps this ritual, which was transformed over time to the asking of forgiveness during Yom Kippur, helped prevent Jews from using scapegoating of people yet also left them more vulnerable to being scapegoated given their admission of guilt. Christianity, on the other hand, may have avoided so much scapegoating since Jesus became the scapegoat for the sins of the people [15].

The psychological repercussions of being vulnerable to scapegoating likely includes insecurity and anxiety, whereas when the scapegoating is in play, the repercussions can range from micro- to macro traumas. More empirical studies of the psychological consequences of Anti-Semitism are still needed, however.

As concluded by the United Nations Educational, Scientific, and Cultural Organization (UNESCO) and the organization for Security and Co-operation in Europe, Anti-Semitism can be expressed as harassment, discrimination, and/or some sort of violence [9]. Often, just the personal expression of Anti-Semitism, such as in Nazi Swastika symbols or Holocaust denial, is added. The Internet, and its potential for anonymity, makes it easier, just a click away, but how to document all those clicks is challenging. Then there are long-standing unsettled questions of whether something is Anti-Semitic or not, such as Christian statements that Jews are going to hell unless they convert. Is that just a Christian religious belief or unintended harassment? Anti-Semitism usually comes from external sources but also can at times seem to derive internally from Jewish people, such as the criticism of some Orthodox that assimilated Jews are thereby not Jewish given the relative lack of their religiosity. Or liberal Jews who make Anti-Zionism comments that can be covers for Anti-Semitism may deny that they are Anti-Semites or even that their comments are Anti-Semitic, as that would threaten their entire liberal identity.

How severe Anti-Semitism is right now is debatable. Certainly, all incidents are not reported for various reasons. On the other hand, when a current incident is a trigger to past trauma, it may feel worse than it is. In addition, Anti-Semitic incidents can be hidden as new symbols are used or just the identification of someone as "Jew" is used where it is otherwise irrelevant. Some interpersonal interactions may be hard to define as Anti-Semitic. Take someone who was Jewish seeing an Arab barber for the first time. When asked about his background by the barber, he said he was Jewish, whereupon the barber pulled his hair twice. That felt Anti-Semitic, but he was not sure and said nothing. Psychiatrists, in our clinical work with patients, are also particularly attuned to what is left out, not said, that should be of obvious importance.

Different cultural groups may define Anti-Semitism differently. Take the case of Anti-Zionism. Zionism for the Jewish people tends to mean having a homeland of our own, whereas Muslims and other groups may view Zionism through the lens of colonialism.

Psychiatry and psychology have also tried to define Anti-Semitism in their terminology over time. That perspective may also lead to other sorts of understanding and recommendations.

Anti-Semitism as a Mental Disease

Perhaps the most prominent proponent of Anti-Semitism being a disease of the mind was Jewish psychiatrist and psychoanalyst Theodore Rubin, M.D. His 1990 book was a psychoanalytic interpretation of Anti-Semitism as a form of psychopathology. He concluded that for the Anti-Semite, Jews were symbols of projected self-hate. Hence, Dr. Rubin used the diagnostic label of a "symbol sickness" [16].

During the development of an Anti-Semite, personal challenges were said to be poorly handled, with envy, self-doubt, externalization of internal conflicts, scapegoating, and identity conflict ensuing. This sort of illness could range from mild to malignant. More generally, he felt that Christian Anti-Semites had ambivalence that Jesus was a Jew and a "conscience-giver," which perhaps relates to the challenge of ethical monotheism.

Dr. Rubin suggested two potential interventions. Using the metaphor of an infectious disease, prevention could occur via inoculation in the form of aggressive early education to counter the misguided view of Jews. Though he recommended nothing specific at the time, Dr. Rubin also thought that medication could potentially help. Coincidentally, that period when his book was published coincided with the emergence of the newer antidepressants, beginning with the release of Prozac, thought to possibly even make the patient better than normal [17]. Since such medications do seem to blunt emotions, including anger and hatred, it therefore makes theoretical sense that medication could eventually be of some use in Anti-Semitism perpetrators.

Dr. Rubin also covered concepts that emerged after World War II, designed for German rehabilitation. One theory considered prejudice as a mass psychosis caused by paranoid contagion. Once again, it was thought to be helped potentially by a vast educational program in Germany, following the advice of the psychiatrist Richard Brickner, M.D. However, renowned psychologist Erich Fromm felt that the medical and educational approach was inappropriate, concluding that Germany's actions were not a sickness but a moral failure that should be called evil.

All attempts to get Anti-Semitism and such related prejudices as racism into the American Psychiatric Association official diagnostic classification have failed. Therefore, for now, Anti-Semitism does not seem to meet any of the current formal criteria for being a psychiatric disorder for any given individual.

Anti-Semitism as a Social Disease

Jewish scholars also played a major role in the development of the field of social psychology, as well as the less robust field of social psychiatry. These scholars were particularly interested in understanding the atrocities of the Holocaust and the nature of Anti-Semitism [18]. Some of their findings included the tendency to conform to your crowd or in-group even if you know that the crowd is wrong, the ease of submission to power in unsettling times, and the belief that the social world is full of unrecognized biases.

The 1957 hit musical *West Side Story* about the conflict between Italian and Puerto Rican gangs, with lyrics by the young Stephen Sondheim, who is Jewish, humorously reflected this concept of social disease in the song "Gee, Officer Krupke." As the character Action (playing a psychiatrist) sings in this brief excerpt:

Yes!
Officer Krupke, he shouldn't be here.
This boy don't need a couch, he needs a useful career. Society's played him a terrible trick,
And sociologically he's sick!

As in the consideration of Islamophobia, the prevalence of Anti-Semitism in some societies suggests a social pathology rather than an individual illness. This sort of pathology could ensue from competition for power and the scapegoating of rivals. This alternative viewpoint arose during and after World War II. Viewing it as such could tie together the passive bystanders in Germany and elsewhere on up to enthusiastic proponents of genocide for the Jewish people.

Proponents at that time of the social pathology concept suggested education, research, and legislation as interventions, though only with cautious optimism. Using the psychoanalytic metaphor, a benignly structured ego needs the assistance of economic, political, and educational reforms.

As far as Anti-Semitism goes, one could have thought that such social reforms were working as Anti-Semitism seemed to have decreased in various European countries and America after World War II. However, Anti-Semitic incidents in those countries escalated in recent years, along with the related Anti-Zionism toward Israel in the Middle East, most strongly conveyed with the message from surrounding countries that Israel should not exist.

Actually, there is no formal diagnostic classification of social "diseases." Given that, perhaps social pathology is a better terminology for now. A more permanent cure of this social pathology still awaits. Perhaps it is also something more that complicates the challenge.

Anti-Semitism as Psychopathology of Everyday Life

One of Freud's most popular concepts is that some psychopathology was part and parcel of everyday life [19]. This concept came out of his study of small deviations from everyday behavior in the form of verbal slips and parapraxes. These included mistaken verbal expressions or behavior, which Freud concluded slipped through from the unconscious to suggest some underlying concern or conflict, similar to what slipped through in dreams. In Freud's terminology, this meant that we all are a bit "neurotic." Over time, the concept obtained some experimental verification [20].

In terms of Anti-Semitism, what little gestures might reveal this particular psychopathology of everyday life? These can look innocent. Nevertheless, off-hand remarks and misunderstandings may cause microtraumas in the Jewish person. Examples could include mentioning that a non-Jew has a surname that is usually thought to be Jewish, or sexual innuendos with a Jewish reference.

Though these Freudian slips may reveal Anti-Semitism, they are not the underlying psychological mechanism. Given that our so-called defense mechanisms presumably function daily, perhaps they are the mechanism and can explain how Anti-Semitism can be so ubiquitous, whether conscious and/or unconscious. These psychoanalytic concepts describe ways that our mind tries to protect our self-esteem and sense of security. They include denial, repression, regression, undoing, projection, sublimation, and reaction formation.

Examination of the conflictual Jewish and Black American relationship that has emerged in recent years suggests that reaction formation may be a cause of Anti-Semitism. Reaction formation is a deep and counterintuitive way of protecting self-esteem, in which a person seeks to repress something unacceptable by adapting an opposite, even exaggerated, stance. In terms of Black Americans and Jewish

Americans, that Jews took the lead in helping Blacks in the civil rights struggles of the 1960s could have made some Black Americans uncomfortable and even ashamed of being dependent on that help. Black scholar Ishmael Reed speculates that this could have stimulated a counterreaction of no longer wanting that help, even extending that to disparaging the source of that help [21].

Similarly, reaction formation could be the reaction to other Jewish knowledge and help. Could there have been some of that in the Christian and Islamic religions as they emerged and developed traditions that seemed to be based in part on the Jewish "Old" Testament, the Torah?

Was this psychological defense mechanism of reaction formation in play with the great opera composer and renowned Anti-Semite Richard Wagner? Wagner definitely had help in getting his floundering career going from Jewish colleagues, especially from his erstwhile colleague, the composer Meyerbeer. Meyerbeer loaned him money and praised Wagner's work, only to later become the recipient of intense and caustic criticism from Wagner.

Another contributor to this idea of Anti-Semitism being some aspect of the psychopathology of everyday life might be the work of Melanie Klein, who also came to live in England to escape the Nazis. Her work did not achieve the renown of Freud but built on it [22]. She had a distinctly uncompromising view of envy and human destructiveness. She worked with young infants and came up with the theory of an infantile paranoid-schizoid position with the potential for later regression. This tendency, reinforced by early trauma or a lack of parental mirroring, leads to unconscious splitting, a projection into good and bad and, in Nazi time, Aryan and Jew. In our time, there seems to be a renaissance of social splitting, with an external world of polarization and discrimination. The goal of personal development and/or treatment was to mature toward the "depressive positive," where one recognizes and feels guilty about the pain suffered by—or inflicted on—the other, which can then lead to concern for the well-being of the other. Without change, it is not uncommon for perpetrators of Anti-Semitism to eventually end up in trouble.

If Anti-Semitism fits under the rubric of the psychopathology of everyday life, then recognitions and interventions would have to be practically integrated into everyday life. In recent decades, a variety of popular implicit bias tests have been developed to identify implicit prejudices like Anti-Semitism [23]. Though they have their critics, these tests help to uncover negative attitudes toward a social group of which the individual may be unaware. These implicit bias tests indicate how common such biases are toward various groups that are discriminated against, including the Jewish people, in various societies.

The Potluck Model of Intercultural Relationships

The United States of America is often described as a desired melting pot. In this model, all the cultures mix together to achieve something more homogenous. The drawback may be the loss of certain cultural and religious values in the assimilation and melting. Even the identification Judeo-Christian implies that other religions and religious values (let alone atheistic ones) are secondary. If the Jewish people are to be considered a "chosen people," that chosenness may lie in the ethical principles of monotheism, although the contributions of other religions and cultural groups, such as their emphases on love, obedience, karma, or suffering, clearly overlap.

A different model might be that of a potluck. In a potluck, which can be traced back to the Middle Ages in Europe, each person or family brings a food or drink item, and collectively, a meal is composed [24]. These dishes might be ethnic food of different cultures. All people need to be nurtured adequately, both physically and psychologically.

Food is just one of the many different contributions that all cultures make to society. Using the metaphor of potluck nourishment for positive intercultural relationships, with the Jewish contribution representing Philo-Semitism, Anti-Semitism would be viewed as a spoiled, or even poisonous, contribution that would be blamed on the Jew and potentially hurt all the contributors.

Interventions

Given that Anti-Semitism is the world's longest running hatred, and is so ubiquitous in societies where Jewish people have lived, any way to end it would also have to be generalizable to people of various backgrounds and cultures and be ongoing.

Since Anti-Semitism can also occur within some Jewish people, who may hate their Jewishness or the Jewishness of others, interventions need to include them. However, caution about conclusions must be included as it may be difficult to distinguish between valid differences of opinion from different religious opinions versus internal Anti-Semitism. Moreover, even if it is a difference of opinion, what takes priority for all? That question has recently taken place with an ultra-Orthodox Jewish community, many of whose children have not been vaccinated for measles, resulting in an outbreak in the secular that can be traced back to them.

Similarly, that Anti-Zionism may be an offshoot and disguise for Anti-Semitism calls for careful attention to the relationships between Jewish people in the United States and Israel. Whereas a unique opportunity exists since this is the first time in history that there has simultaneously been a strong Israel and a strong diaspora, attempts to split that relationship from the conflicts between the political far right and left in both countries fits the historical cycle of putting the Jewish people in the middle and then blaming them.

Many interventions from other perspectives in society have already seemed helpful to some extent. These include the educational, legal, law enforcement, media, political and religious perspectives. In the potluck metaphor, these are cooks of various nourishing meals. Such methods include early childhood education about the Holocaust for both non-Jews and Jews, legal repercussions for hate crimes, media deliberation of how much coverage to give to Anti-Semitic incidents, political leadership that can model cooperation rather than conflict, and religious cooperation over conflict. As with all such interventions, in contrast to, say, studying the benefits of medication through double-blind studies, these interventions, due to the complex variables in society, almost invariably have to be naturalistic or anecdotal and, thereby, without clear proof of effectiveness. Though without expertise in these other areas of knowledge, psychiatrists can make an indirect contribution by being advisers from the psychological standpoint to such interventions.

Perhaps the most striking examples of opposing Anti-Semitism was the courage of the "righteous gentiles" who rescued Jews at the risk of their own lives during World War II. Psychologist Eva Fogelman concluded that the most common quality they had was a familial acceptance of people who were different [25].

The fields of psychology and psychiatry have also seemingly made direct contributions to reducing Anti-Semitism. They include the following: Maslow's hierarchy of needs, where physical needs, safety, and security have to be fulfilled before self-esteem and actualization can flourish [26]; empathy for others, which is best achieved through storytelling [27]; forgiveness [28], which in terms of the Jews and Muslims might go all the way back to the banishment of Ishmael; the harm of defensive self-representation by Jews, whereby counterstereotypic self-representation by minority group members has led to a more negative evaluation by majority group members [29]; new neuroscience research on increasing trust by recognizing excellence in others, sharing success and asking others for help, all of which can increase oxytocin levels in the brain [30]; and more research on how we tend to deny facts and future risks after we mourn and have vigils following a disaster [31]. Leadership that brings people together is essential, although it is noteworthy that Anti-Semitism in the United States has been increasing during the administrations of two very different recent presidents. All these endeavors are capable of reducing Anti-Semitism and the erroneous perceptions involved due to the neuroplasticity of the brain [32]. Storytelling, such as that of Holocaust survivors, is often the best modality [33].

The question, then, is whether there is something new that could be added to these contributions. Given that hate, including hate toward Jewish people, can be conveyed by anger, what about anger management therapy particularly geared to Anti-Semitism? In general, anger management has achieved some accepted success [34], though it does not always accord with expert guidelines [35]. The approach was designed because inappropriate anger is so common and psychiatric treatment so stigmatized, with the result that most perpetrators never got help—which is of course true of psychiatric disorders as well. Now, in situations such as domestic conflict or workplace threats, anger management is often readily available. Techniques include strategies for delaying responding with anger while choosing alternatives.

Hate can be expressed through anger but can also smolder silently and find expression in passive-aggressive ways. Truth can be distorted. Hate, like anger, can have detrimental repercussions on the hater's body and mind, causing insomnia, anxiety, weight gain, and increased blood pressure, and contribute to other chronic illness [36].

These harmful repercussions to both the victims and perpetrators perhaps could be lessened with a spin-off from anger management, which could be called Anti-Semitism management therapy. That could also incorporate some of the principles in cognitive behavioral psychotherapy, founded by Jewish psychiatrist Aaron Beck,

M.D., which helps the patient to reframe misguided thinking. Mentalization-based treatment, mainly developed for borderline personality disorder, may also have a role in increasing making sense of each other [37]. Since medication like the newer antidepressants are occasionally used to modulate anger, they may have a role here, too. Modeling this approach after anger management, the hatred of Anti-Semitism might be alleviated by the following:

- Having the Anti-Semite acknowledge personal hatred
- Coming to understand the source of the hatred, such as fear, insecurity, mistrust, or projected self-hate
- Learning to catch your hatred as it is erupting and take a step back
- Using cognitive techniques to manage the emotion and reframe the misguided thoughts
- Having compassion for one's own weaknesses
- Learning to avoid splitting reactions to others
- Talking to a trusted person who is not part of a hate group, whether a loved one or a therapist, and
- If all the above is not sufficient, considering adding antidepressant medication as a supplement

As in the case of anger management, getting that help would largely depend on the initiative of work colleagues or loved ones. In educational settings, the relevant implicit bias test could help to detect hidden Anti-Semitism. Like diversity training, Anti-Semitism training could also be provided in groups.

For some, the Anti-Semitic beliefs are cultish in their intensity. For that, help in getting out of the cult is the first step, then deprogramming and wraparound services to recover [38].

We do need new methods to change our minds. Early in our evolution, humans tended to band together in tribes in the face of external threats and to be willing to risk self-sacrifice for the sake of the group. That is why it is so easy to mobilize people, including for war, by conjuring up the specter of an external enemy. However, this tendency, so necessary in the age of hunter-gatherers, may no longer be so necessary and useful [39]. Psychological research suggests that once our minds are made up on matters that are important to us, changing them can be very difficult, even when there is danger ahead. One reason is that it is hard to go outside of our identified tribe. Any disloyalty feels dangerous, as if the tribe will kick one out [40]. This fear will intensify in those already anxious about other things. Therefore, when cognitive dissonance is felt about an issue, most people would tend to deny or downplay new information rather than change their worldview to accommodate it. There can be a backlash such that when doubts emerge, for example about Anti-Semitic beliefs, prior beliefs can paradoxically be held even more strongly. Feeling less confident about opinions on controversial issues leads to the same reaction. Moreover, there can also be a negative boomerang effect if teaching people about the biases they hold challenges their self-image [41]. Instead, conspiracy theories that are countered without challenging a person's identity tend to be more effective [2]. Telltale signs of a conspiracy theory are that it is contradictory, it has shaken assumptions, and the evidence against it is used to justify it.

A recent communication, disguised for confidentiality sake, from an anonymous young male Jewish psychiatrist illustrates some of the anguish that can occur when discussing Anti-Semitism, even with fellow psychiatrists:

> I've received a lot of angry feedback whenever I've discussed these issues with psychiatrist friends. It's been incredibly demoralizing and hurtful to me … Based on that, I'm confident in my assessment that this is an important and relevant topic … I think the response people are having is rooted in anti-Semitism itself, or in self-defensive denial of anti-Semitism. And so, it is anti-Semitism that is wearing me down, and fear of anti-Semitism that makes me so reluctant to discuss my ideas publicly. The more I read, the more I realize that the phenomenon I'm talking about is the essence of Diaspora. We have a few generations of assimilation and relative safety, we feel comfortable and accepted, and then it turns out that anti-Semitism is still there. And it is scary and surprising, since it comes from supposed allies, from people we thought shared our values of equality and justice. And they do, just not for us. Somehow, we are still the other.

With any intervention, then, success is more likely if a person

- Does not try to force a particular viewpoint on someone who does not hold it
- Establishes a mutual foundation of respect first
- Asks about how the beliefs came about
- Asks open-ended questions
- Shares one's own experiences about the issue at hand, and
- Most crucially does not show contempt for the other, such as debaters often do, since as in marriages, contempt breaks up relationships [42]

Conclusions

The question of whether Anti-Semitism is a psychiatric disease may still be unanswered. More clearly, it seems to be a social disease of some sort but something even more, perhaps THE "psychopathology of everyday life." Given human nature, then, the question of whether we can cure Anti-Semitism seems more of a rhetorical than realistic one. Certainly, individuals have renounced Anti-Semtism after (re)education, exposure to a new environment, and unexpected kindness from Jewish people. However, more widespread Anti-Semitism that is connected to core religious or cultural beliefs is much more challenging. Even so, progress has been made with some branches of Christianity. For Muslims to decrease their current rise in Anti-Semitism, more may be required, even reformation and enlightenment, as one Muslim who received the Moral Courage Award from the American Jewish Committee concluded [43]. The far left, often atheist, in many countries is another source of rising Anti-Semitism. All of these challenges seem to call for a multipronged global endeavor. There is, however, an apparent positive perspective on Hindus and Jews as it seems that Anti-Semitism has been virtually nil among Hindus, perhaps because the two monotheistic religions grew in parallel but unknown to each other.

Finding other ways to reduce Anti-Semitism should have wider benefits, including reducing the spread and displacement of discrimination against other groups. In so doing, a distinction has to be made between the erroneous beliefs connected to Anti-Semitism versus constructive criticism of Jewish people. Moreover, the Jewish people have to be careful of their own tendency to discriminate, as in the use of the term "goy" as a demeaning slur toward all who are not Jewish.

Though the fields of psychiatry and psychology have long had a strong Jewish presence, concern for Anti-Semitism within them has waned over the last 30 years. To date, the track record of organized psychiatry has been mixed in responding to related social problems of discrimination and prejudice against other groups. Nevertheless, the clinical model of psychiatry can lend itself to a better understanding, prevention, and treatment of Anti-Semitism. The social part of our bio-psycho-social medical model by its very nature includes the social problem of Anti-Semitism, while the psychological part covers how Anti-Semitism is processed in the individual. Perhaps there is even a biological component. Although there are no anti Anti-Semitic medications, some make the case that psychedelics can help heal the trauma from Anti-Semitism, as well as help the perpetrators to feel the unity of all people [44]. Perhaps that had some prophetic aspects as citizens in society are trying very low-dose psychedelics, like LSD, to quell anxiety and fear [45]. Psychiatrists, as we do in evaluations and psychotherapy, should also be particularly adept at recognizing with our "third ear" when Anti-Semitism is covert or left out of relevant discussions [46]. Anti-Semitism occasionally can also be a symptom of commonly treated disorders, like a paranoid disorder.

If we take all the endeavors to address Anti-Semitism and try to weave them together in a tapestry, some of what we may have is as follows:

1. For child development, empathic parents who will also instill an acceptance of those who are different and a global identification with all people to supplement one's "tribal" identity
2. For self-esteem, as much as possible the achievement of basic physical needs, safety, security, and the opportunity for self-actualization for all in societies
3. For hate crimes, effective legal punishment
4. For media, policies to reduce dangerous Anti-Semitic reinforcement, as well as supporting recommendations for things that people like you rarely like (rather than people like you have liked)
5. For political leadership, strategies for the modeling of bringing diverse groups together rather than playing on primitive fears of the other, for when Anti-Semitism gets politicized, its dangerousness escalates
6. For community relationships, both individuals and groups, intermittent and ongoing cross-cultural interactions that challenge scapegoating of the other on both sides
7. For Israel and the USA Jewish diaspora, the avoidance of being divided and conquered by external and internal forces

8. For the victims of Anti-Semitism, opportunities to therapeutically process their trauma and fears

9. For the perpetrators of Anti-Semitism, opportunities to engage in Anti-Semitic management programs

10. For medical professionals, making sure to teach the history of the Holocaust, especially because physicians were particularly vulnerable to Nazi ideologues [47]

This tapestry needs to be made to withstand wear and tear because the need is likely to be ongoing.

Given the longevity of Anti-Semitism, it is essential to be creative and diligent in the quest for a healthy societal potluck. Perhaps mental health organizations can establish an annual prize for the best new idea for reducing Anti-Semitism. For instance, could virtual reality be used to enhance Philo-Semitism and reduce Anti-Semitism? Or could conveying that Anti-Semitism is making the Jewish people stronger have a paradoxical therapeutic effect? Should Jewish leadership reconsider proselytizing? Should a psychiatrist make a journalism tour of countries where Anti-Semitism is increasing to get a better sense of the social scenario than individual patient care allows? Readers of this chapter are very welcome to share ideas, too. Indeed, if the stagnant NASA space program could be accelerated by an open platform for the world to help and 3000 people did [48], then why not do the same for Anti-Semitism? It is not rocket science, is it? Or is it more complicated than rocket science because this is brain science?

References

1. Freud S. Moses and Monotheism. New York: Vintage; 1955.
2. Moyer M. People drawn to conspiracy theories share a cluster of psychological features. Sci Am. 2019;320(3):58–63.
3. Huston M. Implicit biases toward race and sexuality have decreased. Sci Am. 2019;320(4):12.
4. Seeman MV. Psychiatry in the Nazi era. Can J Psychiatr. 2005;50:218–25.
5. Lifton R. The Nazi doctors: medical killing and the psychology of genocide. New York: Basic Books; 1986.
6. Joseph J. The 1942 'euthanasia' debate in the American Journal of Psychiatry. Hist Psychiatry. 2005;16:171–9.
7. Summergrad P, Sharfstein S. Ethics, interrogation, and the American Psychiatric Association. Am J Psychiatr. 2015;172(8):706–7.
8. Marcus K. The definition of anti-Semitism. New York: Oxford University Press; 2015.
9. United Nations Educational, Scientific, and Cultural Organization. Addressing anti-Semitism through education: guidelines for policymakers. UNESCO and OSCE. 2018.
10. Abel D. Freud on instinct and morality. New York: State University of New York Press; 1989.
11. Eissler R. Three instances of injustice. Madison: International Universities Press; 1994.
12. Stern E. Anti-Semitism and orthodoxy in the age of Trump. Tablet. 2019 Mar 12. https://tablet-mag.com/Jewish-arts-and-culture/281547/anti-semitism-orthodoxy-trump.
13. Rosenfeld J. The historic roots of anti-Semitism and how they play out today. Public Source. 2019 Jan 3. https://www.publicsource.org/history-anti-semitism-pittsburgh.
14. Siegel R. Book review: how bad is it? Moment. 2019 Mar–Apr.

15. Rohr R. The universal Christ: how a forgotten reality can change everything we see, hope for, and believe. New York: Convergent Books; 2019.
16. Rubin T. Anti-Semitism: a disease of the mind: a psychiatrist explores the psychodynamics of a symbol sickness. New York: Continnum; 1990.
17. Kramer P. Listening to Prozac: a psychiatrist explores antidepressant drugs and the remaking of the self. New York: Viking Adult; 1993.
18. Simmel E, editor. Anti-Semitism: a social disease. New York: International Universities Press; 1946.
19. Freud S. The psychopathology of everyday life. New Ed ed. London: Penguin Classics; 2002.
20. Erickson M. Experimental demonstrations of the psychopathology of everyday life. Psychoanal Q. 1939;8:338–53.
21. Reed I. Do Jews still believe they're White? And how is it possible that some Jews are still shocked that they're hated in America? Tablet. 2018 Nov 8. https://www.tabletmag.com/jewish-news-and-politics/274414/american-jews-white
22. Rasmussen B, Salhani D. A contemporary Kleinian contribution to understanding racism. Soc Serv Rev. 2010;84(3):491–513.
23. Gladwell M. Blink: the power of thinking without thinking. New York: Back Bay Books; 2007.
24. Mauss M. The gift: the form and reason for exchange in archaic societies. New York: W.W. Norton; 2000.
25. Fogelman E. Conscience and courage. New York: Doubleday; 1994.
26. Maslow A. Toward a psychology of being. Floyd: Sublime Books; 2014.
27. Goleman D, Boyatzis R. Social intelligence and the biology of leadership. Harv Bus Rev Spec Issue. 2019:53–8.
28. Tutu D. The book of forgiving: the fourfold path for healing ourselves and our world. New York: Harper One; 2015.
29. Taylor D, Gardner R. Ethnic stereotypes: the effects on the perceptions of communications of varying credibility. Can J Psychol. 1969;23:161–73.
30. Zak P. The neuroscience of trust. Harv Bus Rev Spec Issue. 2019:44–9.
31. Gorman S, Gorman J. Denying to the grave: why we ignore the facts that will save us. New York: Oxford University Press; 2016.
32. Helmstetter S. The power of neuroplasticity. Cork: Park Avenue Press; 2014.
33. Zak P. Why your brain loves good storytelling. Harv Bus Rev Spec Issue. 2019:60–1.
34. Kassinove H, editor. Anger disorders: definition, diagnosis, and treatment. Washington, DC: Taylor and Francis; 1995.
35. Saini M. A meta-analysis of the psychological treatment of anger: developing guidelines for evidence-based practice. J Am Acad Psychiatry Law. 2009;37(4):473–88.
36. Gaylin W. Hatred: the psychological descent into violence. New York: Public Affairs; 2003.
37. Bateman A, Fonagy P. Mentalization based treatment for borderline personality disorder. World Psychiatry. 2010;9(1):11–5.
38. Hassan S. Combating cult mind control. Newton: Freedom of Mind Press; 2015.
39. Ehrenreich B. Blood rites: origins and history of the passions of war. New York: Metropolitan Books; 1997.
40. Ropeik D. How risky is it, really? Why our fears don't always match the facts. New York: McGraw-Hill Education; 2010.
41. Levy A, Maaravi Y. The boomerang effect of psychological interventions. Soc Influ. 2018;13(1):39–51.
42. Gottman J, Silver N. The seven principles for making marriage work: a practical guide from the country's foremost relationship expert. New York: Harmony Books; 2015.
43. Reis S, Wald H, Weindling P. The holocaust, medicine and becoming a physician: the crucial role of education. Isr J Health Policy Res. 2019. https://doi.org/10.1186/s13584-019-00327-3.
44. Davidson S. The December project: an extraordinary rabbi and a skeptical seeker confront life's greatest mystery. New York: Harper One; 2015.

45. Waldman A. A really good day: how microdosing made a mega difference in my mood, my marriage, and my life. New York: Anchor Books; 2018.
46. Justman Z. My Terezin Diary and what I did not write about: personal history. The New Yorker. 2019 Sept 16, p. 42–9.
47. Ali AH. Can Ilhan Omar overcome her prejudice? Wall Street J. 2019:A11.
48. Lifshitz-Assaf H. Dismantling knowledge boundaries at NASA: the critical role of professional identity in open innovation. Adm Sci Q. 2017;63(4):746–82.

Editors' Conclusions

H. Steven Moffic, John R. Peteet, Ahmed Hankir, and Mary V. Seeman

- Chai!

We began this book with the Chutzpah focus of our Editors' Introduction. It now seems appropriate to end it with Chai. Chai edged out the popular Yiddish phrase Oy vey (or just plain Oy), which expresses exasperation, including a degree of woe is me. It won out because it is more optimistic, though it would be hard to not feel some Oy veh at the resurgence of anti-Semitism. Chai is another popular word in Jewish culture, expressed at many Jewish events. It means life and is synonymous with the numerical value of 18.

Chutzpah, Chai, and Oy veh. Three words that probably couldn't be topped in conveying the Jewish psyche over history: the periodic anti-Semitic traumas and their intergenerational transmission (Oy), the unprecedented continuity of the people (Chai), and the often audacious resilience (Chutzpah), all of which circle back to trying to understand and help the Jewish and human psyche.

The derivative of Chai, "L'Chaim", means "to life"! It is a commonly used Jewish toast in anticipation and hope of all the good things that life can bring. However, uncountable lives have been lost and/or traumatized due to anti-Semitism. Serendipitously, perhaps, as we complete this piece on 9/11/19, 18 years ago on 9/11/01, we experienced a related example of a failure of intercultural and interfaith relationships. An anti-Semitic fringe even blamed the Jews for the bombings. Like

H. S. Moffic
Medical College of Wisconsin, Milwaukee, WI, USA

J. R. Peteet
Department of Psychiatry, Brigham and Women's Hospital, Boston, MA, USA

A. Hankir
South London and Maudsley NHS Foundation Trust, London, UK

M. V. Seeman
Department of Psychiatry, University of Toronto, Toronto, ON, Canada

© Springer Nature Switzerland AG 2020
H. S. Moffic et al. (eds.), *Anti-Semitism and Psychiatry*,
https://doi.org/10.1007/978-3-030-37745-8

the unending war in the novel *1984*, the ensuing "war on terrorism" continues and Islamophobia escalates. Right-wing conservative internal terrorism has for now supplanted other terrorism within the United States.

In the prior Springer book on Islamophobia and Psychiatry, edited and written by many of the same people as this book, we identified 20 important "take home messages", though we trust there were more. For this volume, since we are hoping for more and better Chai, we are listing 18 preliminary conclusions of this volume, addressing the recognition, prevention, and possible innovative interventions from a psychiatric perspective. At the close of the complexity of this big, comprehensive book, these are like aphorisms, a brief and bold approach to some truths, about which readers can deliberate for themselves.

- Anti-Semitism is not only a social problem but a bio-psycho-social-spiritual one.
- That anti-Semitism has persisted for so long in so many countries indicates that it must serve a basic human psychological need that needs fulfillment during certain societal conditions but one that we think can be fulfilled in better and more humanistic ways.
- Like a virus, anti-Semitism can mutate, with different spellings, expressions, and intensity.
- Psychiatrists should be particularly adept at picking out hidden anti-Semitism.
- Ironically, getting rid of anti-Semitism can weaken Jewish identity.
- Jews have often been caught in the middle between the powerful and powerless, caught on a pendulum swinging in either direction depending on societal problems and becoming particularly dangerous when it is politicized.
- Anti-Semitism can be considered to be the canary in the coal mine, a warning of toxic social political problems and psychological processes that are leaking out.
- That Jewish psychiatrists led the development of modern psychiatry in the United States may have brought with it the anti-Semitic side effect of stigma directed against both patients and psychiatrists.
- The Holocaust caused the emigration of many psychoanalysts to the United States, likely delaying the development of biological psychiatry and adequately meeting the needs of the most seriously ill.
- Self-exploration of anti-Semitism by psychiatrists and related professionals can be unexpectedly insightful and therapeutic, a challenge started when Freud seemed to underestimate the emerging horrors of the Holocaust.
- The intergenerational transmission of anti-Semitic trauma occurs through epigenetic as well as parent–child relationships.
- Jewish stereotypes are often reflected in the media portrayal of Jewish psychiatrists and Jewish patients.
- Accepting that others can seem different but still trustworthy is teachable by parents, which was the common factor in those deemed to be "righteous gentiles" during the Holocaust.
- Like interaction of the authors of this book, clinical discussion about cultural competency among those of many different faiths and value systems can reduce cross-cultural, countertransference problems.

- The nourishing potluck meal may be a better metaphor and meeting place for intergroup relationships than the melting pot.
- Anger management techniques may serve as a model for the development of anti-Semitism management techniques.
- A "far out" and way-out-of-the box long shot idea is that micro doses of psychedelics like LSD might contribute to the quest for a cure of anti-Semitism.
- Psychiatry and depth psychology can be the missing "secret ingredient" to get beyond lingering denial of the problem and interventions as usual.

Many of these points may come across as pure Chutzpah. Can there ever be a cure for anti-Semitism or anything close to that? Is it true that anti-Semitism virtually does not exist among Hindus, as claimed in two different chapters, and, if so, why?

It should be noted that the specific content of the chapters is the responsibility of the authors and may, at times, prove controversial. The co-editors, though they have carefully reviewed and edited all of the chapters, may not all agree with all the content. There may be overlapping or opposite conclusions across chapters. Moreover, since the authors vary in cultural background, age, and individual psychology, perspectives are bound to be different, even when similar topics are broached. Most positively, that diversity of approaches adds to the richness of information and insights. Each chapter is meant to stand on its own.

Writing the chapters was often an emotional experience for the writers and editors. Despite occasional fears of retaliation for what is said in this book, several of them have spontaneously and publicly expressed how meaningful the process was for them. For example:

> It has been the most rewarding paper I have ever written. Many other papers that I have written over 50 years have been intellectually interesting and challenging. This paper has invited me to dig very deeply and indeed make discoveries that have never previously crystallized. This is the most "honest" and self-revealing paper I have ever written. I hope it inspires others to take the same journey I have found so rewarding.

For inspiration, one of the editors, Dr. Moffic, by the end of this project, modeling after one of the authors, decided to incorporate his updated Hebrew name, Hillel. Hillel, who lived around the turn of the Common Era, was one of the most important leaders in Jewish history, known especially for this saying:

> If I am not for myself, who will be for me? But if I am only for myself, who am I? If not now, when?

Is anti-Semitism really only about Jews? Or, is it also about our human nature and its hard-wired fears, tenuous self-esteem, and quest for power? If the answer is the latter, human nature is in the wheelhouse of psychiatry and renders all identifiable groups at risk for being shunned, derided, and stigmatized as the "other". As in Cognitive Behavioral Psychotherapy of individual patients, it will take corrective cognitive approaches for societies and their leaders to provide alternative paths for self-actualization. Social forgiveness may be necessary at times when we inevitably stumble along the way. Although anti-Semitism has existed for thousands of years, these psychological tools were not available until recent decades. That development seems to confirm and coincide with the words of Luke Skywalker in the first trailer for the new Star Wars movie, *The Rise of Skywalker*:

A thousand generations live in you now. But this is your fight.

Our fight is this: over the many months of working on this book, many more worrisome anti-Semitic incidents have occurred around the world, and they seem to be significantly increasing year by year. Therefore, there is a sense of urgency and audacity to this project. This should be viewed as a new reality, but not a new normal. Even a psychiatric organization, The European Network for Mental Health Evaluation, cancelled an upcoming conference in Israel, fearing backlash from the BDS (Boycott, Divest, Sanction) movement against Israel. Gratefully, there have been some heartwarming Phiio-Semitic events to counter those, such as the Pittsburgh Post-Gazette giving its Pulitzer Prize monetary award to the Tree of Life Synagogue to help with their post-terrorism repairs and recovery.

Decades ago, the well-known black author, James Baldwin, in *The Price of the Ticket*, warned us to not have a failure of imagination that another Jewish holocaust could not happen in the United States. As the last Holocaust survivors are dying, the power of Holocaust testimonies to contain anti-Semitism out of knowledge, empathy, and guilt may be fading.

The dangerousness of this otherness is potentially a Catch 22 for all of us, as described in a scene in the book of the same name. The protagonist Yossarian speaks to a young soldier appearing before a tribunal. "You haven't a chance, kid. They hate Jews." "But I'm not Jewish", answered Clevinger. "It won't make no difference. They're after everybody." We can make a difference.

Index